D1799400

Care of the Acutely
Ill and Injured

Care of the Acutely Ill and Injured

Edited by

David H. Wilson FRCS
Consultant Surgeon,
Accident and Emergency Department,
The General Infirmary at Leeds

Andrew K. Marsden FRCS
Consultant in Accident and Emergency Medicine,
Pinderfields General Hospital, Wakefield

Proceedings of the Fifth International Congress of Emergency Surgery, Brighton, 1981
which was sponsored by the Casualty Surgeons Association of Great Britain

A Wiley Medical Publication

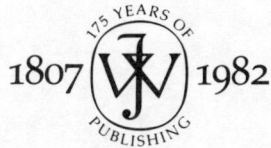

JOHN WILEY & SONS
Chichester · New York · Brisbane · Toronto · Singapore

Copyright © 1982 by John Wiley & Sons Ltd.

All rights reserved.

No part of this book may be reproduced by any means, nor
transmitted, nor translated into a machine language without
the written permission of the publisher.

Library of Congress Cataloging in Publication Data:

International Congress of Emergency Surgery
  (5th: 1981: Brighton, Sussex)
  Care of the acutely ill and injured
  (A Wiley medical publication)
  Includes index.
  1. Surgical emergencies—Congresses. 2. Medical
  emergencies—Congresses.   I. Wilson, David H.
  II. Marsden, Andrew K.   III. Casualty Surgeons
  Association of Great Britain.   IV. Title
  V. Series. [DNLM: 1. Emergency medical services—
  Congresses.   2. Emergencies—Congresses.
  W3 IN372 5th 1981c/WX215 I62 1981c]
  RD92.2.I57 1981 616'.025   82-1836

  ISBN 0 471 10238 5   AACR2

British Library Cataloguing in Publication Data:

International Congress of Emergency Surgery
  (5th: 1981: Brighton)
  Care of the acutely ill and injured.—(A Wiley
  medical publication)
  1. Medical emergencies—Congresses
  I. Title   II. Wilson, David H.   III. Marsden,
  Andrew K.
  616'.025   RC86.2

  ISBN 0 471 10238 5

Printed in Great Britain

CONTENTS

Preface

SECTION ONE

THE ORGANISATION OF EMERGENCY MEDICAL SERVICES

SECTION FIVE

ASPECTS OF WOUNDING

xii

SECTION SEVEN

HEAD INJURIES

SECTION EIGHT

EMERGENCIES IN THE GASTROINTESTINAL TRACT

SECTION NINE

EXPERIMENTAL RESEARCH IN EMERGENCY CARE

PREFACE

The efficient care of patients who are injured or taken suddenly ill
is a subject of increasing importance for the medical profession.
As many of the chronic diseases disappear, violence in society is
increasing and the provision of health care must be adjusted to meet
these changes. Two professional organisations which are striving to
improve the management of surgical and medical emergencies came
together for a three day Conference in Brighton, England in June
1981. This volume contains a large selection of the papers which
were presented by the congress delegates and invited speakers.

The Casualty Surgeons Association was the host for the Congress.
Since it was founded in 1967 this Association has grown in size and
status and now officially represents all doctors working in Accident
and Emergency Departments in the United Kingdom. It also has a
number of overseas members. The "Aims and Policies" include concern
for the provision of physical facilities for emergency patients, for
the training and career prospects of doctors who provide emergency
care and for research and education to improve the level of care.
The Association works in close liaison with all other professional
groups involved in the provision of immediate care and first-aid and
eagerly cooperates in promoting accident prevention.

The International Congress of Emergency Surgery had its first meeting
in Milan in 1973 and since then through its Permanent Committee, it
has sponsored congresses in Zurich (1975), Paris (1977) and Barcelona
(1979) before coming to Brighton. The 1983 Congress will be held in
Belgrade, Yugoslavia.

This fifth Congress was attended by 550 surgeons from 44 different
countries. On the opening day they considered the organisational
and administrative aspects of emergency care. The second day was
concerned with clinical problems, and the subject for the third day
was 'research and the future'.

The delegates shared their knowledge through symposia, plenary sessions
and sectional meetings. Presentations were made through papers,
posters and films and a series of training sessions proved extremely
popular. As at all such meetings a further intangible benefit came
from personal discussions, social contacts and experiencing the
international friendship which the Congress sought to foster.

It has not been possible to print all the papers which were presented.
The selection reflects the wide range of the subjects considered and
the very varied background of the contributors. We trust that reading
them or using the volume for reference will bring to an even wider
audience the universal concern for improved care for the acutely ill
or injured patient.

SECTION ONE

ORGANISATION OF

EMERGENCY MEDICAL SERVICES

Care of the Acutely Ill and Injured
Edited by D. H. Wilson and A. K. Marsden
© 1982, John Wiley & Sons Ltd.

THE CARE OF EMERGENCIES IN THE
UNITED KINGDOM

Miles Irving, MD, ChM, MSc, FRCS (Eng & Ed).

Professor of Surgery, University of Manchester
and Consultant Surgeon, Hope Hospital, Salford, M6 8HD
President of the Vth International Congress of Emergency
Surgery.

I deem it an honour to give this opening address to the Vth
International Congress of Emergency Surgery and I thank the Casualty
Surgeons Associations for inviting me to hold the presidency on their
behalf.

I have chosen as my topic the care of emergencies in the United
Kingdom with two purposes in mind. Firstly, to tell those of you from
other countries how we manage our acutely ill and injured patients
in this country. In this way you can judge for yourselves the efficacy
of the system much of which, in my opinion, is commendable and worth
emulating. However, there are aspects of our service to the acutely
ill and injured which can be considered most unsatisfactory.
Therefore, my second purpose is to use this platform to point out
those areas where I feel the profession, the public, and most of all
the politicians, are impeding the provision of an optimal service.

Many of you come from countries where Emergency Surgery is a specialty
in its own right. This is not the case in the United Kingdom and as
you will hear we have chosen, along with the United States, to appoint
Emergency Physicians, (known in this country as Accident and Emergency
Consultants), to be in initial charge of acutely ill and injured
patients presenting to the Accident and Emergency Departments of our
hospitals.

It is of interest to trace the steps that have led to this position.

I think the United Kingdom can claim the credit for organising the
first comprehensive accident service in the world. My pride in this
fact is increased by the knowledge that it involved those two great
Northern cities, Liverpool - where I received my early training and
Manchester - where I now practise.

In 1888 Sir Robert Jones was appointed consultant surgeon to the
Manchester Ship Canal. This major project linking the Port of
Liverpool with the city of Manchester, employed 20,000 workers on its
35 mile stretch. It took many years to build and exacted a high toll
in serious injury. In one 5 year period there were 3,000 accidents.

1

In order to cope with these emergencies the canal was divided by
Sir Robert into 3 independent sections each with a chain of first aid
stations and each with its own hospital. Each hospital was staffed
with a resident doctor and nurses. The hospitals were linked by a
railway which ran the length of the canal and which was used to convey
the injured to the hospitals. They were also linked by wireless
telegraphy to Sir Robert's Hospital in Liverpool in order that he
could be summoned whenever he was needed.

One would think that this early example of orderly planning of
accident services would have influenced all subsequent development
in the field. Alas, it has not been the case. The rapid expansion
of hospital services at the end of the last century, and in the first
thirty years of this century, resulted in emergency departments
springing up in a haphazard fashion. Such departments often occupied
inadequate accommodation in a corner of the hospital and were staffed
by an experienced and dedicated nursing staff, but often the most
junior medical staff.

When the National Health Service began in 1948 the Ministry of Health
inherited an accident and emergency service in which there was no
discernable plan. That was not to say there were no centres of
considerable excellence in this field. Foremost amongst these was
Birmingham Accident Hospital. This hospital in the industrial midlands
was an experiment designed to improve the care of the injured by
providing continuous cover from consultant surgeons and anaesthetists
supported by a 24 hour radiography and blood transfusion service.

It achieved world wide recognition under its director Professor
William Gissane, who practised in the hospital between 1941 and 1964.
With his inspiration a team of surgeons and research staff, including
a Medical Research Council Industrial Injuries and Burns Unit, was
built up in the hospital. New heights of excellence in the management
of the injured were reached. The demonstration of the extent of
concealed blood loss around closed fractures, the importance of
adequate volume replacement, the problems of venous thrombosis and
fat embolism and the hazards of infection in burned patients were all
thoroughly explored. Hundreds of doctors, including myself, were
inspired either by attending courses at the hospital or working there.

Yet, despite its undoubted success in the management of the injured,
the concept of the "Accident Hospital" staffed by "Trauma Surgeons"
has not gained acceptance, and the experiment has not been repeated
anywhere in this country. In part this has been the result of the
increasing number of patients seen in emergency departments with
medical conditions and acute non-traumatic surgical conditions. Such
patients can only be adequately dealt with in a large district
general hospital in which a broad range of specialities are represented. Along with this realisation, that accident and emergency departments should be an integral part of a comprehensive district general
hospital, has died, at least for the present, the concept of the
trauma surgeon who deals with all aspects of injury.

The problem of how to manage accidents and emergencies has taxed the minds of many people in this country. In true British fashion a multitude of committees have deliberated on the problem and issued their reports.

Surprisingly, these committees have all agreed on the basic method of managing accidents and emergencies and have differed only on the question of manning the departments.

The first committee to consider the matter was the Accident Services Review Committee chaired by Sir Henry Osmond Clark[1]. The committee reported in 1961 and suggested a 3 tier system

>   1. A peripheral casualty service staffed by General Practitioners for the treatment of minor injuries.
>
>   2. A district general hospital accident unit under consultant supervision.
>
>   3. Regional Accident Units serving populations of 1-2 million.

The Department of Health set up a similar inquiry under Manchester Surgeon Sir Harry Platt[2]. This reported in 1962 and suggested a 2 tier system omitting the third tier, the regional accident unit, suggested by Osmond Clark's Committee. The report used the term "Accident and Emergency Department" for the first time. It recommended that these departments should be under the direction of orthopaedic surgeons. The government adopted the principal recommendations of this report.

In 1970 the Accident Services Review Committee issued a further report which indicated that, from the staffing point of view, the orthopaedic cover solution had failed[3]. It revealed that consultant cover of Accident and Emergency departments was often nominal, that recruitment to the specialty was poor and that departments were plagued by low standards of work, inadequate accommodation and absence of planning.

As a result in 1971 the Joint Consultants Committee set up a Committee under the general surgeon Sir John Bruce[4]. He suggested that 32 major departments in the United Kingdom be placed under the control of a new type of specialist, a consultant in Accident and Emergency. Three years later he was able to report that in no instance had an appointment failed to achieve some positive benefit.

By 1976 there were 105 consultants in this new specialty. There are now 136 and in addition there is a training programme at senior registrar level bringing forward the next generation of consultants.

The specialist body representing consultants in Accident and Emergency is the Casualty Surgeons Association which is your host organisation today. It was formed in 1967 with the following stated aims -

"To promote for the public benefit a high standard in the science
and art of casualty medicine and surgery, and to encourage research
into matters relating to the specialty, together with the publication
and dissemination of the results of such research".

The specialty observes that its members are not trauma surgeons and
this point has been emphasised by the designation of the specialty as
"Accident and Emergency Medicine". Accident and Emergency consultants
regard themselves as practitioners capable of dealing with all aspects
of primary care of acutely ill and injured patients prior to the
referral of those patients who need it to the relevant specialty.

Although there are still those who do not like the concept of an all
embracing accident and emergency consultant and still hope for a
service in which the trauma patient is dealt with separately from
other emergency patients (Scott 1979), most of us feel that after a
hesitant and sometimes turbulent start, those accident and emergency
departments under the direction of consultants in this new specialty
are being well managed, and are offering a high standard of treatment.

The seal of approval was set upon the specialty by the most recent of
the reports, the Lewin report$_6$ issued in 1978 by the late Mr. Walpole
Lewin, an Oxford neurosurgeon. He stated that the present system
appeared to be developing in a satisfactory manner. He affirmed
that accident and emergency services should be based upon a 2 tier
system and that all accident and emergency departments should have
effective consultant supervision. He also commented upon the breadth
of training necessary for a consultant in accident and emergency and
emphasised that trainees for this specialty should be drawn from the
ranks of medicine and anaesthesia as well as surgery.

So what of the position today? How does the National Health Service
treat patients who become acutely ill or injured? I have only
mentioned the Health Service for although there is a thriving private
sector in British medicine it does not make a significant contribution
to the care of emergencies.

In the eyes of the public, and most of us who have qualified in
medicine since 1948, the National Health Service is an excellent
way of providing medical care to the population of these islands.
Despite its faults it has provided a fairly uniform standard of good
quality medical practice throughout the country and has relieved the
sick and their families of the worry of the high cost of medical
care. As a system I would not want it otherwise, and apart from one
aspect which I shall deal with, I believe that it serves injured and
acutely ill patients well.

Probably most acutely ill patients are cared for in their own homes
by general practitioners. In rural areas these same doctors may look
after their patients in community hospitals. However the appointments
system introduced in many practices has resulted in an increasing
number of patients referring themselves to Accident and Emergency
Departments for advice and treatment. Indeed Accident and Emergency

Departments now see more patients than all other hospital out patient
departments combined[7]. The management of the majority of self
referred patients in such departments is inappropriate and after
initial assessment and treatment they are transferred back to the
general practitioner.

One of the most successful aspects of our emergency system is the
999 call. Anywhere in this country the act of dialling 999 will
allow the caller to summon one or all of the fire, police and
ambulance services. Any patient injured, or becoming acutely ill
away from home will be collected by ambulance and taken to the
nearest accident and emergency department.

The speed of response and the efficiency of these services in this
country is of the highest quality and I am second to none in my
admiration of the men and women who staff them. That is not to say
there is no room for improvement. We have not really developed the
paramedic concept here, though interestingly the cardiac ambulance
service in Brighton is a notable exception. The concept of a two
tier ambulance transport system with a small number of specialised
paramedics and a larger less skilled transport section has been
recently rejected by the unions in a well reasoned document. However,
I hope that they will constantly reconsider that decision for I
believe that ultimately the best interests of our injured patients
will be served by the development of a highly skilled section of our
ambulance service.

In the meantime that gap is being filled, especially in rural areas,
by general practitioners who have formed themselves into groups who
can respond rapidly to accident calls and provide skilled medical
care at the scene of an accident. These groups have bonded together
into a British Association of Immediate Care Schemes (BASICS).

However, I must express myself as sceptical of the value of such
schemes. The attendance of doctors at the scene of accidents can be
expensive and time wasting especially where there is an efficient
ambulance service. If this sort of service is to continue it should
do so only after carefully planned comparative studies have shown
that it is effective in terms of saving life and lessening the
morbidity of injury.

That is not to say that there is no place for mobile surgical teams
at the scene of major accidents to provide skilled resuscitation,
triage and treatment. Yet in my opinion, and in the opinion of many
other surgeons in this country, the indications for even this type of
activity are very few and far between. The ideal place for a surgeon
to treat his patient is in a well equipped hospital to which patients
should be brought by highly trained ambulancemen, without undue delay.

Increasingly, in the United Kingdom, acutely ill and injured patients
are being taken to such well equipped and well staffed hospitals.
Unfortunately many will still be taken to a small, ill equipped, badly

staffed unit with no consultant in charge and only a junior resident available for initial assessment and diagnosis.

As long as the patients are not desperately ill they may still be reasonably managed in such departments even though they may wait several hours for treatment. Happily in our country the majority of trauma is musculo-skeletal and thus not usually life threatening. Gun shot wounds are rare. I have worked as a surgeon in city centre hospitals in 5 of this country's biggest cities, yet I have never seen a gunshot wound of the chest or abdomen. Sadly my colleagues in Northern Ireland cannot say the same and unfortunately I have seen the effects of 2 terrorist bomb attacks in London. There is no doubt in my mind that these small, ill equipped departments could not cope with such injuries, and by implication that they are not now coping effectively with the seriously injured patient who needs urgent experienced multidisciplinary management.

It is with a sense of shame that I have to admit that nowhere in the United Kingdom is the situation worse than in my own city of Manchester (Fig. 1). Each dot on the map indicates a hospital Accident and Emergency department which receives acutely ill and injured patients. It is hard to believe that there are those who are currently campaigning for an additional department in the area. Only 4 of the departments in Greater Manchester County have Accident and Emergency Consultants in charge.

The distribution of Accident and Emergency Services in Greater Manchester goes entirely contrary to Department of Health Policy and to every report that has been issued on Accident Services. This statement from the Chief Medical Officer in the Department of Health and Social Security is taken from the Lewin report:

"Concentration of Accident and Emergency services in major departments in general hospitals, fully equipped to deal with a wide range of clinical problems on a 24 hour per day basis, has been our policy since the publication of the Platt Report, and remains so today".

Despite this, whenever it is suggested that one of these departments is closed, there is a chorus of protest from consumer groups and local politicians, and some medical practitioners. All these bodies are, in my opinion, guilty of fostering the belief that these small departments have the experienced staff and the facilities to save the lives of the most seriously ill patients. There is not one shred of evidence to support this yet there is ample evidence to the contrary. I believe that if the public was shown the evidence, there would be an outcry as it was realised that they were being denied the standard of care that could save the lives of themselves and their relatives in the event of serious injury and illness.

What is the evidence? Unfortunately there are no adequate studies from the United Kingdom although Yates has produced evidence which suggests that the main danger to injured patients from airway obstruction occurs in small hospital accident departments rather than in the

POST OFFICE TELECOMMUNICATIONS   SECTION 265   SEPTEMBER

Manchester north west   1980

including Bolton. Bury
and some City Centre exchanges

ALPHABETICAL TELEPHONE DIRECTORY

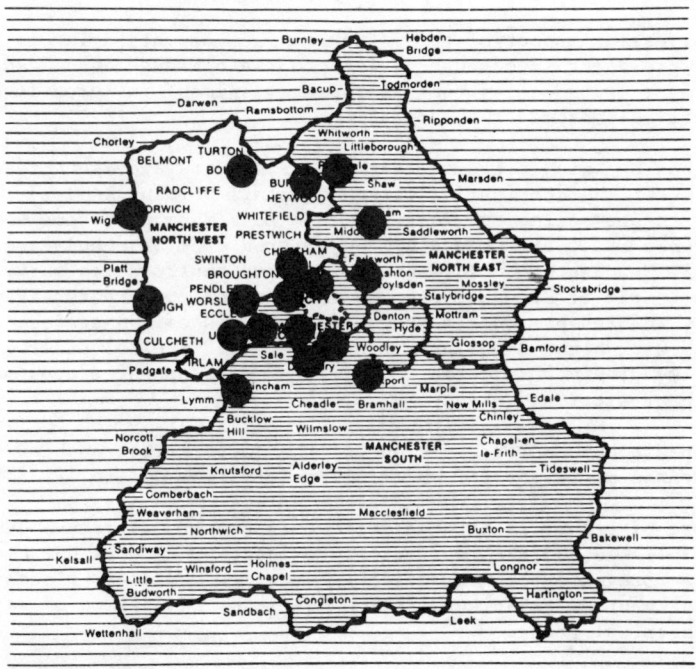

INCLUDES 061 CITY CENTRE EXCHANGES 228/236/245/247/273/829/831/832/833/834/863
PLEASE READ THE PREFACE

Figure 1

ambulance taking the patient to that hospital[8]. Chan et al (1980)[9] studied 327 patients with multiple injuries admitted to a hospital in south west England. They reported that up to 23% of the patients admitted had an injury missed on initial examination. This shows that things have not markedly improved since 1965 when we studied missed injuries in patients with head injury and showed similar findings (Irving & Irving, 1967)[10].

There is however considerable evidence from the United States. One of the most recent studies is by West Trunkey and Lim[11] comparing adjacent counties in one of which accidents are centralised to a single trauma centre, whilst in the other there is a policy of taking the injured to the nearest emergency department. The differences are staggering with only 1% of deaths in the single trauma unit being considered preventable whereas in the other system between 28% and 73% of deaths were considered preventable (Table 1).

The distressing aspect of this study is the patients dying in Orange County were doing so because of inappropriate management of such eminently remediable injuries as ruptured spleen, ruptured liver and extradural haematoma.

The method by which a trauma centre achieves its excellent results is obvious. The combination of senior staff working in good facilities and seeing enough cases to enable them to become well experienced is clearly shown by the figures from St. Paul-Ramsey Hospital, Minnesota[12]. This primary trauma centre which serves the 700,000 people of St. Paul and the surrounding country receives 450 severely injured patients a year. An analysis of 196 consecutive patients with blunt abdominal injury disclosed the 74% underwent laparotomy within 30 minutes. Only 17.3% were operated upon more than 1 hour after admission.

This expeditious approach was one of the factors that enabled them to lower the mortality for abdominal injury from 30% to 18.2%.

This sort of result is attainable in this country if trauma centres are established and the facilities provided. This does not necessarily mean the provision of new buildings etc., rather does it require re-arrangement of existing work schedules and relocation of services within hospital groups.

I must however emphasise that I believe there is substance in the protestation of the politicians and consumer groups when closure of a casualty department is suggested. It is absolutely right that patients with minor injuries, the so called walking wounded, should not travel several miles to a trauma centre. The solution is obvious and is that suggested by every committee that has studied the problem; namely a peripheral service staffed by general practitioners. Such a service could be provided from a community hospital or health centre and should be easily available. After all if rural general practitioners can provide such a service, why cannot the urban and suburban

EFFECTS OF CENTRALISATION OF INJURY MANAGEMENT ON 100 TRAUMA PATIENTS DYING AFTER ARRIVAL IN EMERGENCY DEPARTMENT (WEST TRUNKEY AND LIM, 1979).

	ORANGE COUNTY	SAN FRANCISCO COUNTY
POLICY FOR TRAUMA PATIENT	TAKE TO NEAREST EMERGENCY DEPT.	TAKE TO SINGLE CENTRAL DEPT.
NUMBER OF EMERGENCY DEPTS.	31	1
POPULATION	1.7 million	667.000 (1.6 million during day)
MEDIAN AGE OF RESIDENTS	28	35
AREA	2003 sq Km	127 sq Km
PREVENTABLE DEATHS	73% of Non-CNS related 28% of CNS related	1.1% of all deaths
MISSED EXTRADURAL HAEMATOMAS	8	0
Average I.S.S. for non CNS related deaths with predicted mortality	37 (37%) Ages of majority 10 - 40	45 (63%) Ages of majority 50+
Average I.S.S. for CNS related deaths with predicted mortality	38 (35%) Ages of majority 10 - 40	46.5 (68%) Ages of majority 50+

Table 1

general practitioner. In Greater Manchester this would mean we would
be able to reduce the number of hospitals within 10 miles of the
city centre receiving major trauma to 2 to 3 with a consequent
immediate improvement in standards which would be reflected in a
lower morbidity and lower death rate.

Unfortunately our problems in this area are about to be made worse
by the doctrine advanced by the present Minister of Health, Dr.
Gerard Vaughan, that "small is beautiful". He has issued an
instruction that no new hospital should be bigger than 600 beds, or
800 beds if it is a teaching hospital. This decision would be fine
if such hospitals were allowed to devote their facilities to the
treatment of the acutely ill and injured but the Department of Health
has decreed that such hospitals should contain wards for the old and
mentally ill as well as the medical specialties.

Dr. Vaughan, who is a psychiatrist by training, appears to have
forgotten the multidisciplinary nature of trauma management. Can he
explain how a patient with a head injury, ruptured spleen and bladder,
and fractured pelvis can be effectively managed in a 600 bed hospital
where, as in our own case, 2 of the relevant specialties are situated
in another hospital 4 miles down the road.

It is noteworthy that when the Pope was shot he was not taken to the
nearest hospital but to the 1600 bed Gemelli Hospital with its well
staffed Accident Department. The results are there for all to see.
I am sure the Pope would agree that what is right for him is right
for the rest of us.

What grieves me most about the "small is beautiful" decision is that
it has been made without any scientific evidence to support it. Yet
there is plenty of evidence from the United Kingdom and abroad to show
that large centres with high volumes of specialised work achieve
better results. Luft et al[13] have shown that centres that do more
than 200 vascular operations, per-urethral resections, and open heart
surgery operations each year have death rates 25-41% lower than
hospitals that do fewer operations.

We can but battle on and hope that common sense and sound data will
win the day - there are however, moments when I envy revolutionaries.It
is not only in the question of hospital size that politicians have a
lot to answer for. Doctors are often accused of not being bothered
about prevention of disease. What nonsense! We lay clearly before
the government the dangers of smoking and excessive alcohol consumption yet they refuse to increase significantly the tax on either.
We have shown the relationship between alcohol and road accidents
yet we lag behind the continent of Europe in our penalties, and M.P.'s
refuse to sanction random breath tests all in the name of liberty -
a liberty that is denied to those, often children, who are damaged
or killed by drunken drivers.

Perhaps most criminal of all is the refusal to sanction seat belt
legislation. In 1977 road traffic accidents cost the NHS £44 million.

I presume that by now this will almost have doubled. The evidence that the wearing of seat belts would reduce the number of injuries is incontrovertible[14,15], and has been placed before M.P.'s by every section of the medical profession and by the recent Royal Commission.

Despite this, certain obstructive members of parliament refuse to allow this legislation to be passed on the grounds that it infringes their freedom. Yet presumably these same much travelled gentlemen do not feel threatened by having to wear a seat belt when they are in an aeroplane.

It seems a paradox that on the medical side so much has been achieved in the field of management of trauma and yet our organisation in many areas is such as to prevent these advances being used effectively. However, I believe that slowly but surely we are making progress and I hope that what we hear in this Congress will help us all move along the correct paths more expeditiously.

This paper is reproduced by permission of the Editors, the British Medical Journal.

References

1. Accident Services Review Committee of Great Britain and Ireland
    (Chairman: Sir Henry Osmond Clark) (1965).
    Accident Services of Great Britain and Ireland. Second Report.
    British Medical Association.

2. Standing Medical Advisory Committee (Chairman: Sir Harry Platt)
    (1962). Accident and Emergency Services. London H.M.S.O.

3. Accident Services Review Committee of Great Britain and Ireland
    (Chairman: Sir Henry Osmond Clark) (1970).
    Report of a Working Party on Progress in the Provision of
    Accident Services, British Medical Association.

4. Joint Consultants Committee (Chairman: Sir John Bruce). (1971)
    Report of a Joint Working Party.

5. J.C. Scott (1978) Observations on the care of the injured.
    Injury, 10, 2-4.

6. Joint Consultants Committee (Chairman: Mr. Walpole Lewin) (1978)
    Medical Staffing of Accident and Emergency Services.

7. Wilson, D.H. (1980) The Development of Accident and Emergency
    Medicine. Community Medicine, 2, 28-35.

8. Yates, D.W. (1977) Airway Patency in Fatal Accidents. British
    Medical Journal, 2, 1249-1251.

9. Chan, R.N.W., Ainscow, D. and Sikorski, J.M. (1980) Diagnostic
    Failure in the Multiple Injured. Journal of Trauma, 20, 684-687.

10. Irving, M.H. and Irving, P.M. (1967) Associated Injuries in
    Head Injured Patients. Journal of Trauma, 7, 500-511.

11. West, J., Trunkey, D.D. and Lim, R.C. (1979) Systems of Trauma
    Care. Archives of Surgery, 114, 455-460.

12. Fischer, R.P., Jelense, S. and Perry, J.F. (1978) Direct
    Transfer to Operating Room Improves Care of Trauma Patients.
    Journal of American Medical Association, 240, 1731-1732.

13. Luft, H.S., Bunker, J.P. and Enthoven, A.C. (1979) Should
    Operations be Regionalised? The New England Journal of Medicine,
    301, 1364-1369.

14. Trinca, G. and Dooley, B. (1975) The Effects of Mandatory Seat
    Belt wearing on mortality and pattern of injury of car occupants
    involved in motor vehicle crashes in Victoria. Medical Journal
    of Australia, i, 675-678.

15. Mellbring, G., Dahlin, S. and Lindblod, B. (1981) The Hospital experience of seat belt legislation in the county of Skarabong, Sweden. Injury, 12, 506-509.

Care of the Acutely Ill and Injured
Edited by D. H. Wilson and A. K. Marsden
© 1982, John Wiley & Sons Ltd.

EMERGENCY MEDICAL SERVICES, U.S.A. — THE STATE OF THE ART

Kathleen A. Handal, M.D.

Long Island Jewish-Hillside Medical Center
New Hyde Park, New York, U.S.A.

In the Emergency Medical Services Act of 1973, the United States government provided assistance and encouragement for the development of a comprehensive Emergency Medical Service system throughout the country. The impetus stemmed from the fact that 350,000 cardiac arrests occur annually outside the hospital and within two hours after the onset of symptoms. Added to this is the high number of traumatic deaths annually in the U.S. of 100,000 of 50 million injuries suffered. Regional planning was prescribed to integrate fifteen mandatory components. Manpower, training, communications and transportation being the first four named; facilities, critical care units, public safety agency, consumer participation, accessibility to care, transfer of patients, standard patient record keeping, public information and education, disaster linkage, initial aid agreements being also integrated.

At the state level, laws and licensure govern and protect the Emergency Medical Technicians (EMTs) as he/she administers at the scene basic and/or advanced life support. Minimum state and federal guidelines are integrated with the local regional Emergency Medical Service training committee in setting standards for curriculum and thus allows a uniform state exam. The state also sets requirements for continuing education and license renewal.

The basic EMT completes a minimum of eighty-one (81) hour course, then passing the state licensuring test must continue to fulfill fifty (50) continuing medical education credits and renewal in three (3) years.

In general, basic EMT 1 performs evaluation, extrication, administers basic life support, using the esophageal abdurator airway as a respiratory adjunct and may apply military anti-shock trousers when warranted under protocol.

The EMT may advance to a Paramedic by completing a course of one hundred thirty (130) hours and again successful examination for state licensure. Requirements exist in each state for ongoing yearly education and three (3) year renewal examinations after a formal refresher course.

The Paramedic is trained to be proficient in delivering Advanced Cardiac Life Support (ACLS) through the use of drugs and techniques which include central venous access, endotracheal intubation and defibrillation. Their training allows, after a rather indepth examination via scenarios, to interpret, and whenever possible, transmit their findings verbally and/or via telemetry to the base-hospital physician. The Paramedic may proceed either by direct verbal order from base-hospital physician or by standing protocol to administer life saving defibrillation and/or drugs to the patient. Protocols are developed and routinely revised by the Medical Advisory Committee in each region. They are in algorithm form-specific for life threatening conditions; cardiac, traumatic, psychiatric, pediatric, etc.

The EMT's findings and activities in the field are recorded on regionally uniform run sheets; thus documenting therapy given at scene or enroute for each case. A copy of this form becomes part of patient's permanent Emergency Department record and stays as a legal document of the patient's case. Whenever pertinent attachment of a "hard" copy of patient's EKG that prompted treatment by protocol without communication to the base is attached to the run sheet.

Dependent on the nature of the emergency called in, the dispatch operators, who are themselves Paramedics or nurses will dispatch the nearest Basic or Advanced Life Support Unit or both. Region Systems aim at a response time of less than five (5) minutes for cities in the United States.

As trained, the EMTs communicate and carry out from base-physician; these physicians trained in Advanced Cardiac Life Support, Advanced Trauma Life Support are familiar with protocol for the Emergency Medical Service System. This introduces constant medical control to the system. These physicians are 'checked-off' on the use of telemetry and the workings of console systems. All transactions between EMTs and physician at base are taped from the console at the base-hospital.

The stabilized patient is transported depending on the nature of the emergency to an appropriate facility. This supercedes a patient's preference for a particular hospital. The practice of taking the patient to the nearest hospital holds in situations where base-hospital M.D.s orders have been carried out. However, if patient requires specialized care the Unit will bypass hospitals and take patient to a definitive care hospital. By virtue of their sophisticated level of training the EMTs may render the general Emergency Department's stabilization and triage to rush the patient to an Emergency Department that has been designated by the Emergency Medical Service as being set up, staffed to handle critical patients of the specific nature. The designations of centers are as follows: trauma, burn, re-implantation and neurological.

Copies of the run sheets are reviewed by medical staff as well as the operations for the system and comments made and returned to the squads. Data from these sheets enables placement of units in strategic locations as interpreted by response times. In-field procedures are reviewed as pertains to their frequency of employment, time required and efficiency by the committee of Paramedics and Physicians.

Case follow up is presented by hospital physicians at sessions with units from region.

With this system in place statistics have shown that hundreds of thousands of cardiac and trauma victims have been saved annually.

REFERENCES:

Emergency Medical Services Systems: Program Guidelines, U. S. Department of H.E.W., 1975.

Care of the Acutely Ill and Injured
Edited by D. H. Wilson and A. K. Marsden
© 1982, John Wiley & Sons Ltd.

EMERGENCY DEPARTMENTS: A CROSS-ATLANTIC COMPARISON

Kenneth Lee,
Nuffield Centre for Health Services Studies,
The University of Leeds, UK

and

Geoffrey Gibson,
American Hospital Association, USA

Arguably, it is becoming apparent in both the United Kingdom and the United States that the ability of their hospital emergency departments to render effective and timely acute care to surgical and medical patients is being seriously harmed by the growing number of non-urgent presentations by patients who are either unable or unwilling to secure primary or non-urgent care elsewhere. Although there are profound structural differences between primary health services in the United Kingdom and the United States, seemingly there are surprising similarities in the number of non-urgent presentations in their hospital casualty wards and emergency departments, especially in the inner urban areas. Given these observable differences, what ways have been tried or considered to deal with these issues, and how far can these claim to have been successful?

This paper, after presenting comparative statistics on emergency department utilisation in the United Kingdom and in the United States, makes some specific comparisons between Baltimore, United States, and Leeds in the United Kingdom, with regard to the structure and availability of emergency medical services, the supply and availability of primary care, and offers several hypotheses relating to both structures. Specific institutional comparisons are made between Leeds General Infirmary and Johns Hopkins Medical Hospital as to the diagnostic mix, waiting time, as well as other factors to do with the non-urgent use of hospital emergency departments and casualty wards.

These data sources support the impression already gained, that similarities exist despite the very real differences in the structure and financing of health services in the UK and USA. Among the likely explanations can be included the following: access to medical care for emergency treatment is de facto similar in both countries; the organisation of emergency medical services follows a similar pattern in both settings; health care problems in the city are strikingly similar irrespective of national setting; and, the physical presence of a teaching hospital and the dominating influence it has upon the immediate medical services.

These similarities are most striking in the inner cities, reflecting in many cases that Britain and the United States find located in

their downtown areas some of the worst social and medical problems
combined with some of the poorest primary care services.   In these
circumstances, an emergency department can be said to offer the
inner city dweller an immediate, unfiltered access point to medical
care and also an element of choice as to where to seek help.

The paper concludes by offering suggestions for the future to do
with alternatives that hospital and health authorities may wish to
pursue in either acknowledging or reducing the non-urgent demands
upon their services.   These may include the more imaginative use of
various 'types' of health practitioners; increasing the access and
availability to general practitioners and primary health care
providers; as well as fostering health education interventions to
substitute hospital care by health prevention and promotion.   If
the experience of the two countries is to be taken seriously, then
the structural solution to influencing or changing human behaviour
is unlikely - by itself - to be successful.   Nonetheless, attempts
have been made, and can be made, to face up squarely to the task of
improving access to medical care in a way which simultaneously
improves the efficiency of health care delivery patterns.

Care of the Acutely Ill and Injured
Edited by D. H. Wilson and A. K. Marsden
© 1982, John Wiley & Sons Ltd.

THE EFFICIENCY OF AN EMERGENCY MEDICAL SERVICE
IN MULTIPLE TRAUMA TREATMENT

N. Huten, J. Mesney and J. E.Murat

Emergency Department - University Hospital F 37044
Tours cedex

INTRODUCTION

The difficulties of evaluating all categories of Emergency
Department (E.D.) work (Sadler 1977, Murat 1977,1980) prompted us
to examine cases of multiple injury in depth.

CLINICAL MATERIAL

Of 28,000 patients seen in 1979 in the E.D. of Tours University
Hospital serving a population of three million inhabitants there
were 3,000 with multiple injuries, including 26% abdominal and
head wounds, 14% head and chest, 13% head, chest and abdominal and
9% thoracic and abdominal.

A standardised 17 page record covers every multiple injury
systematically indicating, for example, "follow-up", "autopsy" and
"audit". Drawings are widely used to indicate, for instance,
facial, bony and vascular injuries. No less than 500 items are
checked (97 on the initial clinical examination).

There were 112 cases presenting with more than two injuries, an
arterial blood pressure less than 90 mmHg or a hematocrit less
than 27%. Follow up of these cases revealed delayed initial
diagnosis of 26 lesions in 21 patients.

RESULTS

There was a delay of from 4 to 10 hours in the diagnosis of nine
cases of intra-abdominal bleeding - due, perhaps, to the lack of
routine use of peritoneal lavage in doubtful cases. Six cases
were of ruptured spleen and one of mesenteric arterial damage.
Two diagnoses of hepatic trauma were not realised until 12 to 20
hours.

Ten cases of blunt chest trauma were missed: Initial X Ray
failed to reveal two cases of rupture of the left hemidiaphragm
and two partial aortic tears. Four other cases of chest trauma
(pneumothorax, haemothorax, fractures, flail segment) were
wrongly evaluated leading to complications. Two cases of
myocardial trauma were not revealed until the 2nd and 5th days.

20

N. Huten, J. Mesney and J. E. Murat

In seven cases fractures of the spine were missed and some cases of pelvic and limb fractures were not realised until up to six weeks. Death occurred in a case of aortic rupture and in two cases of pulmonary trauma : there were no deaths from haemorrhage.

DISCUSSION

1. There needs to be a ready availability of experienced surgeons. A practical surgical opinion is required in the Emergency Department as well as on call to the S.A.M.U.
(The SAMU - "Urgent Medical Aid System" is usually directed by an anaesthetist with intensive care qualifications providing care from the accident site to the Emergency Department)

2. Surgeons committed to the Emergency Department should identify specific roles and organise a team approach to defined diagnostic and therapeutic procedures. Some sophisticated operative procedures (e.g. repair of aortic rupture) demand an available specialist expertise.

3. Teaching should be concentrated on practical, clinical problems taught through apprenticeship rather than through the formal instruction of "continuing medical education". It should involve case review and audit provoking such questions as "Could we have done something else better here?" and "What are the basic problems underlying these complications?"

4. A "polytrauma 'check-list'" aids in directing diagnosis and treatment and serves as a useful guide in case-review.

5. Distinct patterns of clinical responsibility require to be recognised with perhaps a specified surgeon responsible for the Emergency Department.

CONCLUSION

"Let the best man do the job" (Allgower 1980). In the management of multiple trauma there is a greater need for a well trained team leader charged with the co-ordination of sophisticated specialties than for a specific specialist in emergency care.

REFERENCES

1. Allgower M., Howard J.M., Borda J.R. and Schatzher J. Trauma Surgery, a speciality - if yes, whose? In "State of the Art of Surgery", 1979/80 p.13-15. Springer Verlag ed 1980.
2. Murat J.E., Vaur J.L., Bernard J.L. and Padeloup J. Guidelines for Hospital Emergency Medical Service in a University Hospital in France. The Am.J. of Surgery 139. 240-243. 1980.
3. Murat J.E. Needs and Practice of Emergency Hospital Departments in France. Curr.Top.Crit.Care Med. 3. 171-175. 1977.
4. Sadler A.L. Jr. Sadler B.L. and Webb S.B. Jr. Emergency Medical Care - The Neglected Public Service. Vol.1 Cambridge. Ballinger, 125. 1977.

Care of the Acutely Ill and Injured
Edited by D. H. Wilson and A. K. Marsden
© 1982, John Wiley & Sons Ltd.

MEDICALIZATION OF PRE-HOSPITAL FIRST AID

J.Metrot, C.Desfemmes, N.Dufeu
SAMU 94
Departement d'Anesthesie Reanimation
Hop. Henri Mondor, Creteil, France.

ABSTRACT

In France the response to a request for medical assistance is
routed through the 'SAMU' Emergency Aid Service which can deploy
an emergency team including, where appropriate, an emergency
physician. SAMU works in close co-operation with the police,
fire brigade and general medical practitioners.

INTRODUCTION

The means of responding to a public request for medical help vary
from sophisticated Emergency Medical Services to a centralised
single call telephone number. In France, in 1967, the first
Mobile Emergency and Resuscitation Units(SMURs) were created
following the initiative of some anaesthetists and emergency
surgeons with close support from the military medical officers
of the Paris fire service and the Marseilles port authorities.
From the necessity to centralise calls and to co-ordinate and
control the response has evolved the national Emergency Aid
Services or SAMUs. SAMU is a public amenity which handles the
communications for medical emergency services, arranges transport
through the SMURs and organises deployment of injured victims to
the Emergency Departments. Being "departement" or even regionally
based, the SAMUs mobilise and co-ordinate several SMURs.

SAMU 94

SAMU 94 was the first SAMU created in Paris's conglomeration in
1972 under the management of the head of the Anaesthesia and
Resuscitation Department of the Henri Mondo Hospital,
Prof.Huguenard. It is based at Creteil, the geographic centre
of the "departement". The Val de Marne SAMU covers part of the
Paris connurbation with 1.3 million inhabitants in an area of
245 sq.kilometres. The population is unequally spread over three
geographic sectors limited by the Seine and Marne rivers. This
is a high risk area containing two motorways encompassing the Orly
Airport, a main marshalling yard, a harbour and power stations.
Within the "departement" are some new developments and recently
created cities - Creteil is one of them.

THE DOCTRINE OF SAMU 94

In order to make the most efficient use of the resources, the
response to requests for assistance can be adjusted.   For example
in an urban population the total annual estimated number of calls
is 6 per 100 inhabitants.   Of these only 10 per cent require an
immediate specialized response - the remainder can be referred to
an available general practitioner and treated at home or transported
by routine ambulance to a care centre.   The sorting of all calls is
the responsibility of a group of doctors referred to as 'emergency
regulator phsicians'.   Telephone and radio calls are centralised
at the SAMU headquarters: four radio frequencies are constantly
monitored and there are about fifty direct telephone links with
hospitals and health authorities.   All calls are recorded.
A Telex intercommunication accelerates message transmission.

MOBILE UNITS

The mobile units are decentralised in order to permit a rapid
response time (statutorily within 15 minutes).   SAMU 94 controls
four "SMURs) based at the west, south, north and centre of the
"departement".   There are seven emergency medical teams, one being
specialised in neonatal resuscitation.   The mobile units take the
form of large resuscitation ambulances or rapid intervention vehicles
with medical equipment packed in suitcases or "Alouette III"
helicopters of the "Securite Civile" or "Gendarmerie Nationale".
SAMU 94 has its own registered heliport in readiness by day or night.
The personnel of the medical teams are in constant radio contact
with the SAMU regulator physician ; the general practitioners have
at their disposal small radio cars - three are fully operational
by day and a permanent on-call arrangement operates at night.

WORK LOAD

In 1980 SAMU 94 processed 20,000 calls.   9,000 required the
assistance of a specialist team either for traumatic (50%) or
medical emergencies.   One quarter of the calls were for mobile
coronary care.   The remaining 11,000 calls were handled by
general practitioners.   SAMU has an additional teaching role
(more than 1000 hours in 1980) for medics, paramedics, first aiders,
police and fire service officers.   SAMU forms part of the disaster
plan and teaches disaster medicine to university diploma standards.

CONCLUSION

An adequate, co-ordinated response for medical assistance has now
been realised by SAMU due to good co-operation between police, fire
and public hospital services and specialist hospital and general
medical practitioners.

REFERENCES

Huguenard P. Desfemmes C. Metrot J. 1978. "Organisation des soins
    medicaux d'urgence dans un departement de la region parisienne".
    7° Symposium Internationnal de Soins Intensifs. Rio de Janeiro.
    Brazil.

Metrot J. 1975. Creation, organisation et activite du SAMU 94. These Creteil-Paris X11.

Huguenard P. Niemeyer E. Herve C. et al. 1981. Justification de l'aide medicale urgente (comparaison de deux series de poly-traumatises avant et apres la creation du SAMU 94). 22° Assises de Medecine du Traffic, Strasbourg.

Care of the Acutely Ill and Injured
Edited by D. H. Wilson and A. K. Marsden
© 1982, John Wiley & Sons Ltd.

BRINGING THE HOSPITAL TO THE EMERGENCY

Dennis B. Dove, MD; William M. Stahl, MDFACS; Louis R.M. delGuercio, MDFACS; Leon D. Star, MDFACS and Louis Abelson, MD. Department of Surgery, New York Medical College, 1901 First Avenue, New York 10029 USA, Medical Office, J.F.K. Airport, Jamaica, New York 11413 USA

INTRODUCTION

John F. Kennedy International Airport (JFKIA) serves the greater New York City Region and handles 27 million passengers annually with 800-1000 take offs and landings every 24 hours. Seventy percent of the airport perimeter is bounded by water and the remaining borders extend to densely populated residential areas. The access roadways to this airport are among the busiest in the metropolitan area. This airport boasted a well conceived cooperative, written disaster plan which had been exercised annually on six occasions prior to 1976.

In June 1976, an incident occurred which involved a B727 aircraft while on final approach. A review of the management of this disaster resulted in the identification of significant flaws in the existing disaster plan. Most prominent among these was the almost immediate hopelessly gridlocked traffic pattern which rendered useless access routes to the airport. Except for the emergency vehicles and personnel on site at the airport, access was delayed until traffic could be unsnarled. Immediate helicopter transport of casualties from the scene was deemed to be impractical for several reasons.

Therefore, in response, the JFKIA disaster plan was modified so as to reflect the concept of "Bringing The Hospital To The Emergency." This concept provides for the assessment, evaluation, resuscitation and stabilization of casualties on site prior to their orderly evacuation to a definitive care facility appropriate to their needs. In order for this concept to be realized, certain conditions had to be fulfilled as follows:

1. Facilities: Facilities suited to these activities had to be identified and secured at the airport. A new piece of equipment known as an Emergency Mobile Hospital was developed. Two such vehicles now stand in constant readiness at the airport and together provide 12 monitored ICU stretcher beds, a 16 stretcher bed burn unit, 2 operating rooms and 60 other stretcher beds. A new modularized version is currently being developed.

2. Personnel: On site personnel recruited from all ranks of airport workers have been trained as Emergency Medical Technicians and Paramedics and respond to a disaster site with the Mobile Hospital.

BRINGING THE HOSPITAL TO THE EMERGENCY

Internal disaster plans are activated at hospitals in the immediate vicinity of the airports and Trauma teams are assembled. Some of these teams by arrangement try to reach the airport by ground transportation, while others maintain a state of readiness at the receiving hospital. Under the auspices of a single area Medical School (New York Medical College) and its affiliated departments of surgery at ten separate hospitals Trauma teams composed of trauma surgeons and critical area nurses are assembled in response to activation of the JFKIA Disaster Plan.

3. Transportation: These Trauma teams are transported by emergency vehicles from the individual hospitals to either of two commercial heliports in midtown Manhattan. Helicopters from the police, coast guard, air national guard, other military units and from four commercial operators converge on these heliports after activation of the same disaster plan component which activated the Trauma teams. The teams are then airlifted to the airport in 8-9 minutes. The helicopters maintain this air link for the transport of additional personnel and equipment as needed at the site.

SUMMARY

Design features of newer widebodied aircraft have provided greater occupant protection and have reduced fatalities. At the same time the increased capacity has resulted in greater numbers of seriously injured persons. Preservation of life in such cases demands maximum preplanned organization for the delivery of precise quality care.

The review of the management of a 1976 aircraft incident at John F. Kennedy International Airport (JFKIA) New York City revealed significant problems with ground access to the site. In response, a new concept of bringing the hospital to the emergency was incorporated into the Airport Disaster Plan. Preassembled Trauma teams are brought by helicopter within 30 minutes to the site.

The principle of bringing the hospital to the emergency, of assembling Trauma teams and transporting these teams to the disaster site is applicable to disaster planning in any other metropolitan area where these facilities exist as at JFKIA and New York City. The use of helicopters for this purpose is ideal since they can be readily scrambled and provide a secure means of bypassing the intolerable situations of ground access to the airport site.

REFERENCES

Abelson, L.C., Star, L.D. and Goldren, A.S. Twenty Years of Medical Support in Aircraft Disasters at Kennedy Airport. Aerospace Med. 44:560, 1973.

Dove, D.B., delGuercio, L.R.M., Stahl, W.M., Starr, L.D. and Abelson, L.C. A Metropolitan Airport Disaster Plan - Coordination of a Multi Hospital Response to Provide an On Site Resuscitation and Stabilization Center. J. Trauma 21, 1981 (In Press)

Care of the Acutely Ill and Injured
Edited by D. H. Wilson and A. K. Marsden
© 1982, John Wiley & Sons Ltd.

DIAGNOSTIC AIDS IN THE EMERGENCY DEPARTMENT

A Sessional Abstract

Anthony Barker, MD, FRCP, FRCS

Saint George's Hospital, London

Every acute emergency coming to an Accident Department demands
decision by the medical attendant. Is the patient's best interest
served by accurate and often time-consuming clinical assessment;
or by prompt action? Full examination with the use of sophisticated
diagnostic methods can result in dangerous delay in the transfer
of the patient correctly labelled but inadequately resuscitated.

There is thus need for the exercise of sound judgement. Will more
complete investigation make a material difference to the patient's
management and ultimate recovery? Or would the patient benefit
from immediate transfer to a specialised department?

This is more than a theoretical question. There is little room
for complacency over our present methods of assessment in the
Emergency Room. Gordon Trinca pointed out in his paper to the
session that, in 1430 victims of car crashes, there was an
overall failure of 40% in the diagnosis of the second - and less
obvious - injury. In some parts of the body this non-recognition
of hidden damage was more common still. Thus, while only 19% of
skull fractures were missed, as many as 60% of haemothoraces
passed unnoticed, and every single instance of small-bowel rupture
went unrecognised at the time of the initial examination.

With such a high level of mistaken diagnosis, it is necessary to
ask 'Why does this happen? Could more sophisticated diagnostic
tools be used to perfect our evaluation of such cases?'. Trinca
identified the main causes of failure. They were, first, that
senior Casualty doctors cannot be in their departments for 24
hours a day, so that many initial assessments must be made by
doctors of relatively little experience. Moreover, these doctors
may be doing their best under the stress of a full waiting-room.
Often the hour is late, and fatigue begins to show. In some
places, even today, facilities are below standard. It is not
that these doctors are incompetent to make the decisions, but
rather that their inexperience may prevent them from asking the
right questions, or from having the appropriate degree of built-
in clinical suspicion. To remember the likely, is the best
protection against error. Good teaching in medical schools

ensures that X-rays are correctly taken of the skull after head
injury, even where there are no external marks of violence, and
most doctors will remember to check the odontoid peg after whip-
lash neck injuries. These are common pitfalls, and are thus
usually avoided. What is not so commonly known is the high
incidence of pelvic fracture in pedestrians knocked down by cars.
Because these fractures are less well known, they may be missed.
And, in the end, there is no substitute for good examination.
Hand and eye remain the best diagnostic aids, in Casualty as
elsewhere.

Although the use of radiology was not the subject of a paper at
the session, its position as the principal diagnostic aid was
recognised throughout the conference. It was usefully dealt with
by Dr McIlrath of Belfast in plenary session, and widely discussed.
Every Accident and Emergency department depends on radiology
daily for the management of fractures and joint injuries as well
as for other conditions both medical and surgical. Perhaps
because it is normally so well and effectively done, and so often
gives the required answer, accident doctors are generally slow
to look forward and ask for the additional help that the radiologists are able to give by reason of the advances in their
discipline. Certainly, most of the departments in this country
are not equipped with more modern instruments. Yet in ultrasound is
an available technique for the diagnosis of gall-bladder disease
and for detecting solid-organ damage and internal haemorrhage.
Venograms, selective angiography and the use of isotopes in the
diagnosis of small-bone fractures have an application to the
Emergency Room. Because of expense and space and the problems of
mobility in patients attached to infusions and monitor leads, the
CT scanner does not appear to have any application.

Mr Pascall spoke of the use of peritoneal lavage in suspected
intra-abdominal injury. Most surgeons who have worked in the
Third World will bear testimony to the use of this procedure in
the diagnosis of ruptured ectopic pregnancy. When positive,
peritoneal lavage can be of much use. But can reliance be
entirely placed on a negative wash?

Of what use is the computer? An expensive Aide-Memoire for the
inexperienced? Or a necessity that no self-respecting Casualty
Officer can afford to be without? Doctor de Dombal reminded us
that with size and price alike greatly reduced, there was really
no reason why even the oldest of us should not try to learn just
how useful these "big, fast, dumb, adding machines" might be in
diagnosis, monitoring and teaching within the Accident Department.
That they can be so useful is certain. Nobody would confuse their
programmed response with a display of wisdom, but it is true that
such an instrument may perform better than inexperience, even as
it can never - by its very nature - come up with the flair of
the widely experienced. Within its limitations, the computer can
help with diagnosis, act as a reminder of forgotten facts, and
behave as a useful early-warning system when the patient is
headed into trouble.

This capacity for alerting the attending medical team to coming danger is shared also by the use of marking systems in patient care. Dr du Feu spoke of Severity Scores which could be deduced from observation on the patient, and especially of the CHOP system devised for the U.S. army medical service. This depends on biological and haematological measurements, pointing the way to timely resuscitation before the onset of collapse.

The Emergency Department remains the starting place for life-saving action, even if, in many instances, the action is completed in specialised departments of the hospital. Getting things going on the right track is the continuing responsibility of the emergency team. To do this with certainty requires that every bit of information that can be obtained about the patient is known and recorded. Diagnostic aids play an important part in gaining this knowledge. They should not be passed over by reason of conservatism, any more than they should be uncritically adopted in response to unthinking trends. Sense and experience have their place here, too: aiding the physician in his choice of the aids which are available to him.

Care of the Acutely Ill and Injured
Edited by D. H. Wilson and A. K. Marsden
© 1982, John Wiley & Sons Ltd.

DIAGNOSTIC AIDS IN THE MANAGEMENT OF THE ACUTE ABDOMEN

E.M. McILRATH,

Department of Radiology,   Royal Victoria Hospital,
BELFAST,   Northern Ireland, BT12 6BA, U.K..

In the past decade, several new techniques have been established in general radiological practice.   Notable among these have been CT scanning and grey-scale untrasound - the latter refined recently by the addition of high definition real-time scanning.   In other established areas such as nuclear medicine, the use of dynamic computerized scanning allows non-invasive angiography and investigation of organ perfusion.   The use of fine needle aspiration, the added sophistication of double-contrast and infusion barium studies are now taken for granted in routine radiological practice.

While many articles studying comparative values of these techniques in routine practice are available, with a few notable exceptions, there has been little comparative study of the various methods available relative to the changing incidence of abdominal emergencies reaching our hospitals.

What, if any, reasons can be given for the apparent lack of use of these new-found tools?   I think the major reason must be the fact that very few accident and emergency departments have specialist radiological consultants attached to, or in charge of, their X-ray departments.   Likewise, the A. & E. departments of many hospitals are remote from the main radiological departments and their sophisticated facilities.   There are exceptions to this rule and one hopes that, with future planning of hospitals, these exceptions will become the rule.

While the cost of CT scanning makes the limited use perhaps explicable, a bigger mystery is the lack of utilization of U/S.   One can presently purchase a high-definition, real-time ultrasound unit for approximately £25,000-£35,000;   this unit is portable, can be used in both the imaging department and by the bedside or in the resuscitation and casualty areas;   U/S does not require a vast amount of operator-training and produces images without access to a dark room.

An image intensifier on a C arm assembly, with suitable trolleys and photofluorography, that is, small film format cameras, is one of the better methods for dealing with multiple trauma.   This particular type of unit, however, costs approximately £60,000, and

there can be no reason other than economic for the failure to
utilize this unit in our A. & E. departments.

Isotopes present a special problem in that the preparation of
isotopes, on a 24-hours' basis, is a rather expensive exercise.
Most targeted isotopes are obtained from a Technetium source, which
is euphimistically known in this country as a"cow". The "cow" has
to be milked by a technician, and the correct dosage of isotope
prepared. While many kits are available to do this,the requirements
of radiation protection mean that the technician would require to be
available for the preparation of the patient doses on a 24-hours'
period, and I doubt the feasibility of this in many centres.

Having outlined the difficulties, it is easy - professionally
if not politically or economically - to produce some answers.

Firstly, the planning of our hospitals in relation to A. & E.
and the imaging departments must be reconsidered.

Secondly, an increase in the number of consultant radiologists
with a particular interest in the A. & E. situation is required and,
fortunately, staffing in the specialty in the training grades now
would appear to give hope that such posts could be filled in the very
near future.

Thirdly, scarce resources must be used adequately.   I think
the day when the scanner belonged to the neurologist and the angiography room to the cardiologist must be past, and that access to
this type of equipment should be available to all members of staff
within the hospital.

<u>The Acute Abdomen Itself</u>:

I hope to deal with common conditions initially suggesting a
format of management in the imaging processes and indicating where
the newer techniques will be of value, but excluding - endoscopy,
diagnostic puncture and the radiology of the urethra and testes.

The order of investigation given represents the experience
available in Belfast, with the resources now available in imaging in
the Royal Victoria Hospital. They may not,therefore, be appropriate
for the centres in which you work, and are given only as a guide-
line rather than a mandatory technique.

Regarding the general considerations of investigating these
patients: I doubt that anyone is likely to disagree with those
outlined below.

TABLE   1

GENERAL CONSIDERATIONS

1.   Sophisticated investigation does not replace an adequate
     history and clinical examination.

2.   Resuscitation to a stable state should precede investigation.

3.   In multiple injuries, priorities must be established and
     monitored for change.

4.   Co-existent disease or medication must be assessed.

Trauma:

I would like to present 100 patients previously reported:

TABLE   2

100 CASES OF ABDOMINAL TRAUMA

Gunshot/Missile Wounds	41
Road Traffic Accidents	36
Other Blunt Trauma	23
Male/Female Ratio	11.5 : 1
Average Age	27 years

Positive radiological findings were present in only 45% of the
gunshot wounds and blunt trauma, and a mere 26% of the road traffic
accidents:

TABLE   3

"POSITIVE" RADIOLOGICAL FINDINGS

TYPE OF INJURY	%
Gunshot Wounds	45.00
Road Traffic Accidents	26.30
Other Blunt Trauma	45.00

Further analysis indicates that many of the positive findings
were in the urinary tracts where a fast, reliable, contrast examination exists.   In 18% the only positive finding was the presence of
a missile within the field of the film which, if excluded, reduces
the positive findings in this group to 27%

I would explain that, in ALL conditions affecting the abdomen, I
would request a chest X-ray as the first imaging investigation.   Not
only are conditions in the chest relevant to the surgeon and anaesthetist, but equally they can mimic conditions causing presentation as
an acute abdomen and, as long as the chest X-ray is adequately taken,
in that the incident beam is at the upper border of the peritoneal

cavity, the chances of showing sub-phrenic gas are good.

TABLE   4

IMAGING   I

Perforation

1. Chest X-ray
2. Straight abdominal X-ray
3. Horizontal beam X-ray
    (a) Erect
    (b) Left lateral decubitus
4. Water-soluble contrast study

I think it is also important that one learns to recognize the
appearances of free-gas on the AP supine film.   This is particularly
true if the patient, for any reason, cannot adequately be positioned
for horizontal beam X-rays.   The supine decubitus X-ray should be
banned under all circumstances, as it makes interpretation of free
intraperitoneal gas extremely difficult, and it is equally useless
in discerning the type of obstruction that might be present in
certain patients.

The supine abdominal X-ray is, in my opinion, almost always
more useful than the horizontal beam X-ray.   I do not find the
erect film as useful as the lateral decubitus views which allow the
air to follow around to the level of the obstruction, and this is
particularly true in the L. colon.

Particularly in Great Britian there appears to be a certain
reluctance to use contrast medium, and I consider this has been a
result of horrific stories regarding the use of oral contrast medium
in large bowel obstruction with inspissation of the barium and an
increased degree of obstruction.   This is entirely unnecessary
because the addition of a small amount of Gastrografin into the
barium mixture holds fluid within the barium and gives excellent
pictures of the large bowel without dehydration of the barium and
possible exacerbation of the obstructive process.

TABLE   5

IMAGING   II

Obstruction

1. Chest X-ray
2. Straight abdominal X-ray
3. Horizontal beam X-ray:
    (a) Erect
    (b) L. lateral decubitus
    (c) R. lateral decubitus
4. Contrast studies:
    (a) Barium enema if caecum distended
    (b) Follow-through or small bowel infusion

While double-contrast barium enemas are now virtually routine
in many X-ray departments, in large bowel obstruction there is really
little necessity to do anything other than a single-contrast enema,
which has some advantage in the sigmoid colon in diverticular disease
and is probably as successful in demonstrating inchaemic colitis as
the double-contrast method.

Small bowel infusion, which has been widely used in the investigation of small bowel disease (particularly by Nolan in Oxford),
lends itself ideally in the recurrent acute small bowel obstruction.
This type of patient frequently requires gastric intubation, and the
appropriate tube can quite easily be passed into the upper jejunum.
The amount of contrast used can be limited; and that the result of
the investigation is evident in a very much shorter time than with
the normal barium follow-through examination.

TABLE   6

IMAGING   III

Gallbladder

1.   Chest X-ray
2.   P.A. gallbladder area
3.   Ultrasound
4.   H.I.D.A. isotope scan

Regarding acute abdominal emergencies related to gallbladder
pathology: again the chest X-ray is important to exclude R. basal
lung or pleural pathology.   Where possible it is better to avoid
doing scout views of the abdomen and take specific gallbladder area
X-rays.   If there are stones present the changes of demonstrating
them on a gallbladder area view are much improved over the scout film.

I do not think there is any place whatsoever for contrast studies
in acute gallbladder pathology.

I slightly prefer U/S to the HIDA isotope scan, which has the
same accuracy and specificity, but requires the preparation of the
isotope by a technician.   The cost of the isotope is considerable
and I think, as the results of the two techniques are similar, then
the cheaper one should be employed.

Weismann, In April 1979, indicated that the accuracy of U/S was
98%, the specificity 100%, the false-negatives were approximately 5%
and there were no false-positive findings.

The point, however, has been made by several authors that, in
acute gallbladder disease, gas in the upper abdomen may obstruct the
visualization of the common bile duct, whereas the HIDA scan almost
always shows the common bile duct.   I believe this is true but it
does not necessarily influence the management of the patient in the
first 24 or 48 hours.   It was also evident that, with the earlier
forms of U/S, gas in the gallbladder area was a great problem,
reducing the number of effective examination by approximately 20%.

The advent of real-time and intercostal scanning has reduced this considerably.

The pancreas remains an organ for which I have a great deal of respect.

TABLE   7

IMAGING   IV

Pancreatitis

1. Chest X-ray
2. Straight abdominal X-ray
3. Ultrasound - Pancreas
                       - Biliary
4. C.T.   N.B.: Complications
5. Occasional contrast studies

I think, again, U/S is extremely relevant in the management of pancreatic disease.   The tail and distal body of the pancreas may be difficult to demonstrate, but if grossly enlarged or there is any accumulation of fluid in the area, they probably will be visualized with some ease, even by a relatively inexperienced ultrasonographer. Equally, U/S allows one to look at the biliary tract to confirm a relationship between biliary disease and pancreatitis.

Should the patient present with the complications of acute pancreatitis, then CT scanning has certain advantages in that it will show extension of the disease outside the area of the pancreas rather more readily than U/S, and may make planned drainage of an abscess easier.

The Glasgow workers have shown that the management of acute pancreatitis by U/S can be exceptionally worthwhile;   monitoring the development of an abscess or pseudocyst, and indicating drainage at the correct time.

In the retroperitoneal area, lesions in the kidney and ureter account for a continuing, significant proportion of acute abdominal admissions.

TABLE   8

IMAGING   V

Kidney & Bladder

1. Emergency I.V.P.
     N.B.: high dose,   tomograms,
                  adequate films
2. β ultrasound or isotope scan
3. C.T. scan
4. Cystogram
5. Arteriogram

At the last count we have carried out slightly over 3,000 IVPs since 1965. Of these, a "normal" IVP was present in only 14 patients with significant renal disease; and in abnormal renal tracts, the IVP was between 95% and 100% specific.

Our viewpoint on contrast dosage is that the required dose is that necessary to produce an adequate examination. Tomography facilities are available in the A. & E. Department, and that adequate early and late films are always taken, and every IVP is supervised by a radiologist. If there is absent or deficient nephrogram, that is a high indicator of compromise of the reno-vascular pedicle and, therefore, the investigation of this finding must be in the short term.

U/S can be useful, particularly in the traumatized kidney. It will also indicate whether a non-functioning kidney is due to tumour or hydronephrosis. The isotope scan with dynamic studies, will also indicate the vascular perfusion characteristics of the kidney.

If doubtful on the urogram, CT scan can be of use in renal trauma and acute renal carbuncle. In our hands, renal masses are, however, better dealt with by U/S. CT scan can also be useful in bladder trauma and one can get spectacularly effective pictures with IV contrast, thus avoiding the requirement for either a cystogram per urethra or by the suprapubic route.

Vascular studies, I feel, are only indicated where there appears to be compromise of the renal vascular pedicle, either by embolization or traumatic subluxation of the pedicle.

In imaging of the liver and spleen or the solid organs, what is known as "conventional radiography" is of virtually no value.

TABLE   9

IMAGING   VI

Liver & Spleen

1.   Ultrasound
2.   Isotope - preferably with perfusion studies
3.   C.T.
4.   Angiograms

Occasionally signs of bleeding in the lower chest or pleura, rupture or elevation of the disphragm and fracture of the appropriate ribs may assist and, although not indicated on this Table, the Chest X-ray is still mandatory.

Again, the first approach should be by U/S - simple, quick, cheap and reasonably effective - although the spleen can be difficult and must be scanned by the intercostal method. Isotope studies with perfusion are, again, a reasonably quick and effective method of studying the parenchyma of these organs. CT, with the newer type of scanner, will be effective; but we have rarely practised CT in major trauma to the upper abdomen, usually because of the availability of U/S and the non-availability of the CT scanner on an emergency basis.

Angiography may particularly be required for the complications of rupture of the liver such as haematobilia or AVM. I really doubt, despite the previous work in the 1960s and 1970s, whether initial angiography is required now for the diagnosis of rupture of the liver and spleen in the acute phase.

Regarding the vascular structures:

TABLE 10

IMAGING VII

Vascular

1. Aorta or I.V.C.
    - Ultrasound
    - Isotope angiogram
    - Digital/Catheter angiogram
2. Branches
    - See solid organs
      N.B.: superior mesenteric embolism
    - Reversible colonic ischaemia

I feel strongly that the isotope angiogram has not been widely enough used. U/S will indicate the presence or absence of an aortic aneurysm, displacement of the cava, the presence in many cases of retroperitoneal haemorrhage; this can also be done by CT, but probably the best study is the isotope angiogram, indicating both the flow through the aorta and its general configuration; both of these techniques - U/S and isotope angiography - can indicate the necessity for standard angiography of any type.

Regarding embolism of the branches: I think the recognition of the type of patient who is likely to have mesenteric embolism or, for that matter, mesenteric ischaemia, is important. Plain X-ray signs such as gas in the gut wall or venous channels, are late and frequently only briefly precede death. If the patient is acutely ill, our practice is not to do angiography, but rather to go straight to laparotomy.

When in training and up to about seven years ago, never a night or week-end went past without the radiologist being asked to investigate GIT haemorrhage. As you will note, it is with great pleasure that I put first on this table - endoscopy.

TABLE   11

IMAGING   VIII

G.I.T. Haemorrhage

1. Endoscopy
2. Double-contrast barium studies
3. Small bowel infusion
4. Angiogram
5. Radioisotope scan

I think emergency endoscopy in the upper GIT haemorrhage is likely to be more successful than barium meals, but it is interesting to compare the figures coming from comparable operators in both fields, rather than to compare the consultant with an interest in endoscopy, to the registrar barium meal which is carried out in many X-ray departments.   I think there is a firm indication for double-contrast barium studies if endoscopy is negative, and stress that they must be <u>double-contrast</u>, be they barium meal or barium enema. There is NO place in GIT haemorrhage for the old-fashioned litres of barium - either per os or per anus.

As stated earlier, I am a protagonist of the small bowel infusion in the study of small bowel pathology.

The role of angiography is difficult to place. Catastrophic bleeding and negative endoscopy and a large amount of barium in the abdomen will render angiography useless.   It may well be that angiography should follow endoscopy if the haemorrhage is of fulminant nature.   On the other hand, I think that many patients who have less severe bleeding can be diagnosed by less invasive procedures than angiography.

Catheter angiograms do allow for Pitressin infusion and therapeutic embolization.

Radioisotope scanning has been used mainly in two fields in GI bleeding - One, of course, is the simple Technetium Pertechnotate scan to indicate the presence of gastric mucosa in a Meckel's diverticulum.   This is a well-known and simple procedure.   Rather less widely used is the infusion of colloid Technetium or labelled red cells, which will leak into the gut if there is frank bleeding into the lumen.   This technique has been used in several centres in the diagnosis of bleeding from diverticular disease from small bowel and from angio dysplasia.   These total, however, a small number of patients, but evidence suggests this is a good, non-invasive, method of locating a bleeding source and one which is, possibly, not widely known.

To summarize, firstly I would like to stress yet again an adequacy of clinical examination and, hopefully, the passage of this information to the radiologist.

I think the chest X-ray is mandatory in all acute abdominal emergencies, straight radiography of the abdomen properly carried out still has a part to play in perforation, obstruction, and in the presence or absence of gallstones.

I think that the emergency IVP will continue to be important.

Advances can be made by a much wider use of ultrasonography and would suggest that this does not need necessarily to be carried out by the radiographer or the radiologists, and that the average surgeon or surgical registrar should be capable of using an U/S machine in the same way as his obstetric colleagues.

A wider use of isotopes is justified.   The HIDA scan is well recognized to be as accurate as ultrasonography.   The isotope angiogram should be in much wider usage, both in the abdomen and elsewhere.

If CT becomes more widely available, and with rapid scanners, it can play an increasing part, but the cost of CT is always going to be a factor; therefore the number of units will be limited, and the demans upon those units will be extensive.

I have tried to indicate, therefore, the use of both conventional and the newer techniques in the A. & E. examination of the acute abdomen. I apologise for the fact that it was impossible to cover the whole field as widely as I would have liked.

I am grateful to the organizers for the opportunity to present a radiologist's view.

Care of the Acutely Ill and Injured
Edited by D. H. Wilson and A. K. Marsden
© 1982, John Wiley & Sons Ltd.

THE COMPUTER IN EMERGENCY CARE.

F.T. de Dombal

Department of Surgery,
St. James Hospital, Leeds, England.

ABSTRACT.

This presentation surveys the use of computers in clinical medicine,
with particular reference to the ways in which this usage will effect
surgeons involved in Emergency Care.   Some aspects of recent
computer science are described which have made small dedicated
systems much more attractive to the non-specialist user (such as the
emergency surgeon).   Specific uses such as monitoring, diagnosis,
departmental information and teaching are reviewed, and future
developments briefly surveyed.

INTRODUCTION.

Until very recently computers have made little impact in medical
care (comparable to the revolutionary impact in other fields such as
banking and business).   Indeed, until recently it might be asserted
that computers did not have much to offer the clinician and what they
offered was difficult to understand and extremely expensive.
However a number of trends in computing science have now made the
computer a much more attractive proposition to clinicians in general
and Emergency Care in particular.   These changes may be listed as
follows:-

Development of Micro Systems.   The "micro revolution" and the
development of the silicone chip have been well documented elsewhere
(Evans 1979).   It is nevertheless, well worth pointing out that one
reason for the increasing use of computers in emergency situations
lies in the fact that systems which previously occupied whole
departments can now be found on an individual doctor's desk.   These
micro systems are not only smaller but quicker and more reliable
than their previous large counterparts.

Cost Reductions.   Equally welcome, the cost of computers has
plummeted in the last twenty years.   Back in the 1960's a computer
of modest storage capacity, a detached house and a Rolls Royce each
cost about the same.   In the 1980's the cost of micro-computers has
fallen so dramatically that many cost less nowadays than a television
set or a car repair bill.   This has made computing a much more
attractive proposition.

<u>Increase in Storage</u>.   For many medical users, the chief trend in
computer science which has opened up new forms of usage, is the vast
increase in storage capacity which has resulted from the development
of the magnetic tape cassette and the floppy disk.   In particular
this latter device, similar to a thin version of a 45 rpm gramophone
record, can currently contain up to one megabyte of information (one
million characters, or 100 items of information about each of
10,000 patients) and costs around $10.   Suddenly, storage capacity
is no longer a problem for the average user.

<u>Ease of Usage</u>.   Another major feature of computer science which has
made life much easier for the medical user is the development of so
called "high level languages" by which the clinician can communicate
with his computer.   In the 1950's communication with a computer was
carried out in "machine code" (e.g. 010110111010... etc).   This was
impossible for the non-specialist user to understand and virtually
ruled out computer use by all but the dedicated professional.   By
the 1960's computer codes had begun to emerge (a good example being
that utilised in the lunar module for guidance and control in the
early Apollo flights).   This code (e.g. 0907 0116 1303 1215 etc)
was easier to understand (just) but still far from clear to the
average clinician.

Nowadays, "high level" languages such as FORTRAN, COBOL and
particularly BASIC, have been developed, which can be readily
understood by even the non-specialist.   Each consist of a specific
series of instructions to the computer most of which are written in
plain English.   For example, if one wishes the computer to print
"Hello", the simple BASIC instruction is this:- "10 PRINT "HELLO".
It needs little imagination to realise the impact which this
development of "high level" language has had on non-specialist users.

<u>Clinical Development</u>.   The last development which has speeded up the
impact of computers in clinical medicine has little to do with
computer science and more to do with the development of the clinical
medicine itself.   In the last 20-30 years hospitals (along with them
Emergency Departments) have become complex places and it has become
far more difficult for any individual to keep track even of what is
going on in his own hospital or department.

This, along with the relatively sudden appearance of small, cheap,
easy to understand, and reliable computer systems has made it almost
inevitable that the usage of these systems should have become more
widespread.   In the coming paragraphs we shall briefly survey some
of the usages in regard of the Emergency Care situation.

<u>USE OF COMPUTER SYSTEMS IN EMERGENCY CARE</u>.

With the current explosion of interest in micro-computers and their
capabilities it is almost impossible to keep track of every computer
application.   New applications are appearing almost daily.
However, as regards the Emergency Department, the major forms of use
can be grouped under the following four headings.

Monitoring.   Computer systems are now widely utilised to monitor
individual patients and it is difficult to argue with the premise
that such monitoring has become already an accepted and "standard"
part of medical Emergency Care.   It is however, necessary to
distinguish rather carefully between three different types of
monitoring systems.

Signal analysis: Computers with a suitable analog-to-digital
conversion system are widely used to interpret signals from an
individual patient.   The signal may be very simple (such as the
patients pulse) or may be very complicated (such as patients ECG or
EEG tracing).   These systems have now proven their value in many
different clinical settings.

Integrated systems: In the next type of system the computer performs
a slightly more complicated task.   As well as recording data from a
patient it analyses the data and produces comment on it.   In this
more complex system the computer will analyse data from several
patients at once and display the results at a central nursing station
often with built-in "error limits".   Thus - at its crudest level -
the computer will flash a light on the nurse's console if a patient's
pulse rate exceeds 120 or drops below 50 beats per minute.

Potentially such systems have considerable value, but they have been
criticised (Moloney 1972) on three accounts.   First, we do not yet
know how to use the machine to best advantage in order to complement
our own human capabilities.   Second, this has led to over emphasis
upon variables (such as the pulse) which can be measured
mathematically - and under emphasis of such variables (as the "look
of the patient") which a computer cannot measure.   Last, the computer
usually fails to respond to "Significant Low Probability Events",
(such as the patient falling out of bed!).

Closed loop systems: Most controversial of all of the monitoring
systems are the "closed loop systems" in which the computer not only
analyses data from the patient, and interprets it, but also acts
upon it - for example, speeding up an i.v. infusion in response to
rising pulse rate or fall in blood pressure.   It is fair to say that
this type of system has been greeted with great suspicion in the
medical profession and whilst simple, cheap, dedicated analysis
systems are likely to become more popular, costly elaborate "closed
loop" systems will (perhaps wisely) be treated with some caution in
the foreseeable future.

Diagnosis and Prognosis.   When the digital computer first appeared
one of the more "easy" tasks predicted for it to carry out in
clinical medicine was diagnosis of patients' ailments.   Needless to
say this early assessment has proved somewhat optimistic, but
recently a number of systems have emerged which appear to offer some
very real value to the clinician - in Emergency Care as elsewhere.

Computerised axial tomography: The "CAT" scan has become a familiar
part of medical life.   Normally such procedures are not undertaken
as emergencies, but on occasion computerised axial tomography can be
helpful in the emergency situation - for example in patients with
obscure abdominal trauma or following head injury.

Dedicated systems: The most widespread use of diagnostic computing
in the Emergency Department however is concerned with dedicated
small systems designed to aid diagnosis in specific areas (such as
abdominal pain, chest pain, jaundice and upper G.I. bleeding).
These systems have all been designed to assist the clinician rather
than replace him and in some areas at least have been quite
successful in improving the diagnostic accuracy of individual doctors.

The evidence for this statement is summarised at some length
elsewhere (de Dombal 1979).   However in respect of acute abdominal
pain, in Leeds the diagnostic accuracy of the first doctor to see
each patient in the Emergency Department in 1971 was 42%.   By 1974
provision of structured data collection forms and detailed computer
feedback had raised this figure to 63% and during the period
1979-1981 the proportion of patients leaving the Emergency Room in
the Leeds General Infirmary with a correct diagnosis had risen to
74%.   Twice as many patients were sent home without needing
admission, leading to substantial and welcome savings in terms of
bed nights and hard cash.

Similar results were obtained in a careful study carried out in
Airedale District General Hospital (West Yorkshire) during the
period 1974-1981.   In these studies McAdam and colleagues also
showed welcome reductions in the negative laparotomy rate and the
rate at which appendices perforated prior to operation.   Others
elsewhere, notably Gunn in Scotland and Boom in Mexico have shown
similar trends.   Variations of the basic system developed in Leeds
in 1971 are now in use in fourteen different countries.

It appears therefore that over the next few years we may expect to
see an expansion of diagnostic systems designed to aid the clinician
in the Emergency Room.   These systems will be small, dedicated
systems.   Some will be computer based, some will not - but all will
act in an adjunctive capacity and will not attempt to remove the
responsibility for decision-making from the Accident and Emergency
doctor.

Record Keeping and Departmental Information.   A further major use
for computers in the Accident and Emergency Department concerns the
provision of a steady flow of information about the working of the
Department so that the resources available may be used to their
best advantage.   Such systems are already in use in several
departments and elsewhere in this volume descriptions will be found
of individual systems.

The information which may be obtained varies from system to system.
Typically, departmental statistics are provided concerning the
type of work load (patient age and sex, type of problem, time of
arrival); patient flow (mode of arrival, action taken in the
Emergency Room, diagnosis and disposal of the patient); and the
doctors performance (referrals for investigation, number of patients
admitted and so on).

Here perhaps more than anywhere else caution is necessary.   It is
quite clear that such systems can be of considerable benefit if
used wisely and sensibly.   It is quite clear also that the

information can be quite "sensitive".   It is vitally important that
data of this kind should be analysed by concerned sympathetic medical
staff rather than by non-medical administrators.   For this reason,
(if no other), it is vital that medical staff concern themselves
with the development of computing systems.

Teaching.   One of the most important uses of computer systems in
the Emergency Room concerns continuing education.   Over the last
five years a large number of teaching packages have appeared,
designed to provide such education for hospital doctors.

The type of computer-aided instruction system which has been
developed varies from relatively simple devices - such as the
provision of multiple choice questions to be answered by the student
(with remedial loops for student errors) - up to quite complex
simulation of patient problems so that the hospital doctor may
practice diagnosis and management.

Perhaps the most sophisticated use of computers has been in the so
called "Delphic Mode" (de Dombal 1979) whereby the computer analyses
a clinicians performance in a series of specific cases, attempts to
develop a hypothesis about the clinician's performance, and feeds
back to the clinician concerned some suggestions for improving
diagnostic or decision-making performance.

The Leeds system (described above) clearly indicates to a clinician
in the Emergency Room (in the event of diagnostic error) whether
this error originated because the clinician failed to ascertain
adequate data from the patient or because the clinician ascertained
the correct information but failed to analyse it correctly.   The
doctor is thus "steered" towards appropriate further training.

These systems, which have developed over the last few years, have
resulted in considerable improvements in patient management and
individual doctor performance.   It seems likely that they will
develop over the next few years into a highly useful series of
packages in other clinical areas.   Indeed the use of computers as
a postgraduate educational device may well become its most
widespread mode of usage in the next five years.

            THE FUTURE.

Computers have therefore, almost overnight, become a part of our
daily way of life - in the Emergency Room as elsewhere.   Future
developments of the computer may be expected, but many of them will
be irrelevant to Emergency Clinical Practice.   For example, the
explosion of computer memory power has already provided us with all
the memory we need.and the advant of hand held computers which
respond to and recognise speech will not prove particularly relevant
to the Emergency doctor.

What will prove relevant is the increasing development of software
packages designed in very specific areas of medicine (such as those
listed above) to assist the Emergency Room clinician in one aspect or
other of his routine tasks.   These packages will become widely
available and will be relatively easy for non-specialist persons

F.T. de Dombal.

(such as clinicians - in the computing sense!) to use. They will depend on small dedicated systems and will, by 1990 or so, be taken for granted.

These developments will happen whether we like them or not. The chief problem which may be foreseen is that they will develop in the absence of a concerned, knowledgable input from the medical profession. If the medical profession ignores these systems, it may expect to see them introduced willy-nilly by administrators, with the backing of the general public, in the name of a more efficient service. If however, the medical profession maintains an interest in their development then we may expect to see (far more quickly and far more readily) the development of systems both valuable to patient care and acceptable to the medical profession.

REFERENCES

de Dombal, F.T. 1979. Computers and the Surgeon - A Matter of Decision, in Surgery Annual (Ed. Nyhus), pp33-57. Appleton-Century-Croft, New York.
Evans, C. 1979. in The Mighty Micro. Gollancz, London
Moloney, J. V. Jr. 1968. The trouble with patient monitoring. Annals of Surgery, 168, 605-619.

Care of the Acutely Ill and Injured
Edited by D. H. Wilson and A. K. Marsden
© 1982, John Wiley & Sons Ltd.

THE VALUE OF A COMPUTERISED A & E RECORD CARD

D.W. Yates

Accident and Emergency Medicine, Hope Hospital, Salford
M6 8HD, U.K.

The basic medical and epidemiological information on all
casualty record cards in Hope Hospital has been stored on computer
since January 1980. The system is being extended to three other
hospitals in 1981 using the same computer and data bank. The record
card is based on the original work of Wilson (May 1977) with some
modifications. There are two flimsy front sheets. The top one can
be used as a general practitioners letter and the second one is sent
to the regional computer centre. The coding boxes have been
realigned into two marginal columns to facilitate data recognition.
The following information is coded for all new patients:

SEX, DATE OF BIRTH
DATE, TIME AND PLACE OF INCIDENT/ONSET
DATE, TIME AND MODE OF ARRIVAL
TIME SEEN, AND BY WHICH DOCTOR
INVESTIGATIONS
DIAGNOSTIC CODE
TREATMENT
NATIONAL INSURANCE CERTIFICATE
DISPOSAL
NUMBER OF REVISITS

The diagnostic code is similar to the one used in Leeds. I.C.D.
codes are considered unsuitable for Accident and Emergency work.
Research boxes are available for use by the A & E department staff
or others in the hospital or the community.

All information on the two flimsy sheets prints through onto the
base card. This forms page one of a folded A4 card. Pages 2 and 3
are for clinical notes and page 4 contains an anaesthetic consent
form and the index to the diagnostic codes.

The following research activities have been facilitated by the use
of the card.

1. Information on the 1980 file has been used to weight cases
according to status on Arrival, Procedures undertaken in the
Department, Diagnosis and Subsequent Management. This weighted case
load or "work load" is much more useful than a mere record of the

of new patients attending and has been used to optimise provision of
medical nursing and administrative staff.

2. An analysis of works injuries showed wide variation in the number
of times patients with identical injuries were seen in the Department
and the length of time off work. This has prompted an investigation
into medical facilities in local industries.

3. Studies on patient flow between hospitals have shown previously
undetected discrepancies in the use of the emergency ambulance
service. Taken together with the "work load" study this information
has been valuable in planning the provision of inner city A/E
services.

4. The facility to record initial and final diagnoses on the record
card improves auditing techniques and identifies areas where mistakes
occur frequently.

The medical information coded from the record card is restricted but
is more accurate than in other hospital information systems. Many
other hospital departments have used the record card as a starting
point to identify patients whom they wish to study in greater detail.

REFERENCES

Wilson, D.H., Gunawardena, A., and Lee, K., 1977. A computerised
    information system for Accident and Emergency Departments.

Care of the Acutely Ill and Injured
Edited by D. H. Wilson and A. K. Marsden
© 1982, John Wiley & Sons Ltd.

A MICROCOMPUTER BASED RECORD SYSTEM IN AN
ACCIDENT UNIT

R. H. Gray,* D. McG. Clarkson,[+] D. H. A. Jones* and
P. H. S. Smith[+]

The Accident Unit* and the Department of Medical
Physics and Bioengineering,[+] C & A Hospital, Bangor, U.K.

ABSTRACT

A Microcomputer System has been developed to upgrade the previous
manual records system. Patient data is input and stored directly
at the reception desk. The computer generates a printed casualty
card which is updated after the patient has been seen by medical
staff.

A logbook of attendances is automatically produced, and the data
can be examined in order to produce various administrative
analyses. Also, the system allows rapid retrieval of our
workload according to various options which include the nature,
type and site of injuries.

INTRODUCTION

Traditional manual record systems do not allow the easy retrieval
and analysis of the out patient workload of orthopaedic and accident
services. This project was undertaken to develop and evaluate
a microcomputer system which could be capable of storing,
retrieving and analysing our accident unit workload.

The role established for the computer in accident unit record
management has tended to limit the degree of direct involvement
of the computer in the day to day operation of the department
(Roberts, Farrer and Harvey, 1977; Dalby, Farrer and Harvey
1974). Patient data, for example, may be entered off-line for
the purpose of undertaking statistical analyses. Typically,
patient information is not input 'on-line' i.e. during the time
of the patient's visit. Also, even for limited applications,
mini computers and even mainframe types have been used. This
has tended to set developments in this field of hospital analysis
more in the field of research at larger centres. The arrival of
the affordable yet often adequately powerful microcomputer has
provided the means whereby computer facilities can be obtained by
significantly smaller units.

The Accident Unit at Bangor is a major accident centre for Gwynedd
and comprises a casualty department, 19 accident beds and an
operating theatre. The unit serves a resident population of 230,000
but this number is regularly and dramatically increased by holiday

makers.   The unit deals with approximately 25,000 patient per year.

EQUIPMENT

The system comprises an 8032 series PET microcomputer, 1.6 Mbyte
Computhink floppy disc drive and a Diablo 1620 daisy wheel printer.
A dual IEEE to RS 232 interface is available to drive up to 2
printers.   The total hardware cost approximated to £4500.

ASPECTS OF DATA INPUT

The input programme is set up daily to display the consultant on
duty, date and time of day, the latter being continuously updated
by the clock within the computer.   Each new patient is
automatically allocated a unique casualty number in the format of
an identifying alphabetic character followed by a four digit
number in the range 1 to 3400.   The casualty number plays an
important role in uniquely identifying each patient and in
subsequent retrieval/updating of data.

Production of Casualty Card. Information relating to patient
identification and incident description (Table 1, left section)
is input directly by the casualty clerk on the arrival of the
patient.   This preliminary information is stored on floppy disc
and is printed on a flimsy attached to the upper portion of the
(as yet) blank casualty card.   The casualty officer, in addition
to writing his general longhand patient diagnosis on the lower
exposed portion of the casualty card, records further relevant
information (Table 1, right section) on the attached flimsy.   This
is in turn used by the casualty clerk to update a given patient's
entry, after which the flimsy is removed and a final definitive
print is made on the upper portion of the casualty card.   If
required, it is possible to code for revisits.

Medical Codes.   A simple set of codes is used which allows up to
three separate injuries to be described.   The type of hospital
emergency (medical, accident/orthopaedic etc) can be coded in up
to 9 ways;   the type of injury (laceration, burn etc) can be coded
in up to 8 ways, and the site of injury (head spine, upper limb etc)
can be coded in up to 7 ways.   In addition, both upper limb and
lower limb can be further subdivided by selection of a single
alphabetic character.

Replacement of Manual Logbook.   The daily logbook is produced
automatically by the microcomputer which prints out entries
between inclusive casualty numbers.   If required, entries of a
specific date only can be printed.   Also up to 1700 entries
may be sorted alphabetically in order to provide a useful reference
for accessing previous casualty cards.

The system has been in operation since December 1980.

TABLE 1   Items of information stored

Presenting Information		Additional Input	
Item of information	Length	Item of information	Length
patient name	25	medical coding	12
patient address	30	multiple injury	1
tel. no.	13	local anaesthetic	1
date of birth	4	cas. officer diag.	37
age	2	follow up	1
GP name	14	unit number	4
GP address	21	clinic date	3
place of incident	1		
location code	1		
referred by	1		
complaint	20		
mode of transport	1		
seen by	14		
revisit (if applic.)	4		

ANALYSIS OF DATA

Aims and Methods   Rather than develop several separate analysis
programmes for specific tasks, a single comprehensive programme
providing 10 analysis functions was developed.   Also, numerous
separate analyses can be specified initially and carried out
without any further operator action.   The resulting modes of
analysis were influenced both by local administrative needs and
the desire to manipulate the available data in a variety of useful
ways.   Up to 6800 records can be analysed in one complete
procedure.   It is possible to select entries to be included in
an analysis on the basis of inclusive casualty numbers and also
on calendar dates or a combination of these.

Options available   Road traffic accidents can be retrieved for
a specific set of data, allowing also 'driver' to be differen-
tiated from 'not driver'.   An analysis of workload on the basis
of age can be calculated, producing for a selected group of
records, the relative number within age groups 0 - 5 years,
5 - 10 years etc.   A separate mode of analysis allows the
retrieval and summary listing of all children under 5.   The
workload of the unit can be rapidly estimated using a routine
which, for e.g. a specified calendar month, can produce details
of numbers of patients treated, including the number of revisits.

The items of input information 'place of incident', 'residential
code', 'mode of referral', 'mode of transport' and 'follow up'
can be conveniently described as the group of 'main coded
categories'.   For a selected set of data it is possible to
summarise the variation of input within each main coded category
in turn.   It is possible, also, for a given main coded category,

to select a specific coded entry e.g. 'place of incident - work'
and for a selected set of data, produce summary listings of all
entries coded as specified.   In all, there are 42 distinct
modes of analysis using this latter option.

<u>Analysis of Coded Medical Input</u>   The system can summarise our
workload according to type of incident, type of injury and site of
injury.   Also, individual or multiple injuries may be retrieved
using appropriate codes.

DISCUSSION

A microcomputer system has been successfully developed in response
to local requirements, and we have made rapid progress in a short
time.   This is to a large extent due to dedicated equipment,
direct involvement of clinicians and rapid response by scientific
staff to the problems as they arise.

Introduction of the system has undoubtedly imposed greater
discipline on collection of information with consequent greater
demands on the reception clerk.   This is offset by the alternative
method of generating the logbook and carrying out certain
statutory functions such as recording road traffic accidents and
recording attendances.

Because the system performs the critical function of casualty card
generation, the hardware has to be reliable.   Technical assistance
must be available to carry out routine maintenance.   Breakdowns
have been rare and of short duration and we are impressed by the
robust quality of the equipment.

The initial software development was estimated to have required
6 man months of effort.

REFERENCES

Dalby, B. C. S., Farrer, J. A. and Harvey, P. W., 1974. Casualty
activity analysis coding and computing, in <u>Computer Programs in
Biomedicine 3</u>, pp 254 - 266.   North Holland Publishing Co.

Roberts, J. M., Farrer, J. A. and Harvey P. W., 1977. The use of a
computer system in the study of the attendance profile in a
district hospital casualty department.   Comput. Biol. Med., 7,
pp 291 - 299.

ACKNOWLEDGEMENTS

To the Gwynedd Research Committee for a grant used to purchase
computer equipment and to Mrs. Linda Roberts, Receptionist, for
her valued and patient cooperation.

Care of the Acutely Ill and Injured
Edited by D. H. Wilson and A. K. Marsden
© 1982, John Wiley & Sons Ltd.

A NEW (INTERNATIONAL) MEDICAL RECORD FOR THE
EMERGENCY DEPARTMENT

R. Riva, R. Azzoni, E. Bossi, C. Ronzani

Emergency Traumatological Service,
1st Surgical Clinic - University of Milan
Policlinico Hospital

An emergency medical record form has been devised at the
Policlinico Hospital of Milan. By virtue of its design, it can
be understood by doctors in other hospitals and could be recognised
internationally.

Its main design criteria are:

1. Simplicity in usage and completion especially with regard to
   the first pathological findings.

2. Provision of adequate clerical and identification data.

3. Comprehensibility by an overseas reader.

4. Linkage of specialist information with treatment instituted
   in the Emergency Department.

5. Facility for information retrieval for statistical review.

6. Provision of an adequate medicolegal clinical record.

The record comprises a folder in which is stored additional specific
sheets.

The front page of the folder - A (Fig.1) summarises identification
information together with therapeutic data thus allowing "at a
glance" understanding of the main features of the case. Two items
are worthy of particular note:

(a) there is provision for two addresses and telephone numbers
    (as frequently patients become injured away from home and
    information has to be transferred between hospitals).

(a) adequate space is available for a record of tetanus immunity
    status.

The last page of the folder is made up of instructions for the
proper use of the form.

The middle pages of the folder allow space for History; Clinical
Examination; Operation Notes and Histological Diagnosis.

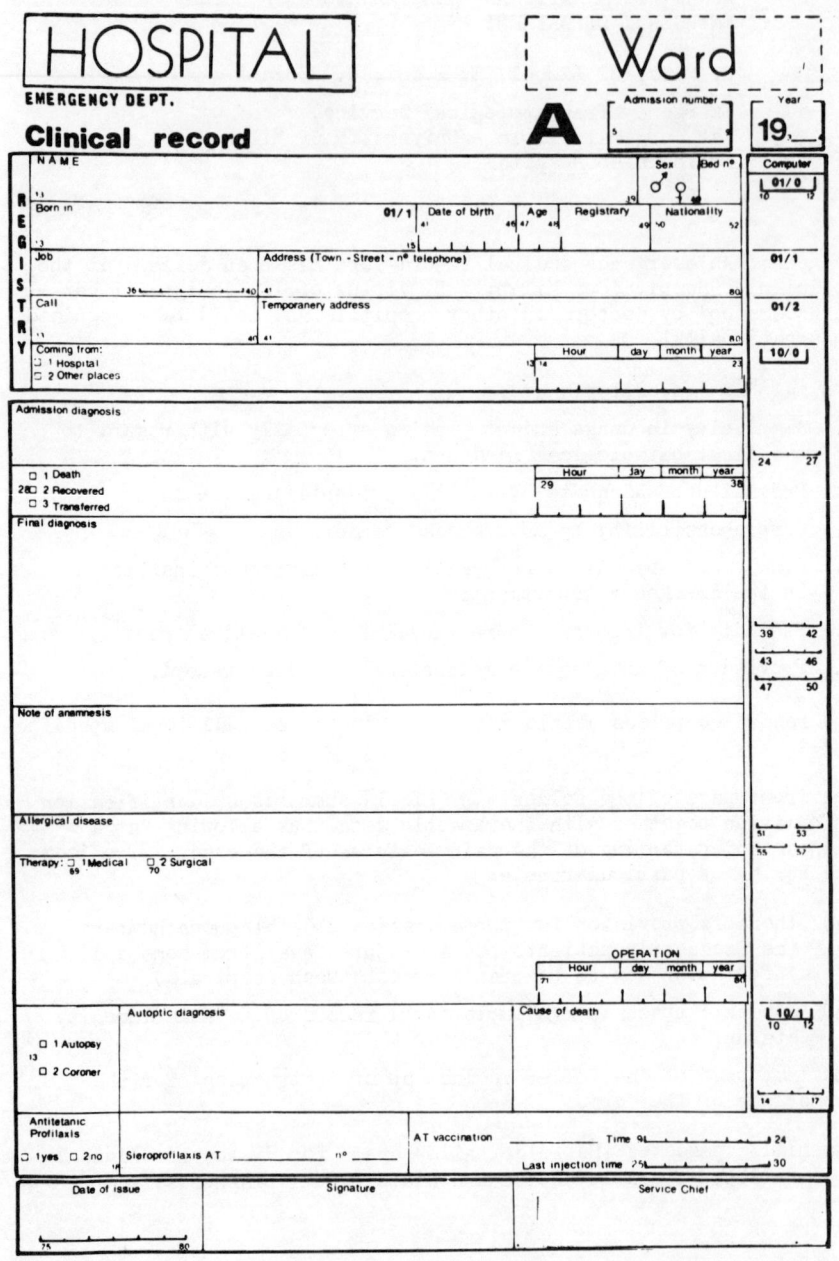

Figure 1

Included in the folder are specialist record sheets, e.g.:

FIRST MEDICAL EXAMINATION - Page B (Fig.2)

This annotates the diagnostic and initial therapeutic procedures
performed in the Emergency Room.

A numerically coded list of pathological items and injuries is
displayed on the right hand side of the sheet.   Numbers from
this list are marked onto a series of schematic figures representing
the main body areas.   This pictorial description is readily
translatable into other languages.

Space is left at the foot of the page for a working diagnosis
and the surgeon's name.

On the reverse of the sheet is a monitor record and a detailed
check list of laboratory and radiological tests requested.

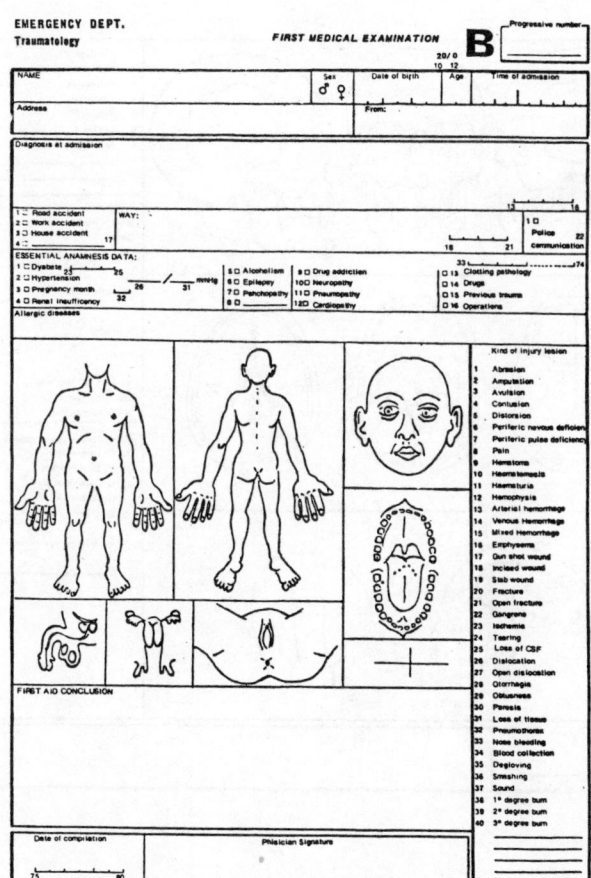

Figure 2

LABORATORY DATA - Page C

In diary form is a record of haematological and chemical pathological data

NEUROSURGICAL - Page D (Fig.3)

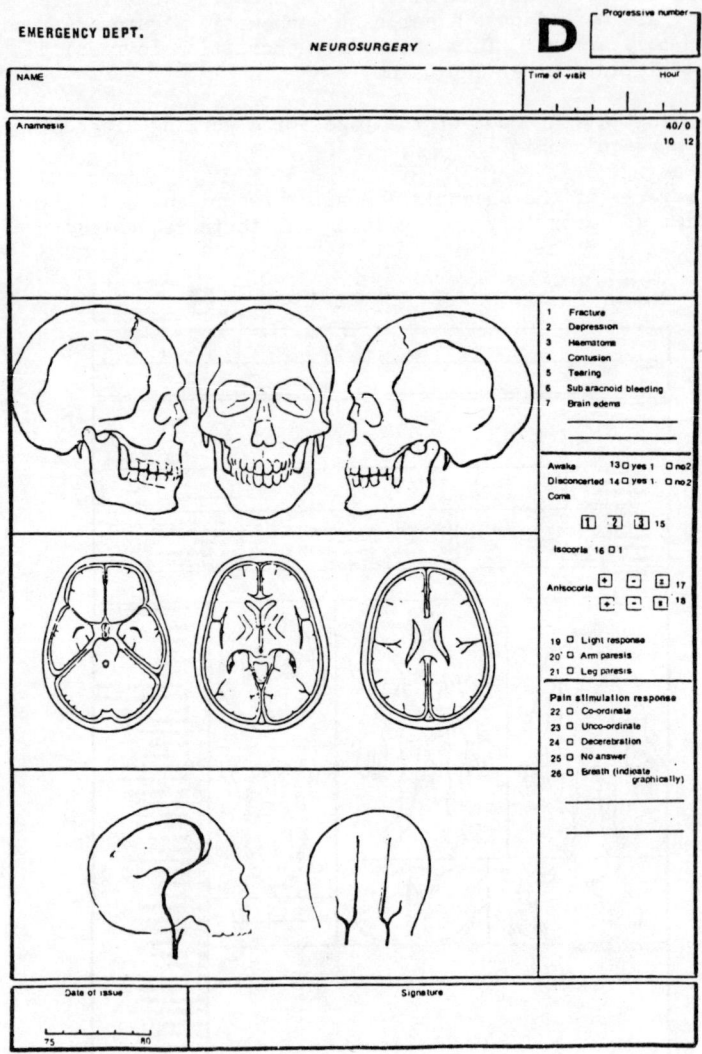

Figure 3

RADIOLOGY - Page E (Fig.4)

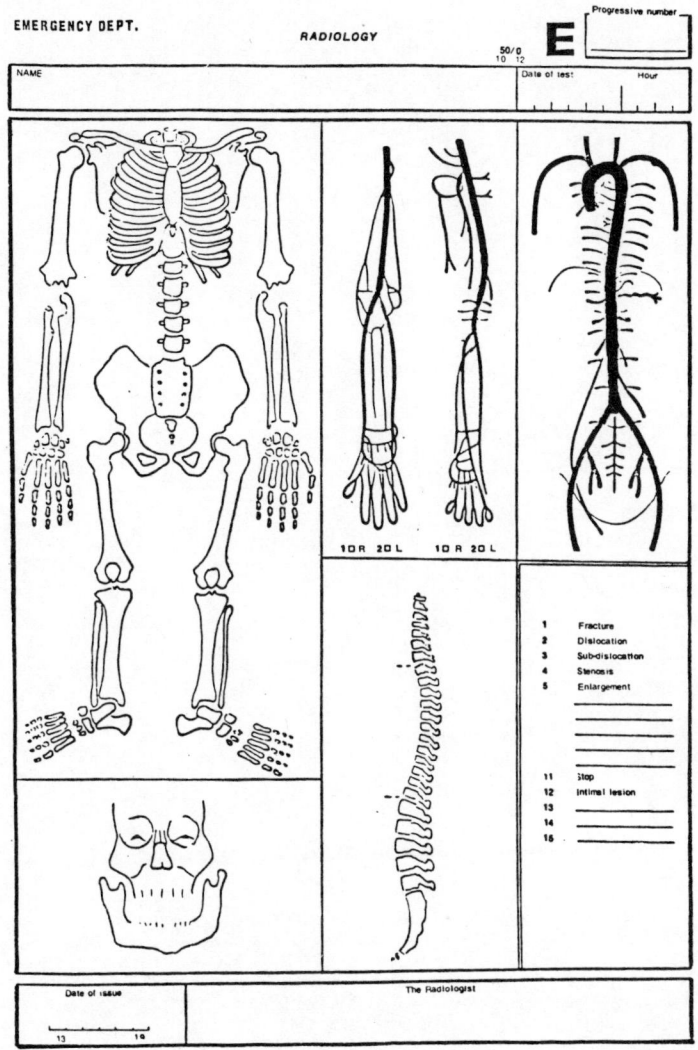

Figure 4

The specialist sheets have been drawn up in collaboration with
the specialists working at the hospital.

The authors have presented a copy of this record form to all
delegates attending the Congress in order to obtain feedback and
suggestions for improvement towards an international adoption.

Care of the Acutely Ill and Injured
Edited by D. H. Wilson and A. K. Marsden
© 1982, John Wiley & Sons Ltd.

COMPUTERISED MEDICAL RECORDS IN A SURGICAL
EMERGENCY DEPARTMENT

J. Micheels, M.Th. Pire, M. Lamy

Dept. of Anesthesiology
University of Liege,
Hopital de Baviere, Liege, Belgium.

ABSTRACT

A prospective study using computerised records was run for three
months in our Emergency Department. Six thousand cases were
investigated. Of these 3020 were surgical cases which were
analysed with reference to:

a) epidemiology
b) demography
c) organisation and method in the unit.

MATERIAL AND METHODS

Six thousand patients were studied including 3020 surgical cases.
Each patient had a special two-sheet coding form completed in the
Emergency Department. The medical information service prepared
punched cards and from these information was transferred to magnetic
tape. Analysis was performed on a computer IBM 370/158 using BMDP
programmes from The University of California.

RESULTS

a) Epidemiology

1. The commonest emergency at all ages is the simple domestic
    accident. Children in the home are at greatest risk aged
    about three years.

2. The incidence of accidents involving two-wheeled vehicles rises
    with age reaching a peak with teenagers.

3. The incidence of public accidents remains static at all ages.

4. The young, active male demands proportionately more emergency
    care than the rest of the population.

b) Demography

1. 98% of cases requested advice of a medical nature (only 2% of
    cases were social or, in some other way, irrelevant to the
    service).

2. Of the population examined only 48% required the services of
    a hospital department and 50% could have been treated at home.

3. There were 3.5% cases actually in danger of death.   44.5% were
    deemed 'real emergencies' though not in danger of death.

4. Only 1.7% of patients called their family physician before
    presenting ; 22% used the "900" (Belgian emergency telephone
    number) system :   76% were self-referred.

c) Management of the Department

1. The weekly case load follows a stable pattern with a demonstrable
    need for nursing staff at week ends.

2. There is a poor correlation between the hourly patient load and
    the on-duty hours of the nursing staff.

3. The peak hourly patient load equated with the predictable hourly
    patient load i.e. 0.01% of the activity of one year ($\frac{100}{365 \times 24}$)

4. 80% of patients are discharged home, 1% died in the emergency
    department and 19% are admitted (11% to the surgical unit and
    3% to the Intensive Care Unit).

CONCLUSION

This analysis serves to demonstrate the benefit of computerised
records in an emergency department, with a clearer knowledge and
understanding of the emergency department's function other functions
could be studied in this way, for example cost analysis of medical
activity; analysis of medical students' role in emergency
situations etc.

SECTION TWO

PREHOSPITAL CARE

Care of the Acutely Ill and Injured
Edited by D. H. Wilson and A. K. Marsden
© 1982, John Wiley & Sons Ltd.

RESUSCITATION ON SITE.
INTRODUCTORY REMARKS.

P.S. London

Birmingham Accident Hospital

Interest in and practice of resuscitation where an accident occurs
are already widely spread in the world and they are increasing. As
a result, to question the usefulness of what I prefer to call
medical or otherwise advanced first aid will suggest either
ignorance or a refusal to face facts. In inviting others to present
the case for and against this practice I am not seeking to question
its justification so much as to challenge some of the assertions
that have been made since the need for skilled first aid was stated
in 1967. I challenge particularly the assertion that in Britain
more than 1,000 lives could be saved each year were highly skilled
first aid readily available after road accidents. The estimate
arose from German sources and it has been given a new lease of life
by the application of Mr. A.H. Dooley of his index of care, which is
derived from the ratio of immediate to later mortality rates both
with and without medical first aid. These estimates of a 20-25%
saving of life are more or less speculative and bear no resemblance
to the figures of about 5% which come from studies by Mr. Hoffman,
from whom we shall be hearing, by myself and by my colleague, Dr.
Sevitt, who studied fatal road accidents in Birmingham and, like
Mr. Hoffman, found more reason to improve medical attention in

hospitals than to provide it outwith them.

Can these figures be reconciled and, if not, can the differences be
explained? The weakness of Dooley's case lies in the presumption
that the improvement in results achieved by the organizations he has
studied can be applied to the country as a whole. This is clearly
not so and for two particular reasons. The first is that only about
1,500 of the 20,000 or so general practitioners undertake to provide
medical aid where an accident happens; their distribution is uneven
and their numbers have not shown much increase for a few years and,
at least in Mid-Anglia, about one third of calls for doctors to
attend accidents went unanswered. In his study of the Mid-Anglia
General Practitioners' Accident Service Mr. Silverston has shown
also in how few cases has a doctor had to do more than any other
first aider and also that he is not always the first to arrive.
This is one of the reasons why I do not consider the widely used
term immediate care to be properly used in this connexion. It may
be provided immediately after the doctor arrives but this will
usually be at least minutes after the accident. I use the words
first aid because they are the most appropriate when used in their
literal sense.

This is the outline of the case that medical and other skilled first
aiders must answer and the subsequent speakers have been asked not
merely to describe their organizations but to give facts and figures
of what they do.

Care of the Acutely Ill and Injured
Edited by D. H. Wilson and A. K. Marsden
© 1982, John Wiley & Sons Ltd.

EVIDENCE "FOR" IMMEDIATE CARE

Rosemary H. M. Adams, F. R. C. S., F. R. C. S. E.

Chairman, Research Committee,
British Association for Immediate Care.
Consultant in A/E Department, Norwich.

I am speaking for the Research Committee of the British Association for Immediate Care, a committee which came into being in 1977, one year after the formation of the Association.

As you may know, the Immediate Care Schemes in the U. K. arose from a great need in the pre hospital care of the injured and those otherwise afflicted in emergency situations; the main necessity was medical care at the roadside.

This work, started more than 10 years ago, was not, and indeed is still not, a fully recognised activity of the National Health Service, but since the formation of the Association the D. H. S. S. has accepted responsibility to the extent of providing our central administrative costs.

The 70 Immediate Care Schemes which now exist were all started voluntarily and are registered as charities. Even the Hospital Flying Squad Immediate Care Schemes started as financially independent bodies.

As well as roadside care the Schemes include mountain rescue, cave rescue and sea and air rescue services. In 1979 the doctors attended 5, 500 incidents, 4, 000 of them were road traffic accidents.

72% of our work is concerned with road traffic accidents. Fatalities from road traffic accidents in Great Britain in 1979 numbered 6, 352 - these were equally divided between urban and rural areas.

We know that approximately 55% of the victims die instantly.
Ruffell Smith's figures (1970) show that in rural areas $\frac{2}{3}$ die within
the first 25 minutes.   We are therefore concerned in the first
instance in trying to save the lives or improve the condition of
seriously injured and very seriously injured people.

The cause of death in most cases is multiple injuries, head and
chest injuries especially if combined, having the highest mortality.
There is little time for action.

Time is the most important factor of all, because the essential
part about Immediate Care is bringing the time of treatment from
the Casualty Department to the accident scene.   If treatment is
given at the scene, and assuming that morbidity increases with
time, then scope for benefit from Immediate Care will be greater
the longer the distance and time between scene and hospital.

Time being all important, who arrives first at the scene of
accident? and how long does it take to get there?

Our research in this country shows that in the urban districts the
police arrive first, in the semi rural districts the police and
ambulance arrive within a short time of each other.   In the remote
rural areas the doctor is usually first on the scene.

It has been laid down by the D. H. S. S. that an ambulance should
reach the accident within 20 minutes.   This is the mean time,
including long distance journeys.   In actual fact since the siting
of accident ambulances in chosen parts of the county, the arrival
time of the ambulance is frequently within 12 minutes.

The mean time of arrival of a doctor at an accident is between
5 and 10 minutes.   One of the hospital Flying Squads, Bath
Hospital, has a mean arrival time of 7. 6 minutes.   Doctor's
arrival time is effectively speeded by good radio communication
which now exists in most Immediate Care Schemes.   When he
arrives the doctor and/or his ambulance colleagues will establish
an airway, correct hypovolemia, and relieve the patient's pain and
prepare him for transport.

It is extremely difficult to evaluate Immediate Care.

In the absence of a direct method of quantifying morbidity, the
objective evaluation of Immediate Care has been intrinsically
difficult.

We have based our work on the method developed by Alfred Dooley
in the study carried out for the Medical Commission for Accident
Prevention in 1975-76.

This represented the practical outcome of a probablistic approach,
that is, that a given accident environment should result in a pattern
of injury and morbidity associated with finite levels of immediate
and later deaths, later deaths being influenced by the effectiveness
of Immediate Care.

If care is effective it will surely reduce the number of people dying
later.   Results are expressed as a Care Index:-

$$\text{Care Index} \quad = \quad \frac{FI + FL}{FL}$$

where FI = Immediate deaths - within 10 mins

and   FL = Later deaths - 10 mins to 30 days

Working on the Road Accident After Care Scheme in N. Yorkshire
started by the pioneer of Immediate Care Schemes Dr. Ken Easton
in 1967, a Care Index of 2.92 was calculated against a norm of 1.96
for a comparable area of rural Yorkshire.   (Dooley's Paper R.C.S.
Annals 1978).   These figures represented an overall Care Index.
Correcting the figures for age 15-54 on roads in a speed limit of up
to 60 mph we have a Care Index of 4.50 compared with 2.10.

	C.I. overall	15-54
R.A.A.C.	2.92	4.50
Rest Rural N. Yorkshire	1.96	2.10

Correction for age is made - because of the relatively small
numbers of the young and old, and because these are particularly
high risk cases.

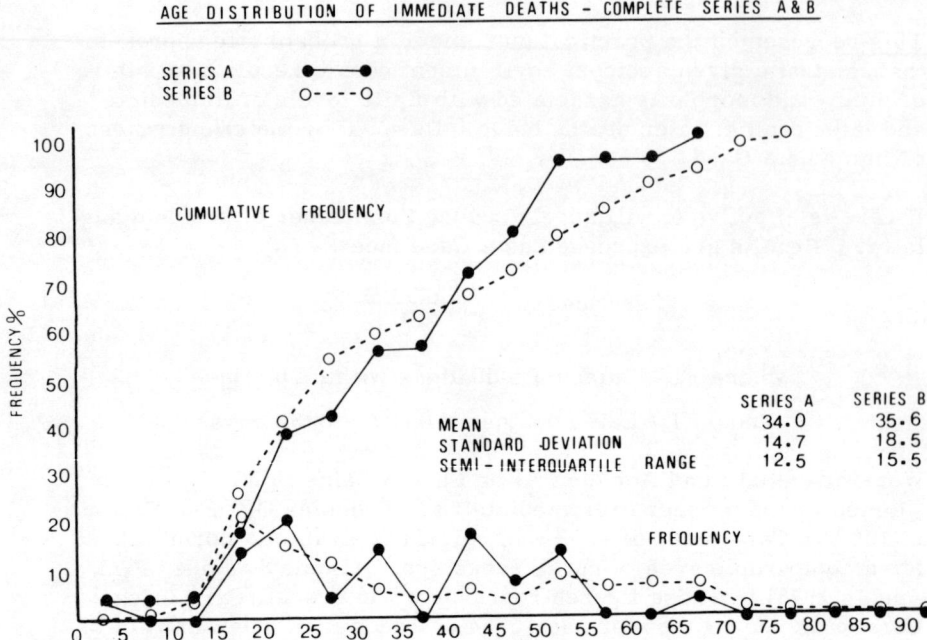

AGE DISTRIBUTION OF IMMEDIATE DEATHS - COMPLETE SERIES A & B

A rise in Care Index from 2 to 3 implies a reduction in later deaths of some 50%, which in relation to the total deaths means we can prevent something of the order of 20% of total R.T.A. deaths, a figure very close to that calculated in America and Israel where efficient Emergency Medical Services exist.   This accords well with Frey's studies of road traffic fatalities in Michigan, where it was calculated that 18% of patients were salvagable.

Evaluations are difficult to carry out in that they involve time consuming data collection and analysis. They rely on police reports giving the time of the accident, location, type of road user, type of road, speed limit, etc. on ambulance activation records, doctor mobilisation records, on A/E Department and hospital records and post mortem reports. The problem is aggravated by the continued delay in linking police, ambulance and hospital records, and in computerising the latter.

Evaluations are only feasible where the confines of the Immediate Care scheme correspond to the county boundaries.

The following table shows some of the results we have obtained. u sing again the original "norm" from N. rural Yorkshire.

Care Index corrected for age 15-54

"Norm"	2.10	
Norfolk	2.63	(1977)
	3.27	(1978)
	3.70	(1979)
Cambridge	4.00	
N. Wales	2.70	
S. Wales	2.40	
Dyfed	2.63	
RAAC	4.50	

Few though they are, we feel these figures are significant and indicate a considerable saving of life, and corresponding reduction in morbidity.

It is not a coincidence that two of the best schemes in the country have a high Care Index.

Many Immediate Care Schemes with a good record of care cannot carry out evaluations because of the complexity of their data collection. To cite but two examples, we have Saffron Walden and N. Hampshire.

N. Hampshire has three counties, three police forces, three ambulance services and admits to five hospitals.

We feel that the Care Index figures could be further improved if the standard of Immediate Care were better in hospitals.   Jennett and Yates(1977) have both shown conclusively that lives are lost unnecessarily in the A/E Department, and in transit of patients from that Department to other wards or other hospitals.
Dr. Hamish McLeod in a recent article on Immediate Care makes a plea that Accident Departments should make it their prime task to continue the Immediate Care which has already been started at the roadside, before launching into detailed examination and investigation of the patient.

If lives are to be saved this is to be done mainly by correction of hypoxia and hypovolemia.

Howard Sherriff, a member of the Research Committee, has just completed a retrospective study of fatalities from road traffic accidents in the Cambridge area over a period of seven years. This comprises some 330 cases.   Detailed post mortem reports indicated that one third of the cases died from blood loss and 7-10% of these could have been saved by adequate infusion.

We are currently carrying out a study on the use of Haemaccel in emergency work in the field.   Immediate Care doctors taking part return a questionnaire plus a Patient Information Form with full details of the victim's injuries.

In 52 cases, half the victims were trapped, the majority for periods of over 30 minutes.   In 80% of cases infusion was started within 30 minutes, in 10% it was started within 15 minutes. The seriously injured patient can reach hospital in a stable condition: this supports the argument for aggressive Immediate Care.

I would like to cite three cases in detail, cases in which recovery would have been unlikely without immediate resuscitation.

1.   The first, a road traffic accident.   The driver of a lorry was crushed, his leg was mutilated and the source of arterial bleeding.   He was trapped for $1\frac{3}{4}$ hours.   A two-line i. v. infusion was set up.   Three litres of Haemaccel were given and blood was sent by police car for cross matching.   After a 40 minute ambulance journey the patient reached hospital in a stable condition.   His leg was amputated and his life saved.

2.   A car driver's vehicle ran under a lorry.   It burst into
flames and was extricated by the fast thinking of a following lorry
driver who rammed his vehicle under the bumper of the first lorry,
raising it up and allowing release of the car.   The driver was
literally welded into his molten manmade fibre clothing.   He
suffered 65-70% burns.   Infusion was started and blood sent for
cross matching.   After a 22 mile journey he arrived in a stable
condition and eventually made a good recovery.

3.   A young woman sent home from hospital after a termination
of pregnancy developed severe haemorrhage on the 5th day.   The
obstetric flying squad was not available, neither was her G. P.
An Immediate Care doctor was called.   She was on the 7th floor
of a block of flats and the lift was out of order.   She was unconscious from blood loss.   So severe was this blood loss that
she required six units of Haemaccel and four units of O negative
blood before she could be carried downstairs.   She recovered.

These are three out of dozens of cases I could relate to you.
They could all have been Road Traffic Accidents.

Although my brief is to limit observations to the British experience
of roadside care, I must in all fairness to Immediate Care doctors
point out that 28% of the emergencies they attend are cases other
than R. T. A. s, occasional drownings, electrocutions, industrial
accidents and a large number of cardiac cases.   Here the evidence
for Immediate Care is overwhelming.   Ventricular fibrillation is
what kills the patient and this must be corrected within four
minutes.

Pantridge in 1969 showed that if cases could be treated within this
time they could survive.

MANAGEMENT OF VENTRICULAR FIBRILLATION OUTSIDE HOSPITAL

PANTRIDGE 1969

126 PATIENTS CARDIAC ARREST

    55 PATIENTS RESUSCITATION STARTED WITHIN 4 MIN'S

        48 PATIENTS HAD V.F.

           39 PATIENTS SURVIVED

27 LEFT HOSPITAL ALIVE AND WELL

Douglas Chamberlain here in Brighton started a coronary
ambulance scheme in 1971. This effectively saves 12-15 lives
a year. It is another example of the necessity and the success
of Immediate Care.

Numbers of lives saved is what we are really being asked to prove,
but if we can save some lives and improve the condition of others,
above all relieve suffering, even though this is in a dying victim,
then surely we have made a case "For" Immediate Care.

REFERENCES

Dooley A, Lucas B G B. The evaluation of emergency care.
Annals of Royal College of Surgeons 1978; 6 : 451

Frey C. et al. Resuscitation and survival in motor vehicle
accidents. Journal of Trauma: 9 : 4

Jennett B. Preventable mortality and morbidity after head
injury. Injury; 10 : 1

Pantridge J F, Adgey A A J et. Lancet; June 1969

Ruffell Smith. Time to die from injuries received in road traffic
accidents. Injury; October 1970

Yates W. Airway patency in fatal accidents. Brit Med J
November 1977

Care of the Acutely Ill and Injured
Edited by D. H. Wilson and A. K. Marsden
© 1982, John Wiley & Sons Ltd.

FACTS BEHIND THE FLYING SQUADS – THE ROADSIDE
RESUSCITATION SCHEMES IN THE U.K.

Mr G G Bodiwala MS FICS FICA

Leicester Royal Infirmary (University of Leicester)
Leicester

ABSTRACT

A survey was carried out to find out the information on Roadside
Resuscitation Schemes from the hospitals accident & emergency
centres. 80 replies were received from 195 questionnaires sent. 47
centres are running Roadside Resuscitation Schemes in the U.K., out
of which I would consider 20 are active with 10 to 100 calls a year.
All these departments have Consultants except two. Majority are
provided transport by ambulance services and have established their
own Radio links. Call out system is pretty similar to most centres.
They have a role to play in the Major Disasters.

Only 13 centres do not wish to have Flying Squads at all. There are
60 G.P. Schemes available as well where 15 of them have hospital
Flying Squad in their areas.

INTRODUCTION

R.T.A. is the biggest killer between the age of 4 and 44. Last year
6000 were killed on the roads of Britain. In the United Kingdom,
the schemes which participate in the resuscitation of road accidents
victims, are run by Doctors and Nurses in the hospital and Doctors
in the general practices. However, emergency services e.g. ambulance
mainly, police & fire brigade do have their roles in these.

METHOD

A survey was carried out by sending questionnaires to 195 accident &
emergency centres in the country. Questions were asked on the total
attendances, medical and nursing staffing and provision of a team
for roadside resuscitation. Also information was obtained on the
organisation, transport, communication, liaison with emergency
services and responsibility in Major Disaster events. Points were
also covered on insurance and funding of the schemes.

RESULTS

More and more accident and emergency centres are recognising the
importance of Flying Squad. Now there are 47 Flying Squads in the
U.K. and 15 of them have G.P. Schemes along with them.

TABLE 1.   F.S. 1980/81

47   F.S.
 6   Plans for future
 2   No plans but willing to provide a team
 3   No (because G.P. schemes exist)
 7   No (because of the Metropolitan area)
13   Definite No
 2   Have since left A/E responsibility

Out of these 47, 20 have active squads attending 10 to 100 calls a
year. All the departments have Consultants in charge of Accident &
Emergency except two and their average new patients attendances per
year is 30 – 40,000 patients. 80% of the centres have either
registrars or senior registrars middle grade cover too.

TABLE 2.1.   Transport

 6   Special vehicles
27   Ambulance transport
 8   Police cars
 6   Own

TABLE 2.2   Funded by

 2   Public donations
 2   Public donations and A.H.A.
 2   A.H.A.

Majority i.e. 27 centres have transport provided by the ambulance
services. 6 centres have been able to establish their own Flying
Squad vehicles either funded by Public Donations, or Area Health
Authority or combination of two. Only one centre has special
drivers appointed to the squad to drive their vehicles. 8 centres
have co-operation from police, who take the team out at the scene.

TABLE 3.   Radio communication

28   yes   18 own channel
15   no

                11 own Hand Sets

                Telephone line with

35   Ambulance
10   Police
 2   Fire Brigade

Communication has always been vital. Still only 28 centres out of 47
have been able to establish their own radios. Most of 47 have
telephone links with ambulance if not through radios. Only 10

TABLE 3.   Radio communication (cont.)

centres have seen the importance of establishing links with police
and 2 centres with Fire Brigade.

FIGURE 1.   F.S. call-out

Ambulance
Police
Fire Brigade
G.P.
Industry
Airport

The call-out system is pretty similar to all centres as shown in
figure 1. However 6 centres wish to have their teams called out
by ambulance services only.

All 47 schemes have major role to play in the event of a major
disaster but only 15 carry out regular exercises. Once again
only 24 have insurance cover for their teams.

TABLE 4.   33 No F.S.

6   Plans for future
2   No plans but willing to provide a team
3   No (because G.P. schemes exist)
7   No (because of the Metropolitan area)
13 Definite no
2   Have since left A/E responsibility

Out of 33 centres who do not have schemes, 13 do not see any function
provided by the flying squad. 6 expressed to establish one in future
and 2 are willing to provide team if required. 10 centres do not see
any need as in their areas G.P. schemes already exists. 7
Metropolitan areas do not see any need for one.

G.P. schemes and finance

It is worth mentioning that there are approximately 60 G.P. schemes
run in this country - mostly a one man show in the event of a single
accident. Hospital schemes do not have seperate funds or budget
available for it but usually general practitioners are supported
financially in their schemes by organising sponsor walks, jumble
sales and Red Cross or other social clubs. They use their own
vehicles and have established communications of immediate care
schemes like LIVES in Lincoln. Also some of these General
Practitioner Schemes have good liaison with the hospital schemes
and in actual fact 15 of them have associated with their hospital
flying squads.

MR G G Bodiwala

DISCUSSION

Since first Flying Squad was established by John Collins in Derby
in 1955, 47 have emerged. There is a recognition by 47 that a
role is there to be played by a Specialist at the roadside
resuscitation. This message has been taken over by the General
Practitioners who have established 60 schemes. The problem of
staff, transport, communication and training should be considered
in more details for future establishments.

Care of the Acutely Ill and Injured
Edited by D. H. Wilson and A. K. Marsden
© 1982, John Wiley & Sons Ltd.

ON SITE RESUSCITATION

E. Hoffman

Middlesbrough, UK

ABSTRACT

Routine medical aid at the site is not likely to lead to a significant reduction
in early mortality. Upper airway obstruction and inhalation are important
fatal complications, generally occurring within the first few minutes
following an accident. The ability of members of the general public to
provide early respiratory assistance would be a great advance in emergency
care at the site.

INTRODUCTION

Knowledge of what happens to road accident victims after they are injured is
scanty. Most information on fatalities is retrospective and comes from
post mortem reports, but pathologists are often only concerned with the
forensic cause of death. A study was made based on clinical observation
following casualties from the accident site until their discharge or death
(Hoffman, 1976). Information was collected from forms which were
completed by ambulancemen, the police, casualty officers and pathologists.
Hospital notes were also reviewed. Details were obtained on 2,392
surviving hospital admissions and 344 deaths. The main emphasis was on
preventable deaths.

MEDICAL AID AT SITE

To assess the value of medical aid at accidents, the length of survival, type
of injuries and management of those dying at the scene and during transit
was investigated. Of the 344 deaths, 159 were said to have died instantly.

Necropsy reports suggested that a proportion of these probably lived for some minutes, because they died of complications of their injury. Thus immediate effective first aid could be of great importance.

Thirteen (3.8%) of the casualties died later at the site and 19 (5.5%) during transit. Of the 13 casualties dying at the scene, 9 did so within 10 minutes, before the ambulance could arrive. The 32 casualties who died before admission sustained severe multiple injuries. There were 22 cases with brain damage (all but 3 with other injuries), 14 had a haemothorax (5 of these with a ruptured aorta), 14 a haemoperitoneum, 6 a torn heart, 6 a flail chest, and 6 fracture dislocation of the cervical spine with cord damage, while in 2 massive inhalation of blood was present. Even a skilled doctor at the site could not have prevented death, except perhaps in 2 cases in which early intubation and assisted ventilation might possibly have saved life. One of these patients inhaled blood from a fractured base of skull and the other had bilateral rib fractures and died later in hospital. On present evidence, routine medical aid at the site is not likely to lead to a significant reduction in early mortality, but its influence on morbidity is more difficult to assess.

Currently most hospital based flying squads and general practitioners in immediate care schemes, only attend accidents when called by the emergency services because they cannot cope, or the casualties are trapped. In my series 5% of casualties were trapped. As medical aid in such cases has proved of considerable benefit, all district general hospitals should provide an "on call" flying squad service.

EARLY FATAL COMPLICATIONS

Of the 191 who died before admission, 168 did so within the first 10 minutes before the emergency services could arrive. Death in these cases was either due to injuries not compatible with life, or to two major complications respiratory difficulties or blood loss. Respiratory obstruction is the more immediately life threatening, as it can lead to irreversible brain damage within 3-5 minutes. It occurs mainly in the unconscious, and is due to upper airway obstruction or to inhalation. As 76.6% of fatalities were unconscious at the site, and 62.7% were still unconscious on admission, the prevention of these complications is of great importance.

Upper Airway Obstruction in the deeply unconscious may be due to the tongue falling back or to displacement of fractured facial bones. When casualties at the site were first seen by ambulancemen, 38.9% of those dying later, had an obstructed airway. This suggests that early respiratory aid by lay persons present at accidents may well determine whether some seriously injured will survive. It would be of great benefit if the general public knew how to clear the throat and maintain a free airway.

Casualty officers found on admission, that the breathing of 10.7% of the hospital fatalities, was still obstructed. Ambulancemen succeeded in clearing the airway in the majority of cases, but they should have done even better, and greater stress should be laid on teaching them respiratory resuscitation.

It is often stressed that in the unconscious, efforts at airway control may produce cord damage, as an unsuspected cervical injury may be present. In a group of 53 head injuries who inhaled and died within 5 minutes after injury, there were 10 spinal fractures; 8 of these cervical with cord damage, 9 also had chest and 7 abdominal trauma. A combination of brain and cervical injuries is known to have a bad prognosis, and thus in head injuries respiratory resuscitation should always be given priority.

Inhalation. Unconscious patients are in danger of asphyxia from inhaled blood, vomit or foreign material. Of the 344 deaths inhalation of blood was found in 114, of vomit in 18 and in 1 case chips from a shattered windscreen led to suffocation at the accident site. Inhaled blood originated from 3 areas: maxillo-facial fractures (30 out of 41, i.e. 73.1%), skull fractures (50 out of 199, i.e. 25.1%) and lung injuries (34 out of 122, i.e. 27.8%). Positioning in facial and skull fractures is an effective preventive measure, but little can be done to avoid aspiration from a lacerated lung.

In the pathologists' opinion inhalation was the cause of death in 7 (2%) cases, contributory in 27 (7.8%) and irrelevant in 89 (25.8%).

Aspiration was frequent in casualties who died soon after injury; 59.6% of those inhaling blood and 38.9% of those aspirating vomit died instantly or within minutes. This shows that knowledgeable bystanders are most likely to save lives by posturing an unconscious casualty at the earliest opportunity. Members of the general public should be taught how to turn an unconscious patient on to his side with the head and trunk in the neutral position. One half of all fatalities with inhalation occurred in car occupants, their positioning is usually not feasible and extrication should be left to the emergency services.

Lay Assistance at Accidents. The general public were the first on the scene in 39.1% of accidents. The necessity to educate the public in respiratory resuscitation has been stressed at a number of international meetings, most recently in Oslo in 1979. In this country not enough emphasis is laid on emergency lay help before the arrival of the ambulance.

Schools and teachers colleges are the most obvious places to teach this subject. The assistance of the mass media should be enrolled to make the public aware of the need to acquire basic resuscitation skills. These must include a knowledge of how to protect themselves and the victims from further accidents. Drivers, who of necessity are the first on the scene, should be required to pass a practical first aid test before obtaining a driving licence. Such an examination is already obligatory in West Germany and Australia.

REFERENCE

Hoffman, E., 1976. Mortality and morbidity following road accidents.
    Annals of the Royal College of Surgeons of England, 58,   233-240.

Care of the Acutely Ill and Injured
Edited by D. H. Wilson and A. K. Marsden
© 1982, John Wiley & Sons Ltd.

'ON SITE' RESUSCITATION - THE EVIDENCE FOR AND AGAINST

H.B. STONER
MRC TRAUMA UNIT, UNIVERSITY OF MANCHESTER, MANCHESTER, U.K.

and P.S. LONDON
BIRMINGHAM ACCIDENT HOSPITAL, U.K.

DISCUSSION

I do not think we have sufficient data to decide whether 'on site' resuscitation, in addition to first aid, is worthwhile in the treatment of the injured. Nor do I think that there is a single answer to this question. We are concerned with two aspects of resuscitation, the preservation of the air-way and fluid replacement. The answers to these questions seem to me to depend very much on geography. What would be appropriate in rural surroundings might not be in an urban situation. Geography may also be a factor in the type of trauma which has to be treated.

In urban Britain where most of the injuries are musculo-skeletal and where the injured are usually brought to hospital by competent ambulance men within 30 minutes, on-site resuscitation could be counterproductive, particularly as it has been shown that airway management on the way to hospital is satisfactory. In country areas where it may take a long time for an ambulance to reach the patient and transport him to hospital there could be a place for on-site resuscitation. However, before one embarks on elaborate schemes every effort should be made to discover if they would be worthwhile. This will not be easy. Sophisticated statistical techniques will be needed to demonstrate any advantage since the number of lives which could be saved by these methods is probably small.

CLOSING REMARKS AFTER THE INDIVIDUAL CONTRIBUTIONS

It is difficult to sum up such widely ranging accounts except in the most general terms.

It stands to reason that the sooner a seriously injured, or ill, person receives aid and the better the quality of that first aid the better the chances that preventable changes will be prevented and that the risks of complications and death will be reduced. The extent to which such reduction is possible varies with place and time. In towns, the speed of response and delivery by the emergency services leaves little place for doctors unless casualties are trapped and need resuscitation,but where the population is sparse doctors are likely to be more numerous than ambulance stations and consequently more likely to be able to treat casualties before ambulances can arrive. A well organized accident service is one that can provide good medical aid at the place of accident when this is necessary.

Care of the Acutely Ill and Injured
Edited by D. H. Wilson and A. K. Marsden
© 1982, John Wiley & Sons Ltd.

THE EMERGENCY MEDICAL TECHNICIAN – THE CURRENT
SITUATION

M. H. Hall

The Royal Infirmary,
Preston, Lancashire, U.K.

INTRODUCTION

In 1976 the Department of Health recommended that at that time there
was no firm evidence which would warrant introduction of a National
Advanced Training Scheme and that no further schemes of this nature
should be introduced until further research into their value became
available.

At a Seminar held at the National Health Service Training and Study
Centre in Harrogate on the 7th and 8th June, 1979, papers were presented in which the provision of more sophisticated care at the scene
of an accident were discussed.

The meetings were attended by senior representatives from the medical
profession, the Ambulance Service, the Department of Health, the
Hospital Administration Services and the trade unions.

Statistical evidence was presented from the Brighton and Hove Scheme
that out of 524 known calls to known cardiac emergencies, 55
defibrillations were attempted and 23 patients were admitted alive
to hospital. The overall number of calls attended in the first year
totalled 2,483. The details were given of the training required and
an estimated figure of £10,000 per year was given as the cost of the
scheme.

Details were also given of the course in coronary care which was
provided at the Royal Sussex County Hospital.

Dr. Baskett presented details of the training and service programme
for paramedics but no statistical details were provided about the use
made of these personnel in the Bristol area.

Dr. Easton presented details of the General Practitioner Scheme,
which has been operational for many years in the Yorkshire area, and
pointed out that there were, at that time, 73 Immediate Care Schemes
involving 1200 voluntary doctors in operation over about one-third of
the United Kingdom.

Details of a research programme carried out on Cardiac Ambulance
Schemes in the Nottingham area was presented by Dr. Hampton who

concluded that there was little future for mobile care units though
he did give qualified support for emergency ambulances carrying
defibrillators staffed by personnel trained to an advanced level.
He considered that this might lead to a tierd ambulance service and
felt that future evolution in this direction should be by experiment
with a very critical evaluation of the results obtained by such
schemes.

Mr. Lea presented a paper on the Leeds Scheme and indicated that 15
months' experience had not provided any evidence to indicate significant patient benefit arising from the Scheme.

Since the Harrogate meeting there has been proliferation and expansion of Advanced Training Schemes in various parts of the country.
Many are of high quality and use a training programme similar to
that advocated by Dr. Baskett.   These are run in close association
with the Basics' Organisation and others have developed in association with the Emergency Medical Technicians Association which works
in close collaboration with the Basics' Organisation.

The Standing Medical Advisory Committee of the Department of Health
has not felt it is in a position to make a formal recommendation
either way about the value of these schemes and because of national
pressure to introduce these schemes more widely the N.S.C. has felt
it appropriate to consider the matter in considerable depth in order
that the full implications of the introduction of these schemes may
be considered.   In considering such schemes it is important to bear
in mind that the Ambulance Service is part of the Health Service and
is therefore subject to the overall supervision by the Department of
Health and that any schemes that are operational at the present time
are run on a voluntary basis by the authorities who have the immediate operational control of the service.

The schemes do not have the support (nor do they have the disapproval)
of the Department and because of their fragmented nature there is no
standardisation throughout the country and the whole picture is
becoming increasingly confused by a failure to appreciate the major
implications that the widespread introduction of these schemes would
have for both the structure and function of the Ambulance Service,
and, though to a lesser extent, the Hospital Emergency Services.

DEFINITION

The term 'Advanced Training of Ambulancemen' has come into use without a clear cut understanding of the significance of the term.   It
tends to mean all things to all men and there must be concern that in
their enthusiasm the proponents of this scheme tend to overlook the
great importance of adequate basic training for all personnel. Basic
training has undergone significant changes in the past few years and
is now reasonably standardised throughout the country though, again
because of the manner of controlling the Ambulance Service, there are
still variations between the training given to the personnel in
different regions.

The point must be made whether or not it is justifiable to introduce further training until such a time as basic training is on a satisfactory level in all areas.

Much of the advanced training appears to be concentrated on the care of coronary patients but there is a direct conflict of views in this field.   The Brighton Scheme appears to have worked extremely well in that area but research in Nottingham, and to a lesser extent in Leeds, suggested that there were no significant benefits to the patients.   Whether or not this is a direct result of the geographical structure of the Brighton area and the type of population when compared to Nottingham and Leeds, is not known but the influences of these facts on the results must not be ignored.

In the writer's own experience of a Hospital Emergency Team, which has been operating for 20 years, no benefit has been seen to patients in the acute arrest situation and in those patients who arrest in the Emergency Department where conditions could not be more favourable, the results are extremely depressing when compared to the results obtained by defibrillation in the Coronary Care Unit.

Few figures have been published which would give help in assessing the benefits of further training in the accident situation but the Bristol training, which covers all types of emergencies, is therefore more appropriate than that concentrated purely on the cardiac patient and the rest of this paper will be directed towards considering training which covers all types of emergencies.

Any definition of further training must include the importance of the primary diagnostic skills of the individual, the use of complex electronic and other equipment and the maintenance of the skills that have been acquired as a result of the training.   Neither the medical or nursing professions make use of the term 'advanced'. The problem does not arise in medicine because the training provided takes the development of such skills into account when the doctor is working his way through the training programmes which are appropriate for his chosen field.   In contradistinction the nursing profession is now significantly concerned about the 'extended role of the nurse'. Official approval is now being given to nurses being trained for and undertaking certain tasks which, in part or in whole, have hitherto been reserved for medically qualified personnel.

For example nurses working on Coronary Care Units regularly defibrillate the patients, in Kidney Units nurses are responsible for the supervision of home dialysis and in other fields the role of the nurse is gradually expanding into the medical field whilst the medical field is expanding in new directions.

The writer would prefer that ambulancemen should be trained for 'the extended role of the ambulanceman'.   This term should be understood to cover the selection of appropriate personnel to undergo instruction in anatomy physiology and diagnosis to enable them to undertake procedures which have hitherto been reserved to the medical and nursing professions.   It must also include the recognition that training to ensure that these skills are maintained is of equal importance to their acquisition.

a)   The choice of personnel for further training is important. The academic and diagnostic requirements need an academic ability which is not necessary for the normal performance of ambulance duties.   It would therefore be necessary to develop a method of assessing the ability of persons to undergo training of this nature.   It is also important that any person undertaking further training should have had some years experience of the normal work of the ambulance service in order that they may have had the opportunity to develop some degree of diagnostic skill as a result of their normal work with sick or injured patients.

b)   The training programmes at present in use vary between 40 and 200 hours and there is a wide variation in both the content and depth of the courses.   The absence of a clearly defined objective in many of these schemes makes comparison almost impossible and there is no national uniform examination standard in existance to assess the proficiency of the candidates at the end of their training.   There is also no nationally agreed opinion about the content of the training, for example, should the training include intravenous therapy or the use of drugs and there is no standardisation of electronic equipment throughout the country.

c)   Extra skills are not required every day;   even doctors do not have to intubate or defibrillate every day and the maintenance of these skills, when they are only used infrequently, is important.   Therefore refresher courses will be required at least annually.

It is possible, using simulaters, to practice with electronic apparatus every day but intubation, which is comparatively easy in the simulated situation, becomes increasingly difficult the more important it is that the patient should be intubated and therefore hospital training would be essential for this aspect of training.

If intravenous therapy is considered appropriate for this training hospital attendances would also be necessary since this skill cannot be practiced on a simulater.

NATIONAL STANDARDS

National standards are set by official bodies in medicine, nursing and the professions allied to medicine, i.e. radiographers, chiropodists, etc.   These bodies have statutory powers to control the training.   On completion of the training and the passing of an examination persons are placed on the Register and the controlling body of the group has the power, under certain circumstances, to remove that person from the Register.   These professions also have bodies which control the professional standards of those persons who are on the various Registers.   They are therefore very largely

self-regulating with the over-riding concern being the well-being
of the public.   In contradistinction the Police and Fire Services
are hierarchical bodies in which there is a direct day to day control
of the various individuals from the top to the lowest level in the
service.   Such a situation exists at the present time in the
Ambulance Service and if there is to be an acceptance that further
training should be introduced consideration will have to be given to
the setting up of some forms of regulatory body.   Such a body must
be of a statutory nature.   Control of training and standards are
essential for the protection of the public and this can only be
achieved with an official body.   An ad hoc committee, however well
intentioned, has no statutory powers, cannot control effectively the
members and may not necessarily represent the wide range of persons
who should have an involvment in the on-going committment towards
the service.

If the Ambulance Service wishes to become a more professional body,
similar to that of the nurses, then this approach will be essential.
There are many advantages in becoming a professional organisation but
it does carry equally great responsibilities towards those whom it
serves and this is something that only the members of the service
should decide for themselves.

EVOLUTION

The importance of evolutionary changes in the care of the patients
has received little attention when extending training is considered
for ambulance personnel.   Nevertheless it is one of the most
significant features in deciding whether or not further training
should be instituted.

At the beginning of the last war the first-aid manual used by first-
aiders and those involved in the care of the injured was very largely
based on methods that had developed during the first world war.
They were complex, unnecessarily detailed, and provided detailed
instructions for treating each particular fracture.   There was little
attempt to standardise the treatment of injuries of the upper or the
lower limbs.   The treatment of poisons was highly complex and
respiratory problems received a totally inadequate degree of space.

Until the early part of the last decade the first-aid manuals available lagged far behind the medical approach to the care of the sick
and injured and consequently the training of the professional first-
aider, as examplified by the ambulance personnel, had to develop
along its own lines which were developed by those members of the
medical profession who were responsible for their training.

The normal first-aid manual is adequate for the occasional first-
aider but for the professionals in this field it became necessary to
ensure that the handling of the patients was compatible with the
advances that were being made in the medical field, particularly in
respect of the recognition that a functioning airway and circulation
were essential for the survival of the patient.

In hospitals significant changes were occurring in the management of
patients with respiratory and cardiac problems. The development of
the defibrillators in the 1960s meant that patients with cardiac
arrest could now be treated. It also meant that the care of the
airway had reached a level where it was unacceptable for any patient
to have their recovery prejudiced by inadequate attention to this
important area.

The writer can recall, with clarity, giving instructions at this time
in external cardiac massage when orders had been given by the local
Medical Officer of Health, who was then the Director of the local
Ambulance Service, that the ambulance personnel were not to undertake
this procedure. Fortunately this situation did not last for long
and external cardiac massage became part of the repertoire of all
the ambulance personnel in the locality.

Initially in hospital these techniques were limited to the senior
staff but gradually the success of these techniques, together with
the demonstration that they could be used successfully by all medical
staff, ensured their wide availability in all departments of the
hospital until, at the present time, a unit dealing with emergency
patients is not considered to be properly equiped unless the necessary apparatus for cardiac and other resuscitation is available.

In Coronary Care Units where cardiac arrest is a relatively common
occurrence it has become routine for nursing staff to undertake
defibrillation, thus a technique which was initially regarded as
suitable only for senior medical personnel has now become part of the
routine work of nurses in certain fields of the profession.

Intubation is still not carried out regularly by nursing staff;
there is little need for this procedure as a primary treatment in
coronary care units and in the Emergency Department because of
certain technical problems it still tends to be restricted to the
more senior members of the unit or the doctors who have had special
training in this procedure.

There is, however, an increasing desire that this technique should be
introduced as part of the extended role of the nurse for those members
of the profession who work in areas where this skill may be needed.
Thus over a period of about 15 years a technique has been developed
which has now become part of the routine work of nursing staff in
certain fields of hospital medicine. It has been demonstrated that
this technique can be safely used by trained nursing staff and junior
doctors and on these grounds the writer can see no reason why it
should not be possible to train ambulancemen of adequate academic
ability in the use of this technique.

Suitable training aids are available, the apparatus has been
simplified and the maintenance of skill in the use of apparatus is
straight forward. Intubation and intravenous therapy are rather
more difficult; this skill is not used by many nurses, or junior
doctors, training aids are not a substitute for patients and the
maintenance of this skill is more difficult. Nevertheless there are

certain situations where a patient, who has been intubated, may stand
a better chance of recovery than if this procedure had not been
carried out.

The development of skills required to put up intravenous fluid lines
are more difficult and can only be gained by familiarity, nevertheless failure to put up a drip may well not have any prejudiced effect
on the patient's chance of recovery.

INFLUENCES OF GEOGRAPHICAL CONDITIONS

In considering the necessity to have trained paramedical personnel
available at the scene of an incident, much will depend on the local
geography. If the main Accident and Emergency Department is in the
centre of a close-knit township where the distance between the
periphery and the hospital is small there would appear to be little
point in spending time undertaking paramedical procedures. Provided
the patient's airway is functioning satisfactorily the journey to
hospital will not take more than a few minutes and delay in reaching
the hospital may result in the use of essential medical procedures
being delayed.

In contrast different circumstances apply in more rural areas. For
example mid-way between Carlisle and Newcastle, in the Highlands
of Scotland or in the West country, particularly during the holiday
period, significant delays may occur before an ambulance can arrive
at the scene of an accident and the journey to the nearest Accident
and Emergency Department may be prolonged. In these circumstances
the patient's recovery may well be prejudiced if the airway cannot be
properly maintained or if replacement fluid therapy is delayed and it
is under these circumstances where paramedical services may be of
considerable value.

HOSPITAL OR GENERAL PRACTITIONER SCHEMES

Many areas are served by groups of doctors who are prepared to attend
the scene of an accident with a full set of equipment. In other
areas hospitals are also prepared to supply a medical and nursing
team to attend incidents. Hospital teams may be called out as a
primary measure or alternatively they may be called out if the
ambulance personnel consider that further help is needed. In the
more rural areas, General Practitioners may be first on the scene and
if either of these types of medical schemes are in operation in any
district there appears little point in training ambulance personnel
to the level required for undertaking any extra procedures.

The Emergency Team provided from the writer's department is primarily
a skilled back-up team for the ambulance personnel. There is little
point in training ambulance personnel to a high basic level and then
calling out medical personnel for an accident. To do so would be
uneconomical in all ways but as a back-up facility for the ambulance
personnel it has worked well for many years and because the distances
involved are small, at no time has there been any indication that
patients would have benefited if extended treatment had been given

initially by members of the ambulance service.

In the past few years there has been a significant increase in the
number of calls to patients who are suffering from cardiac arrest.
The results from these cases have been uniformly disappointing and
subsequent assessment in the post-mortem room has not revealed any
patients who might have been saved by on-site defibrillation.

It is interesting to note that in a recent case of cardiac arrest
which occurred in a local market, initial first-aid treatment was
given by a Policeman.   When the ambulance arrived the treatment was
taken over and the Policeman drove the vehicle to the hospital.   The
patient was successfully defibrillated and so far his progress has
been satisfactory.   In another case treated by the writer and a
colleague in the Emergency Department over a period of about 45
minutes, more than 24 shocks were administered after which the
patient made a very rapid and complete recovery.

Both these cases illustrate the points that if adequate ventillation
and external cardiac massage is used, the time factor is of considerably less significance than is normally assumed and that if basic
first-aid is properly carried out recovery will not be prejudiced.

It is essential, if extending the training of ambulance personnel is
to be introduced in to a district, the place of any existing schemes
must be carefully considered before it's introduction.

EQUIPMENT

The cost of equipping a single vehicle is comparatively small at about
£2,000.   The most expensive item is the cardioscope/defibrillator
which is around £2,000.   The cost of intubation and intravenous
equipment should be less than £100.   There is, however, little point
in equipping a single vehicle in any one station and in an area where
there are several stations;   if three in each station are equipped the
cost would become significant.   For a Regional Health Authority
responsible for a large section of the country, the expense would be
considerable and apart from the initial capital cost there would be
an on-going cost for the maintenance of the equipment, for the
provision of training and for the renewal of solutions and plastic
items of equipment.   An idealised approximation of the cost of
introducing such a scheme in the Preston area would be about £70,000.

MAINTENANCE OF SKILLS

It is difficult even for medical and nursing professions to maintain
skills which they are not often required to use.

Training aids are available for defibrillation.   The aids for training in intubation are not adequate and to remain expert in this
procedure it would be necessary for the personnel to attend in an
operating theatre in order that they might intubate live patients
under an anaesthetic.   Skill in intubating unconscious patients with
foreign matter in the larynx is very difficult to acquire, easy to

lose, and there is no satisfactory answer to this problem. Unfortunately the more urgent it is to intubate such a patient the more difficult it is likely to be and it is for this reason that such a large amount of attention has to be given to the maintenance of the airway during primary training.

A possible way in which these skills might be maintained would be to station an ambulance vehicle at the local Accident and Emergency Department and allow the men to work in the unit as part of the staffing of the unit. They could go out to emergency calls when appropriate but when they were not busy they would be able to work with the other members of the department, thus benefiting by constant exposure to hospital disciplines.

This approach could possibly be further extended by working a larger number of ambulance vehicles from the hospital. Unfortunately the design of new hospitals does not take this into consideration but it has much to commend it and would result in the Ambulance Service developing much closer links with the Accident and Emergency Services.

To some extent this is linked with the development of a two tier ambulance system and as consideration of this is not the primary purpose of this paper it will therefore not be considered further.

The development and maintenance of intravenous fluid line therapy skills would have to follow a similar course to that used by the medical and nursing professions in developing the necessary techniques. This is primarily a matter of observing how the drips are set up and later putting them up on patients under supervision. In this area alone, of all these extra skills, there is a very valid argument that could be advanced for allowing ambulance personnel to set up drips. Frequently by the time the patient reaches hospital the veins have collapsed and it can be extremely difficult to set up a drip. It might well be that if drips were set up, even a few minutes sooner, there would be less difficulty getting the drips going and whilst this is not a significant argument in whether or not ambulance personnel should be allowed to set up this apparatus, it is a point which must be taken into consideration.

OTHER ASPECTS

If ambulance personnel acquire extra skills it would not be unreasonable for these skills to have a financial reward. The acquisition of these skills should not, however, be seen as a means of increasing their pay. If the medical and nursing professions only introduced new techniques on such grounds no advances would ever be made. The professional approach is that if any extra skills are of a benefit to the patient they will be used irrespective of the financial aspects. The writer cannot recall any member of either of these professions receiving other than professional recognition for the development of new methods of treating a patient. It is this aspect of the care of patients that forms part of the professional commitment towards them and would need careful consideration by members of the Ambulance Service if they were to seek professional status.

In the medical profession salary rises with experience and transfer
to a higher grade depends on the acquisition of knowledge and
experience appropriate to that grade.   Movement to a higher grade
is always open to competition.   This would not be appropriate in
the operational side of the ambulance service but it would not seem
unreasonable for persons who acquire extra skills to be promoted to
a higher level in the structure of the service.   This again is linked
with tiering of the service and will not be considered further.

The other feature which has not hitherto received significant
attention is that working on emergency ambulances is primarily a
young man's job.   It is very noticeable that among the older men
their physical ability falls off after about 55 and if members of
the service are given extended training the possibility of their
having to move from the emergency field would have to be considered.
Should this occur, it would be inappropriate for their salary to
drop though they would no longer be dealing with matters of urgency.
It is, in the present structure, difficult to see how this conflict
can be resolved.   Nevertheless it is the writer's opinion that the
age limits of the front-line members of the ambulance service will
have to be considered at some time.

CONCLUSIONS

In this paper the writer has attempted to prepare an unbiased view
of some of the major difficulties that would arise if extended train
-ing were to be introduced into the ambulance service.   It is
essential that an informal attempt be made to evaluate whether or
not training of this nature would benefit the patient.   Purely on
an evolutionary basis it is difficult to see how extended training
can be rejected but equally there would be little point in introducing such training in an area where the services are at present
considered adequate for the needs of the population.   The writer
considers that a suitable training scheme should be introduced in
the part of the country where there is a reasonably valid assumption
that benefits would follow such a scheme.   Such an area should be
geographically widely spread where hospitals are few in number and
where transport to the hospital may be difficult and/or prolonged.
Careful assessment should be made of all stages in the programme.
The results of training, both theoretical and practical, should be
monitored at each stage and a very carefully controlled trial should
be carried out on the results of the training.   If a suitable area
was picked it would be possible to make a controlled study in one
section, on patients who had received treatment by these techniques
and in the other where these techniques were not used.   In this way
it might be possible to finally establish if these schemes could
legitimately be supported by the Department of Health as being of
significant benefit to the patients or whether the benefits were so
small that there was little point in introducing them on a wider
scale.

Care of the Acutely Ill and Injured
Edited by D. H. Wilson and A. K. Marsden
© 1982, John Wiley & Sons Ltd.

OPTIMISING PARAMEDIC SERVICES IN THE UNITED STATES

M.Gifford
Denver, U.S.A.

As the role of the Emergency Medical Technician becomes more
standardised it becomes important to review the purpose for which
the grade was established, namely to reduce morbidity and mortality
in cases of accident or sudden illness at the lowest socially
acceptable cost.   We must examine, in turn, the training,
equipment and environment affecting the work of the E.M.T.   These
three factors are inter-related to the extent that developments in
one area must take into consideration the state of the other areas.

TRAINING

This varies from the 40 hour "First Responder" course through the
81 hour "EMT-B" Basic Course to the 15 Module, 500 hour "EMT-P"
Paramedic Course.   Many places offer intermediate training
extending this to nurses or even physicians.

The cost of training dictates the variety of programmes available
- not all communities can afford (or choose not to afford) paramedic
services.   Is there then some other way of making an impact upon
the mortality rate in that community - some innovative intermediate
training programmes are offering impressive data which seems to
support this concept.

EQUIPMENT

Equipment, likewise, varies with the funds available but seems to
be more dependent on local medical bias.   The American College of
Emergency Physicians is currently developing a recommended list of
equipment for Advanced Life Support Vehicles.   The many "gadgets"
designed primarily for prehospital care will require further data
to validate their usefulness and/or cost-effectiveness.

ENVIRONMENT

Environmental considerations must include the psychological well-
being of the EMT as well as the service arrangements for delivery
of prehospital care.   The latter should include private ambulance
services, fire department services, police department services,
third city services and/or volunteer rescue units.

The EMT as the first-line of organised emergency medical care must
be encouraged to develop as a professional person.   There is no
best or only way to provide good pre-hospital care.   Each system

must examine its strengths and weaknesses to determine the best
combination of personnel, training, equipment and environment for
that system.   In order to continually provide optimal usefulness,
the EMT System must not only offer good patient care but also
support the individuals involved.

The EMT's are making an impact.   They must feel that they are
making that impact for emergency prehospital care to continue at
its highest level.

Care of the Acutely Ill and Injured
Edited by D. H. Wilson and A. K. Marsden
© 1982, John Wiley & Sons Ltd.

THE EMERGENCY MEDICAL TECHNICIAN IN FRANCE
- A NURSE SPECIALISED IN ANAESTHESIOLOGY.
LUXURY OR NECESSITY?

P.Parent, C.Desfemmes, N.Dufeu, et al.

SAMU 94. Departement d'Anesthesie Reanimation.
Hopital Henri Mondor, Creteil, France.

ABSTRACT

In France the specialist anaesthetic nurse forms part of the
medical team on board the mobile emergency and resuscitation
units. Her role is described and discussed.

INTRODUCTION

Ten years ago, in France, a decision was made to medicalise first
aid services and the first SAMU's (Emergency Medical Assistance
Services) were created. SAMU's accepted control of the emergency
mobile resuscitation units (or S.M.U.R.'s) which were designed to
take the facilities of the hospital into the community. As the
frequency of life-threatening emergencies became established so
did the necessity to employ staff competent to deal with those
emergencies.

The ideal team comprises:
1. An emergency physician (trained in anaesthesia)
2. An ambulance driver (holding a first aid qualification)
3. A nurse specialised in anaesthesiology

Is the presence of the third member of the team - the nurse -
really justified?

THE SPECIALISED NURSE AND THE S.M.U.R.'s

Prehospital emergency care is attractive to young members of the
nursing profession. In practice there are considerable difficulties - an abnormal, unfamiliar or even hostile environment;
lack of direct managerial support and difficult or strained
working conditions and practices. Periods of anaesthetic
training will familiarise the nurse with resuscitative
techniques and equipment but basic training in emergency care
will have been provided earlier in the Emergency Department.
Once the nurse has mastered necessary skills in the intensive
care area, operating theatre and resuscitation rooms will he/she
be able to participate in the S.M.U.R.'s with any measure of
efficiency. A preferable level of training is for the nurse to
have specialised in anaesthesia and resuscitation for two years

following three years of general training.   After this period the
nurse can be said to be 'specialised' to work in an S.M.U.R. - a
criterion of admission in our own SAMU.

JUSTIFICATION FOR THE PRESENCE OF A SPECIALISED NURSE OUTSIDE THE EMERGENCY CONTEXT

(a)   Maintenance of Resuscitation kits
        Ambulance Equipment
        Mobile Emergency Cases and Specialist Apparatus
        e.g. Cardiac Monitors
        Emergency Drugs
        Medical Gases

(b)   Special Duties within the S.M.U.R.
        Incubation procedures
        Aseptic procedures
        Isolation procedures

(c)   Teaching

JUSTIFICATION FOR THE PRESENCE OF A SPECIALISED NURSE WITHIN THE EMERGENCY CONTEXT

(a)   Maintenance of all equipment within its proper place

(b)   Technical aid to the emergency physician
        - within a resucitation procedure
        - through monitoring
        - through notekeeping
        - with regard to patients identification and property

CONCLUSION

If it be accepted that it is a necessity to regroup around a
patient in distress the same surroundings and expertise as in a
hospital then the role of the S.M.U.R. nurse appears to be
justified.   This nurse, however, must have a high degree of
technical competence and, specifically, be trained in anaesthesia
and resuscitation.   Nevertheless these duties should not be
restricted to the S.M.U.R. but the nurse should be able to feel
equally at home and to practice within different parts of the
hospital emergency service.

REFERENCES

Ministry of Health. Ordinance nr 72 105, 24 January 1972.
  Article nr.8 "Creation d'un certificat d'aptitude aux
  fonctions d'Aide Anesthesiste.
Vial R.: L'Aide Anesthesiste. Assist.Pub.Act. 15. 13-15.
Medeji T. 1977. L'enseignement des infirmiers (eres) Aide-
Anesthesistes. Rev.Soins. 22. 55-59.

Care of the Acutely Ill and Injured
Edited by D. H. Wilson and A. K. Marsden
© 1982, John Wiley & Sons Ltd.

THE CLASSIFICATION OF DISASTERS

William H. Rutherford* and Jan de Boer**

*Accident and Emergency Department, Royal Victoria Hospital,
 Belfast, Northern Ireland.

**Surgeon, Het Nieve Spittal, Warnsveld, Netherlands.

One of the difficulties in the field of disaster medicine is that the
basic definitions and classifications are still a matter of personal
opinion and preference. If disaster medicine is to be the subject of
scientific debate, then the fundamental questions of classification
must be answered. Otherwise nothing more than anecdotal exchange is
possible.

About a year ago, we decided to attempt to collect a number of
emminent authorities, and invite them to sit on a working party to
struggle with these fundamental matters. We were fortunate to secure
as a sponsor the International Trauma Foundation. The group met in
Brighton on 21st and 22nd October, 1980.

Proposals had been circulated in advance of the meeting. These were
debated and amended. Following the meeting a further draft was
circulated to all members, and on the basis of comments a final
report was prepared. This report was submitted to the International
Congress of Emergency Surgery in Brighton on Wednesday, June, 10th,
1981.

Dr. Jan de Boer explained the main features of the report, copies of
which were in the hands of all the delegates. The chairman of the
session asked the conference to indicate whether it was prepared to
accept the proposals. The report was accepted unanimously.

TEXT OF REPORT

INTERNATIONAL WORKING PARTY ON THE DEFINITION AND CLASSIFICATION OF
DISASTERS

Sponsored by the International Trauma Foundation.

Membership of the party:-

W.H. Rutherford, Chairman, Royal Victoria Hospital, Belfast, U.K.
Dr. Jacob Adler, Shaara Zadek Hospital, Jerusalem, Israel.
Dr. Peter Baskett, Frenchay Hospital, Bristol, U.K.
Dr. Jan de Boer, Het Nieve Spittal, Warnsveld, Netherlands.

Professor Jo Brismar, Department of Surgery, Huddinge, Sweden.
Dr. Rudolf Frey, Department of Anaesthesiology, Maintz, West Germany.
Dr. Olafur Jonson, Borgarspitalinn, Reykjavik, Iceland.
Dr. Stanley Miles, International Trauma Foundation, Salsbury, U.K.
Dr. Ronald Stewart, University of Pittsburg, U.S.A.
Dr. Henryk Zielinski, League of Red Cross Societies, Geneva,
Switzerland.

CONTENTS OF REPORT

Document A - Recommendations on definition or classification of
disaster.
Document B - Argument in support of recommendation.
Document C - Appendix.

DOCUMENT 'A'

DEFINITION AND CLASSIFICATION OF DISASTERS FOR THE PURPOSES OF DISASTER MEDICINE

DEFINITION OF DISASTER

A disaster is a destructive event which, relative to the resources
available, causes many casualities, usually occurring within a short
period of time.

There are two main types:

(1) Simple   - where the structure of the community remains intact.
(2) Compound - where the structure and function of the community is
disrupted.

The response to the disaster may be:

(a) an extraordinary mobilization of emergency services.
(b) activation and co-ordination of national and international
 agencies and resources.

CLASSIFICATION OF DISASTERS

(1) By effect on the surrounding community
(a) Simple   - where the structure of the community remains intact.
(b) Compound - where the structure of the community is disrupted.

(2) By cause
(a) Extreme or violent acts of nature, such as floods, volcanic
eruptions, earthquakes, tropical storms, tidal abnormalities and land
and snow avalanches.
(b) Sudden artificial catastrophies, such as fire, explosions,
transportation wrecks (on land) and contamination from escaped gases,
chemicals or other harmful elements.
(c) Calamities not occurring on land - maritime disasters

(d) Illness or disease of epidemic proportions.
(e) Famine, malnutrition and related illnesses.
(f) Acts of hostility, or armed conflicts, both internal and international, in which the civilian population is threatened or affected.

(3) By number of casualities.
(a) Minor   - 25-99 casualities live or dead, or
                10-49 casualities requiring hospital in-patient
                treatment.
(b) Moderate- 100-99 casualities live or dead, or
                50-249 casualities requiring hospital in-patient
                treatment.
(c) Major   - Over 5,000 people affected, or
                Over 1,000 casualities live or dead, or
                Over   250 casualities requiring hospital in-patient
                treatment.

Proforma for collecting this information:

1	2			3	
	Patients admitted to hospital				
A	A	B	C	A	B
Dead before arrival at hospital or clearing station	1. Total injured 2. Total ill but not injured 3. Total unknown diagnosis	Died within one month	Survived over one month	Injured or ill but not requiring hospital admission	Affected by disaster but not injured or ill

(4) By nature of pathology
     (It is accepted that this type of analysis may only be possible
in simple disasters of minor and moderate size. Where possible, it
should follow these rules).
(a) Injured
(b) Emotionally shocked
(c) Other pathology - by ICD classification
The injured should (if possible) be further subdivided. For each
casualty show -
(i   ) Show each body region separately (as for ISS)
(ii) Classification, nature of injury, ICD in each region.
(iii) AIS of worst injury in each region
(iv) ISS

Note: Ignore all injuries with AIS of 1 unless this leaves patient
with no diagnosis, when a single No. 1 AIS injury may be entered.

(5) <u>By time while cause operating</u>
(a) Short   -   less than 1 hour
(b) Medium -   1 - 24 hours
(c) Long   -   over 1 day

(6) <u>By time of rescue procedures (primary treatment) at site</u>
(a) less than 6 hours
(b) 6 - 24 hours
(c) over 24 hours

(7) <u>By area</u>
(a) Radius - less than 1 km
(b) Radius - 1 - 100 km
(c) Radius - over 100 km

(8) <u>By location (for simple disasters only)</u>
(a) Rural
(b) Urban

(9) <u>By ease of evacuation (for simple disasters only)</u>
(a) No obstruction to quick evacuation of site
(b) Evacuation of casualities from site difficult

<u>DOCUMENT 'B'</u>

<u>COMMENTS</u>

<u>Definition</u>

This definition is drawn up from the point of view of disaster
medicine. Hence the crucial importance of casualities. Governments
may sometimes be faced with large destructive events very like
compound disasters which may produce few if any casualities. If
possible, a separate term should be used for such an event (e.g., a
natural catastrophy or a major emergency). Similarly, major
pollution accidents should, if possible, not be called disasters when
there are no casualities.

Dividing disasters into simple and compound is the beginning of
classification. Often a failure to distinguish these two types of
disaster causes confusion in medical writing and speaking. Therefore
the distinction has been included in the definition.

In practice a disaster and the response to a disaster are very closely
related, and the presence of a typical response is one way of
identifying a disaster. Usually a simple disaster has a response,
limited to the extraordinary mobilization of emergency services,
especially the primary emergency services (see appendix).

A compound disaster necessitates the activation and co-ordination of
national and international agencies and resources. Agencies refer to
government departments, relief organizations, etc. Resources refer

to the staff and material which the agencies control (see appendix).

Classification

(1) The effect on the community
The importance of this distinction has been noted above. A typical
simple disaster is a railway accident. A typical compound disaster
is an earthquake.

(2) By cause
No special comment needed.

(3) Size
The rationale for the three sizes is that the small disaster is
large enough to be of significant interest at hospital and municipal
level, but maybe not large enough to create regional interest. The
medium sized disaster is conceived as often creating problems at
regional or provincial level. The major disaster is conceived as a
national or international event.

It is appreciated that in some situations, a very few casualities may
create very great problems because resources are not available, and
in centres with great resources, even quite large numbers may not
present great difficulty. There is a sense in which a disaster is a
relationship between demand and resources rather than a simple matter
of size. However, there seems no simple way of defining this
relationship in a clear enough way to form a proper criterion for a
register. We therefore admit the drawbacks of this classification by
numbers of casualities, but accept it in preference to the prospect
of no register, as at present.

From a medical standpoint those people sufficiently seriously injured
to require hospital treatment, yet still alive and therefore capable
of treatment, are the most crucial of all. This classification
emphasises these types of casualty. Those immediately dead and those
with minor injuries not requiring hospitalization are much less
important. While in many major disasters, hospitals may be wrecked
and the numbers needing such treatment unavailable, usually these
disasters will clearly have over 1,000 casualities. For simple
disasters of minor and moderate sizes, exact figures will be expected.
For compound major disasters the best available estimate will be
acceptable.

(4) The analysis of the types of injury will only be possible in
developed countries, and maybe only for simple disasters of minor and
moderate size. However, medically this information is of great
importance, and therefore a framework for its collection is given.
Where an attempt is being made to describe the pathology of the
casualty, the analysis should be set out in the framework given here.
AIS stands for 'Abbreviated Injury Scale', ISS for 'Injury Severity
Score' and ICD for 'International Classification of Disease'.

(5) Time when cause operating
Most simple disasters will be instantaneous, but many compound

disasters may continue to be caused over a considerable time scale.
The actual time over which the cause operated should be given. The
classification into instantaneous, short, medium and long may require
revision in the light of experience.

(6) The rescue operation (primary treatment) time
In most simple disasters of minor or moderate size, the time of
primary treatment will be the time until the site is cleared and all
casualities brought to hospital. In a compound disaster, the primary
treatment is the initial first-aid and resuscitation which takes
place at the site. Final treatment refers to major surgery, whether
done in a normal hospital or a field hospital, which may be set up in
the disaster site.

In some compound disasters primary treatment time may be hard to
estimate, but its importance is obvious and it would seem worthwhile
attempting to make the measurement. Again the actual time should be
given, and the subdivisions of this time may require amendment.

(7) Area
No special comment needed.

(8) Location
In simple disasters the problems facing the emergency services are
very different in an urban and rural setting.

(9) Ease of evacuation
This distinction may correspond with the time of rescue procedures
and primary treatment, but some sites (underground disasters,
maritime disasters) provide very special problems, and this attempts
to highlight them.

The value of an inventory of disasters

Once the definition and basic criteria for classification are agreed,
it will be possible to monitor the occurrence of disasters, to see
whether (as some suspect) with increasing world population and
increasing technology using concentrated energy, disasters are
increasing. It will also be possible to compare different disasters,
and the classification should ensure that like is being compared to
like.

We would hope that one of the international bodies would undertake
the compilation of such a register. It would be dependent on
national governments supplying information, and this would entail
national governments keeping registers of disasters within their own
frontiers, ensuing the same rules.

With an agreed definition of disasters and basic rules for classification, it will be possible to approach the field of disaster
medicine in a scientific way. Without definition and classification,
disaster medicine is a mere anecdotal medical interest.

Other information, like the number of hospitals involved, the size of these hospitals, the number of operating teams and operating theatres, the average operating time, the amount of blood and other fluids used for infusion, may be added to the present scheme either for special reports, or at a later stage of development. The prime necessity now is to agree on the minimum basic criteria on the basis of which a useful register may be started.

DOCUMENT 'C'   APPENDIX

Emergency Services

(a) Primary

> Police
> Fire
> Ambulance Services
> Hospitals
> Regional Medical Administration
> Rescue Services or teams

(b) Secondary
> Armed Services
> General Practitioners
> Social and Welfare Services - Government
>   - Voluntary
>
> News Media

NATIONAL AND INTERNATIONAL AGENCIES INVOLVED IN DISASTER PLANNING AND MANAGEMENT

(1)   International and national (regional and local) branches of organisatious such as Red Cross, United Nations Relied Organisation, World Health Organization etc.

(2)   Meteorological services - radar, aircraft reports such as U.S. project STORM FURY, etc., providing advance information on danger areas and the likely scale of the calamity.

(3)   Authorised national disaster co-ordinators of planning services.

(4)   Food and agricultural authorities and suppliers of provisions.

(5)   Public works (electricity, gas and water supply authorities).

(6)   Transportation services - private and government.

(7)   Education

(8)   Finance

(9)   Commerce

(10) Public Health

(11) Civil Defence

(12) Individual helpers not connected with specific organisations, including 'able' victims of the disaster.

(13) Those able to provide food, clothing, accomodation, etc., not only for the injured or ill victims of the disaster, but for their relatives should the need arise.

Care of the Acutely Ill and Injured
Edited by D. H. Wilson and A. K. Marsden
© 1982, John Wiley & Sons Ltd.

**DISASTER MANAGEMENT
A Review of the Hospital Paperwork**

**L J Martin
Accident & Emergency Department
St Stephen's Hospital, London**

INTRODUCTION

The purpose of this short paper is to look at the specific
documentation required for a major accident procedure, and to
suggest some models based on practical experience at a London
hospital. I shall examine this documentation under three
categories (Fig 1) - first the written procedure itself its
format and distribution, secondly the clinical documentation issued
at the triage point and that used for initial clinical assessment,
and thirdly, documentation sent to the Control Room showing the
disposal of patients.

DOCUMENTATION

1.. Major Accident   Format
     Procedure
                         Distribution

2.   Clinical   At triage
     Documentation
                        Initial assessment
                        and treatment

3.   At disposal

Figure 1

FORMAT

Twelve years ago our Major Accident Procedure looked like this
(Fig 2) - a large collection of papers of which every member of
staff was supposed to have a copy. Experience shows however, that
faced with a document as big as this, few people read it and fewer
still remember anything about it. Most copies found their way to
the back of a cupboard and gathered dust. The written procedure was
periodically reviewed, minor alterations were made, and some new
ideas were introduced but it remained substantially the same
document and was never effectively tested.

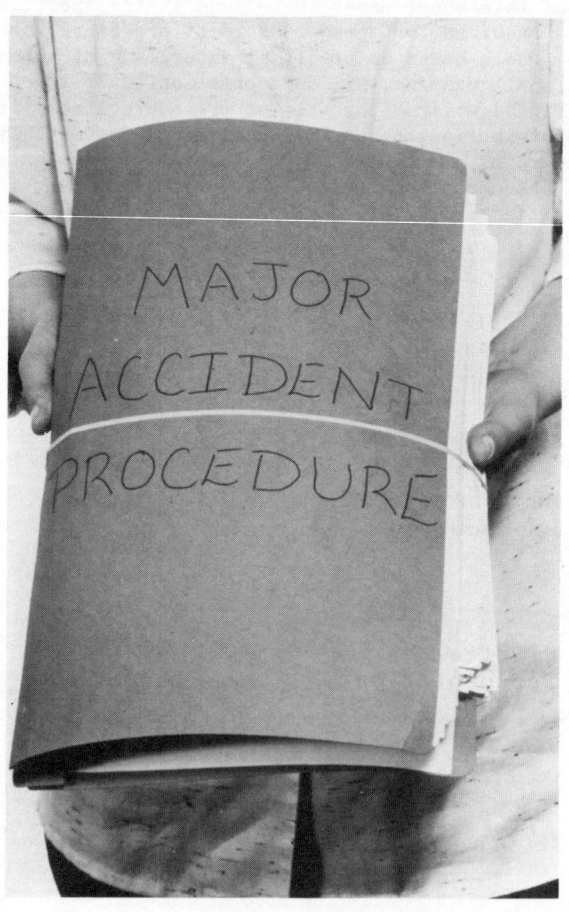

Figure 2

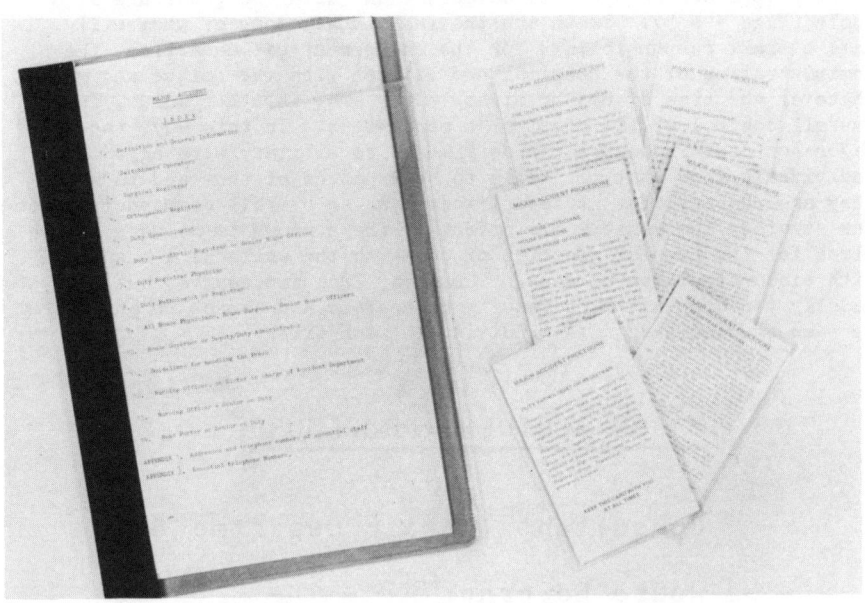

Figure 3

DISTRIBUTION

In 1973 with the beginning of several bomb explosions due to
terrorist activities in this country, it was decided to develop a
new format and method of distribution for our Major Accident
Procedure. The result was this (Fig 3). The new procedure is slim,
attractive and simply numbered. All medical staff and all key
personnel in nursing, radiology, administration, portering and
catering, are required to read a copy of the procedure on appointment
and to sign a declaration that they have done so. They are then
given one of the Action Cards shown in the illustration, and they
are required to carry this card with them at all times. Each card
is specific to the individual's appointment and gives him or her
precise instructions as to what to do in the event of a major
accident and to whom he or she is responsible.

On the back of each card is a list of essential telephone numbers
such as the receiving ward, Control Room etc. On being informed
that a major accident has been declared, the individual responds by
reading the instruction card and acting accordingly. In two major
bomb incidents and at the Iranian Embassy siege, we have found this
procedure to work very smoothly.

A few people are required to be conversant with the procedure as a
whole (Figs 4 & 5). These are the individuals some of whom will
have overall responsibility for the management of casualties, the
administration of the hospital and liaison with the police and media,
whatever the time of day or night. They are, in other words, in
overall control of the hospital's management. In this way, the
Major Accident Procedure can be likened to military strategy.
Individuals know what is likely to be expected of them and to whom
they are responsible. A few officers and an overall commander direct
the strategy and monitor its effects. There seems to me very little
place for the popular practice of covering the walls of a hospital
with elaborate coloured maps. These may look impressive, but are
usually too complex to be readily understood and cannot in any case
be seen by more than a few individuals at a time.

MAJOR ACCIDENT PROCEDURE

Consultant - A & E Department

House Governor

Deputy House Governor
+ Assistants

Figure 4

Unit Nursing Officer - A & E Department

All Sisters - A & E Department

Senior Nursing Officer - Hospital

Senior Nursing Officer - Night duty

Figure 5

CLINICAL DOCUMENTATION

I turn now to the documentation of patients. In the general
confusion, great care must be taken not to misidentify patients.
The seriously injured may be unable to identify themselves, and our
experience in Central London has had the added problem that with
large numbers of foreign nationals being involved, language
communication is sometimes difficult.

We use the system illustrated here (Fig 6) which is initiated at the
triage point, ie the entrance to the Accident & Emergency Department
where the ambulances off-load. A tear-off number is attached to each
patient entering the Department, preferably to an upper limb, using
the attached rubber band. The identically numbered envelope of
documents is then placed with the patient or given to the patient to
hold if conscious. The same number is already written on each of the
contents which include the clinical assessment form, anaesthetic
record, anaesthetic consent form, X-ray request form, haematology and
pathology request forms, disposal form for the Control Room, an
envelope for the patient's valuables and a large polythene bag for
the clothing, together with a check-list. Actual identities are
entered in the Accident & Emergency Register by clerical staff as
details become available, using new and separate pages for all major
accident patients. Meanwhile, urgent investigations are done using
the numerical identification system.

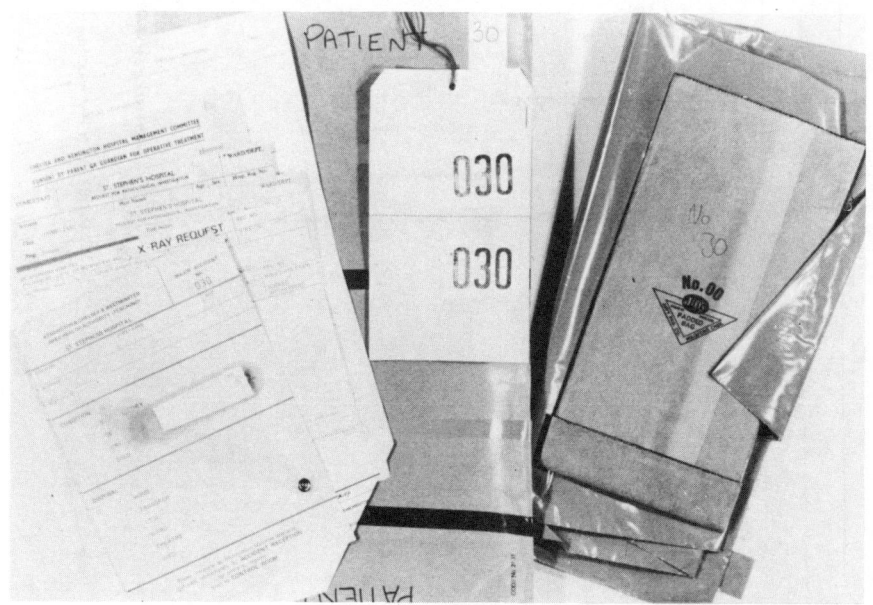

Figure 6

For clinical assessment we use a single folded form, the pages of which are illustrated here (Figs 7,8,9 & 10). This form, which at other times is our standard assessment record for multiple injuries, combines the initial medical and nursing records.

SURNAME	FIRST NAME	D.o.B.	SPECIAL CONDITIONS Allergies/Diabetes/Epilepsy/Haemophilia/Other/Steroids	No.

INITIAL ASSESSMENT

Continuous observation chart

Time / Pulse / Resp. / B.P. / Pupils (R)(L)

AIRWAY:

Dentures

F.B.   Vomitus   Suction

Intubated Yes/No   Tube size   Check length

OBVIOUS HAEMORRHAGE:

Wounds (specify)

Body orifice (specify)

MODE OF INJURY:

1. **R.T.A.** Car Driver / front seat passenger / rear seat passenger
              Motor cyclist / pillion rider
              Cyclist
              Pedestrian

2. **Fall:**   Height:

3. **Burns:** (chart)   Agent:

4. **Other**

LEVEL OF CONSCIOUSNESS:

Conscious Yes/No   Loss of consciousness – how long?

Response to pain

Gag reflex   Cough reflex

PHYSICAL EXAMINATION: (Specify fractures, wounds, tenderness etc.)

Head:

                                                C.V.S.

Chest:

Abdomen:

Pelvis:

                                                R.S.

Spine:

Arms:

                                                C.N.S.

Legs:

URINE   (Note time)   Routine testing

Use chart to show wounds and burns

CHELSEA & KENSINGTON & WESTMINSTER A.H.A. (T) SOUTH SECTION

ACCIDENT & EMERGENCY DEPARTMENT

HOSPITAL

Figure 7

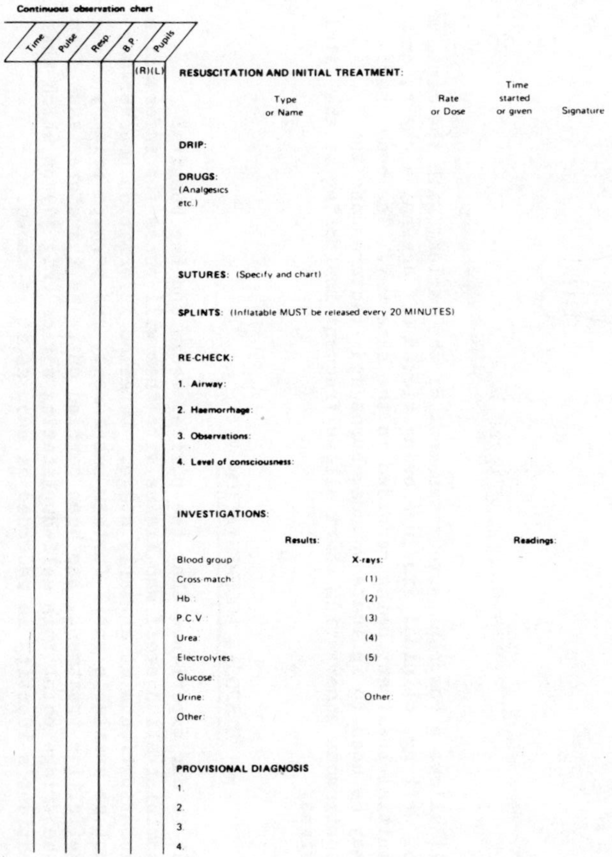

Figure 9

Continuous observation chart

Time	Pulse	Resp	B.P	Pupils (R)(L)

RECHECK

FURTHER NOTES:

DISPOSAL:
Operating Theatre
I.T.U.
Transfer to ward
Direct to ward
Discharged
Died

Figure 8

Continuous observation chart

Time	Pulse	Resp	B.P	Pupils (R)(L)

RESUSCITATION AND INITIAL TREATMENT:

Type or Name	Rate or Dose	Time started or given	Signature

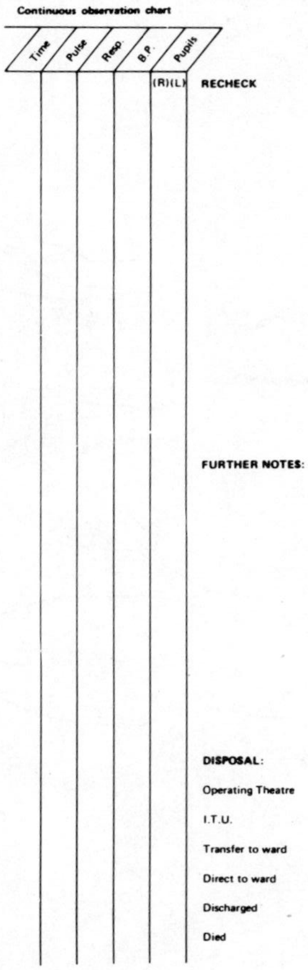

DRIP:

DRUGS: (Analgesics etc.)

SUTURES: (Specify and chart)

SPLINTS: (Inflatable MUST be released every 20 MINUTES)

RE-CHECK:
1. Airway:
2. Haemorrhage:
3. Observation:
4. Level of consciousness:

INVESTIGATIONS:

Results: Readings:

X-rays:
Blood group (1)
Cross match (2)
Hb (3)
P.C.V (4)
Urea (5)
Electrolytes
Glucose Other
Urine
Other

PROVISIONAL DIAGNOSIS
1
2
3
4

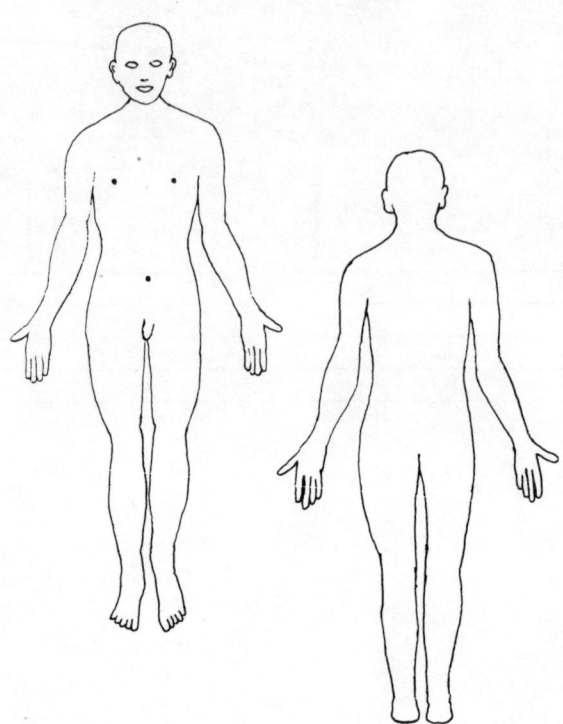

BODY CHART FOR WOUNDS AND BURNS

Figure 10

It allows a comprehensive assessment of the patient with the minimum
of writing, clinical findings being ticked off against a chart, and
initial treatment being recorded in the same way. The body chart
may be used to indicate wounds, burns and fractures and the
continuous observation chart allows frequent monitoring of the vital
signs.

DISPOSAL DOCUMENTATION

It is our experience that the police, media and the hospital
administration staff who liaise with them will press for information
about patients at an early stage. Detailed information however may
not be available until further assessment, and perhaps primary
definitive treatment, has been carried out. We therefore issue from
the triage point this self-duplicating notice (Fig 11) on which the
patient's identity is recorded as soon as it is known.

KENSINGTON & CHELSEA & WESTMINSTER AREA HEALTH AUTHORITY (TEACHING) ST. STEPHEN'S HOSPITAL		MAJOR ACCIDENT NUMBER	
SURNAME	FORENAMES	SEX	AGE
ADDRESS			
NEXT OF KIN			
CONDITION MINOR INJURY SERIOUS CRITICAL DEAD			
DISPOSAL HOME THEATRE I.T.U. WARD (NAME) TRANSFER (HOSPITAL) DIED			
AUTHORISING SIGNATURE:			

*Please complete and pass immediately to ACCIDENT RECEPTION for entry to register,t then to CONTROL ROOM.

Figure 11

It gives an indication of the seriousness of the patient's condition according to triage estimation, together with a note of the disposal of the patient. This information is passed to the Administrative Police Control Room which is next door to the Accident & Emergency Department (Fig 12) and is housed in the Out-Patient Waiting Hall in the Medical Records Department. This doubles as an administrative Control Office for the hospital administration and has the advantages of space, seating and several telephones. It also contains the Transport Office so that contact can be maintained with ambulance control.

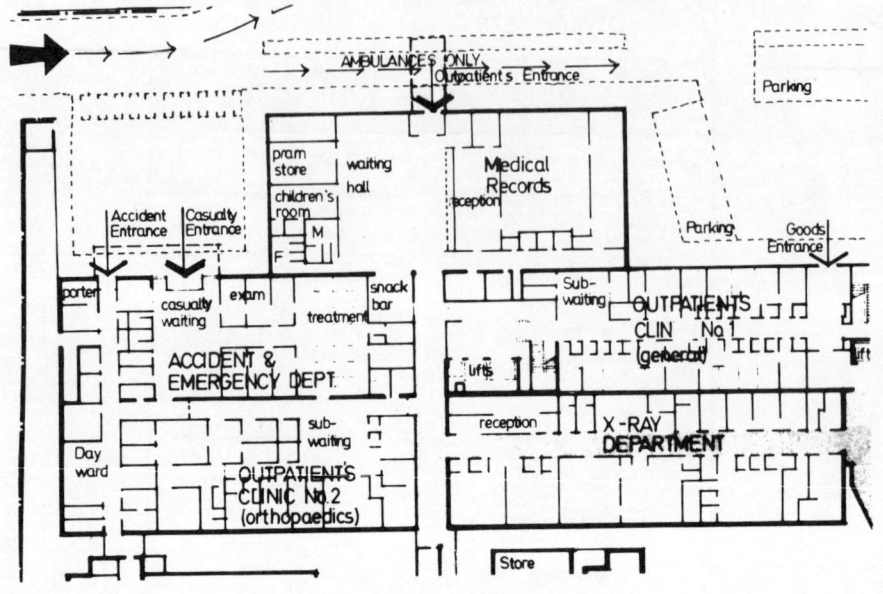

Figure 12

My overall message is "keep it simple". It can be difficult enough
to manage a major incident without submerging oneself in a sea of
paper work.

Care of the Acutely Ill and Injured
Edited by D. H. Wilson and A. K. Marsden
© 1982, John Wiley & Sons Ltd.

NATIONAL PLANNING FOR DISASTERS IN DIFFERENT COUNTRIES

B. Brismar

Department of Surgery, Huddinge University Hospital,
S-141 86 Huddinge, Sweden

The definition and classification of disasters have previously been far from uniform (Rutherford, 1973). This is clearly evident when studying the national planning for disasters in different countries. Depending on the structure and level of development of the respective societies, and on the political conditions and geographical location, the term disaster can have different implications (WHO, 1980). An event which in one country is regarded as a disaster may for another country be something which is a relatively normal, frequent occurrence with which the population has learnt to live (Huller et al., 1970, Boyd, 1975, Klinghoffer, 1978, Duffy, 1979, Henry, 1980).

As an overall definition, however, a disaster may be said to be an event which by its nature or magnitude, places urgent and extreme demands on personnel and material resources. A catastrophic situation may also arise when the demands upon resources are normal but when the supply of resources in the form of manpower or material necessities is stopped, for example as a result of political conflicts (Norberg et al., 1981). This is a disaster hazard which as far as medical care is concerned emerges as increasingly threatening the more technologically advanced the medical services become, with increased dependence upon imported goods due to a changeover to disposable articles and plastic products and with greater vulnerability resulting from a need for large supplies of electricity, water and gas for technical purposes.

In several countries, therefore, by reason of the political situation, it has been considered appropriate to couple the national planning for disasters with the planning of preparedness for war or blockade. For this reason the planning has been placed under the control of the military or civil defence authorities. This is the case, for example, in Israel, South Korea and Switzerland, where major war experiences or threats of war have been decisive for the formulation of the disaster plans.

Israel has been involved in four wars during the last 30 years - in 1948, 1956, 1967 and 1973. Furthermore, in recent years the country has been in a constant state of preparedness on account of frequent terrorist attacks. Their medical care has therefore been organized with a view to being able to cope with mass casualties at

any time (Adler, 1978). As emergency departments with facilities
for operations are the most vital part of a general hospital, considerable efforts have been made to protect these against inter-
ference with their running and against bomb attacks. In several
hospitals protected underground units have been built as a supplement to existing emergency departments. Several of these have their
own supply of electricity from reserve generators, water from their
own drilled well and in some cases an oxygen supply from their own
factory within the hospital premises. The emergency departments
are built with large triage areas and open treatment areas to facilitate the reception of a large number of casualties simultaneously.

In South Korea also, the threat of war has been decisive in the
formulation of the disaster plans. Every year a nationwide Command
Post Exercise (CPX), lasting one week, is carried out to prepare
for war or other disaster situations. As a part of the CPX a medical emergency plan is designed. According to this, priority is given to disaster or war casualties, while the treatment of other
patients depends upon the possibilities. In the event of a disaster
the hospitals are mobilized to care for severely injured persons,
while the existing inpatients are sent home to the greatest possible extent. If necessary, according to the plan, designated
schools or other buildings are to be requisitioned for medical care
purposes. The mobilized hospitals are also responsible for organi-
zing mobile medical teams and despatching them to take care of casualties at the scene of a disaster or to add to existing medical
care personnel in affected areas. The mobile team consists of a
doctor, two nurses, two laboratory technicians and a chaffeur. They
have access to a lorry and extensive emergency care equipment. To
tackle a massive outbreak of casualties, the mayor of Seoul will
maintain a fleet of ambulances and will allocate ambulances to mobilized hospitals and health centres.

Switzerland, a neutral country which has been spared from war for
more than 100 years, also experiences the threat of war as a highly tangible risk of catastrophe. The ravages wrought by the Second
World War in neighbouring countries has led to highly developed
disaster and defensive preparedness among the population. In rural
areas there are several protected civil defence installations. Beneath a number of large general hospitals protected medical care
units have been built and the hospitals have stores of essential
supplies sufficient for several months of use in the event of a
blockade. As a rule the hospitals also have possibilities of providing their own supplies of water and electricity.

At the same time Switzerland keeps up its old tradition of maintaining efficient rescue and disaster service - a necessity in view
of the geographical structure of the country, with its great mountain ranges and roads that in winter are rendered impassable. By
the development of a well functioning helicopter organization the
rescue time in mountain accidents, for instance, has been considerably reduced and owing to the large radius of action of the helicopters the patients can be transported directly to specialised
trauma or burn units.

Two other European countries - <u>Northern Ireland</u> and <u>Italy</u> - do not perhaps experience the threat of war as the most imminent risk of a major disaster, but here the frequent terrorist attacks present the medical care authorities with special problems. As the terrorist outrages usually in densely populated areas with short distances to hospitals, these hospitals are often forced to receive a large number of severely injured persons at very short notice or with no notice at all.

One example is the severe bomb attack in Bologna, Italy, on the 2nd of August 1980, when 291 persons were injured, 73 of whom died instantaneously (Brismar et al., 1981 a). The majority of the casualties were taken to the two largest general hospitals of the city. No actual disaster plans existed, either for the whole region or for the individual hospitals. Instead, as a result of the massive efforts of voluntary workers and the good inprovisation capacity of these hospitals they managed to maintain the flow of patients through the emergency department to the operating theatres, intensive care unit and wards without any queuing problem. A well functioning emergency care system with experienced personnel was found in Bologna to be a fundamental prerequisite for coping with the casualties. It was emphasized, in fact, that this system could in no way have been replaced by a disaster plan, however sophisticated.

Within the industrialized world we are also affected yearly by other types of man-made disasters of varying magnitudes. These include accidents involving public transport and industrial catastrophes. To meet the needs in such situations we in <u>Sweden</u>, for example, have designed regional disaster plans in the different counties (Brismar et al., 1981 b). These serve as a framework of instructions for coordination of the rescue activities within each county, where regional alarm centres control the activity and coordinate the tasks of the police, the fire service and medical services. In addition, for the individual hospitals plans are drawn up for the internal activity in dealing with a mass casualty situation. It is also an obligation of the hospitals to be able to send out mobile medical teams on request to the scene of a disaster in order to assist in the rescue work.

The activity in situations with mass casualties has been greatly simplified in Sweden, as in many Western European countries and the USA, by the development of the ambulance service from being merely a means of transportation to becoming an emergency care unit on wheels. This means that the ambulance system is now able to serve as an extended arm of the medical care services in the event of a catastrophe.

In summary, we find on examining the planning for disasters in different countries that the plans are, quite naturally, designed in accordance with what are considered the most prominent disaster hazards. The medical care problems that arise in different types of catastrophes often have much in common, however, and publication and exchange of experiences from disaster areas are therefore

of great importance. The work undertaken by the international working party on the definition and classification of disasters will
facilitate such communication.

REFERENCES

Adler, J., 1978. Abtransport und Behandlung der Verwundeten im Okto-
    ber-Krieg 1973. Wehrmed. Mschr., 7, 196-199.
Boyd, N.A., 1975. A military surgical team in Belfast. Annals of
    the Royal College of Surgeons of England, 56, 15-25.
Brismar, B. and Bergenwald, L., 1981a. The terrorist bomb explosion
    in Bologna, Italy, 1980. - An analysis of the effects and inju-
    ries sustained. Submitted for publication.
Brismar, B. and Norberg, K.A., 1981b. Disaster planning in the Stock-
    holm region, Sweden. Medical teams for qualified first aid. II:nd
    World Congress on Emergency and Disaster Med., Pittsburgh.
Duffy, J.C., 1979. Disaster at Sea: Problem and Prospects. Military
    Med., 144, 616-618.
Henry, S., 1980. Mississauga Hospital: largest evacuation in Cana-
    da's history. CMA Journal, 122, 582-586.
Huller, T. and Bazini, Y., 1970. Blast Injuries of the Chest and
    Abdomen. Arch. Surg., 100, 24-30.
Klinghoffer, M., 1978. A pre-triage plan for mass casualty care.
    Occupational Health and Safety, 47: 6, 32-35.
Norberg, K.A. and Brismar, B., 1981. Medical care at emergency hospi-
    tals in conventional war. Essential features of the planning
    of the Swedish National Board of Health and Welfare. II:nd World
    Congress on Emergency and Disaster Med., Pittsburgh.
Emergency care in natural disasters. Views of an international se-
    minar. 1980. WHO Chronicle, 34, 96-100.

Care of the Acutely Ill and Injured
Edited by D. H. Wilson and A. K. Marsden
© 1982, John Wiley & Sons Ltd.

EXPERIENCE WITH A SURGICAL RESUSCITATION TEAM IN THE
SOUTHERN ITALIAN EARTHQUAKE, NOVEMBER 1980

G. Sinigaglia, E. Bossi and R. Riva.

Emergency Traumatology Service, 1st Surgical Clinic,
University of Milan Policlinico Hospital.

Recent geological studies have classified more than three quarters
of the Italian territory as a "seismic area". Serious earthquakes
have been recorded throughout the whole of the long history of our
country. Entire towns and their surrounding countryside have been
destroyed, some of them on several occasions. Pompei is a classical
example of these repeated major disasters. In AD79 it was completely
obliterated by an earthquake and a simultaneous eruption of Vesuvius.

When evaluating calamities of this proportion it is very important to
recognise that, apart from floods or disasters caused by gas or
chemical agents, they all have one common feature so far as human
suffering is concerned, ninety per cent of the victims sustain
traumatic injuries and a very high proportion of them require
resuscitation. This fact must influence the planning and preparation
of emergency medical help in the following ways:-

a) Medical teams capable of treating large numbers of casualties
    must reach the site of the disaster with the shortest possible
    delay. The first 24-48 hours is of vital importance.

b) To achieve this the teams and their equipment must be well
    organised and thoroughly prepared before the disaster occurs
    and the equipment must be extremely mobile.

c) This implies selection and training of highly competent doctors,
    nurses and support staff who are able to handle the logistic
    problems of the situation as well as the medical tasks which
    face them.

d) To work effectively each team must have complete autonomy and be
    able to function independently for 6-7 days - (its specific
    usefulness will expire after such a period because both staff
    and supplies will be nearing exhaustion).

The basic task of a surgical resuscitation team at the centre of the
disaster is to sustain life for the largest possible number of
casualties. For the most seriously injured they must control
haemodynamic shock and prepare patients for safe transfer by the

fastest means possible to permanent medical facilities on the borders
of the disaster area.

These principles form the guidelines for the constitution and selection of the emergency medical team. The professional skills and
expertise must reflect the operational policy of the exercise and we
have found it necessary to have a team of fourteen people to fulfil
these requirements:-

> 2 Emergency traumatology surgeons
>
> 2 Emergency general surgeons
>
> 2 Anaesthetists - resuscitation
>
> 1 Hygienist physician
>
> 1 Veterinarian
>
> 2 Theatre nurses
>
> 3 Male nurses trained in first aid and traumatology
>
> 1 Technician experienced in setting up and running
> equipment and devices

The presence of a hygienist physician and a veterinarian is very
important. The first is able to manage the most serious sanitary
and public health problems, the latter, in a rural area, can attend
to the urgent needs of domestic and farm animals.

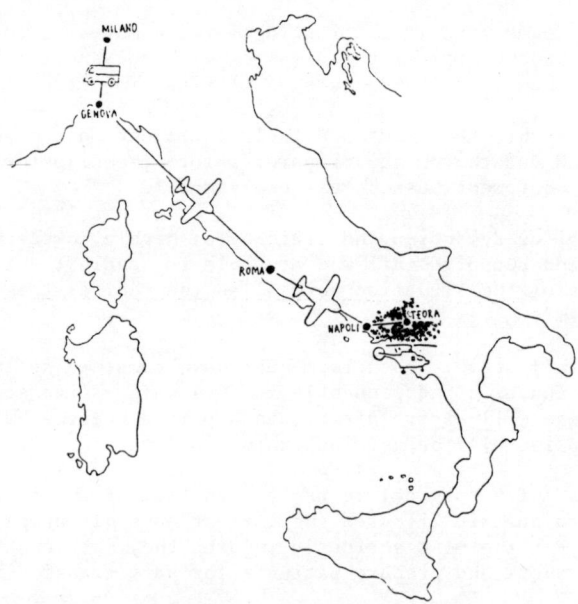

Itinerary of the Emergency Unit
and zone of disaster

We wish to emphasise the importance of all members of the team coming
from one hospital. This allows the team to have experience in
working together before they arrive at the scene of the disaster and
also enables all the members of the team to be familiar with the
equipment.

On Sunday evening, November 23rd 1980, a serious earthquake occurred
in the region of Campania and Basilicata in southern Italy. For a
long time the Institute of Emergency Surgery of the University of
Milan has been prepared to respond to the urgent medical needs of
people involved in such a major disaster and it is appropriate that
we report on our recent experience to an International Congress of
Emergency Surgery.

Previously, on the occasion of an earthquake in the El Asman district
of Algeria, the team and its equipment had been ready to move into
the disaster area. Through the Italian Foreign Affairs Ministry, the
Algerian Government received our offer of immediate medical help.
It was agreed that we should travel by air to the disaster zone but
then a few hours later, the Algerian Government cancelled its request.
However, the experience of mobilising the team and equipment proved
useful and when the disaster of November 1980 occurred we were able
to leave for Southern Italy within four hours.

Milan Airport was fog-bound so we started our journey by road to
Genoa with the equipment loaded on trucks. Here we transferred to a
military G222 freight plane but this could only take us as far as Rome
because Naples Airport was also closed by fog. At dawn on the morning
of 25th November we left for Naples where this time the personnel
and equipment were transferred to three helicopters of the Italian
Navy. After a 40 minute flight we landed in the disaster zone at
Teora in Irpinia.

This area, which is 3000 feet above sea level, had not been reached
by any other emergency medical team when we arrived. Approximately
2500 people normally live in the village and the surrounding farms.
85% of their homes had been destroyed. On the afternoon of November
26th the weather conditions deteriorated, with continuous rain and
awful cold. Soldiers and Firemen formed rescue squads seeking people
who were trapped. Survivors were extracted from beneath the debris
36, 48 and even 72 hours after the earthquake.

With our medical skill and the equipment we had brought with us, we
were able to give a good level of care to many patients who had
multiple injuries, shock, or crush syndrome. The worst casualties,
after surgical resuscitation, were flown by helicopter to a large,
undamaged hospital on the border of the disaster zone.

Our unit was not planned and equipped with the intention of performing major surgical operations, but rather to stabilise a patient's
condition so that they could be safely transported to a base hospital.

This plan conforms with the modern concept of avoiding major surgery
in circumstances where full aseptic conditions and absolute technical
security cannot be assured.

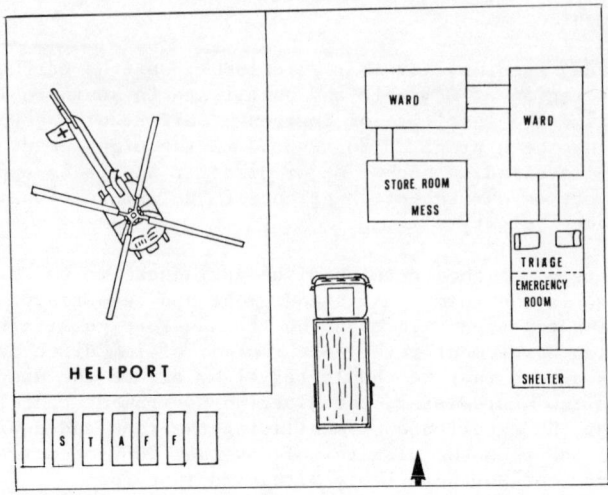

Scheme of deployed Emergency Unit
in tents and Emergency Shelter

As a result of this experience we wish to propose the following
criteria for an emergency surgical resuscitation unit:-

1.   There should be at least one unit, comprising personnel and
     equipment in every Region of the country. The unit should be
     composed of staff from the most important hospital complex in
     the Region so that they can train and maintain their equipment
     together.

2.   The unit must be fully self-sufficient and be able to leave for
     the centre of activity with the minimum of delay. On arrival
     it must be able to set up and commence full activity almost
     immediately.

3.   The unit should have supplies and provisions to able to function
     for 6-8 days. At the end of this period of time the supplies
     will be exhausted, the personnel fatigued and the nature of the
     emergency will have changed, so the unit should then withdraw.

4.   The personnel must be trained and prepared to work in very close
     and strict collaboration in extremely difficult environmental
     conditions and without the opportunity of prolonged breaks for
     rest or relaxation.

Our unit is now in permanent readiness to work in these conditions
and to accomplish its tasks in a swift and efficient manner either
in Italy or abroad.

Care of the Acutely Ill and Injured
Edited by D. H. Wilson and A. K. Marsden
© 1982, John Wiley & Sons Ltd.

HELICOPTERS IN MEDICAL CARE

CHAIRMAN   Dr. J.K. Gosnold, Hull, England

        Since the advent of Emergency Surgery, transport either of
the doctor to the patient, or the patient to the doctor, has always
been of extreme importance.

It was therefore of little surprise that, despite the hour, a
session of interest to an interested audience emerged.

Contributions were presented to the Symposium by:-

        Dr. P. Hrouda, Creteil, France

        The Role of the Helicopter in the
        SAMU 94 Department

        Dr. A.E. Cram, Iowa City, U.S.A.

        The Role of the Helicopter in Rural
        Emergency Systems

        Dr. D.B. Dove, New York, U.S.A.

        The Bringing of the Hospital to the
        Emergency

        Dr. G.P. Rossi, Milan, Italy

        A Study of the Organisation of an
        Aeromedical Rescue and Transport
        Service in a Composite Geographical
        Region

All the presentations served to compare and contrast the usefulness
of the helicopter as a means of transport in the urban situation and
in the rural situation, and as a means of transporting the patient
from either a peripheral centre, or the site of accident, to a
centre of excellence; or, in the more major disaster, of
transporting a hospital team with operating facilities to the heart
of the incident.

Several factors emerged as definite advantages to the use of the helicopter, mainly the speed of service and the ease of access to the incident, even in the urban situation. Dr. Hrouda impressed the audience by his description of the use of crossroads in the French cities as being useful landing sites for the SAMU 94 Helicopters, possibly a pointer for the removal of flower beds from the middle of English urban roundabouts! Certainly his attendance times impressed upon us the usefulness of the helicopter as a means of bypassing the urban traffic jam.

In a much more rural situation the presentation by Dr. Cram stressed the extreme importance of the helicopter as a means of rapid transfer of patients in a critical condition from the peripheral centres to the central specialist centres in Iowa City. Despite the occasional inability to use the helicopter in extreme weather, it was pointed out that the same weather would also prevent the use of roads for transport and that the helicopter would be of immediate use after the cessation of the storm whereas roads would not.

Dr. Cram did confirm the feeling of everyone present that although a rapid efficient mode of transport, the helicopter was not the ideal place for treatment of the patient.

Dr. Dove then proceeded to convince the audience that the helicopter could also be used in the alternative role of transportation of treatment facilities to the scene. Certainly, in the major disaster, e.g. the Jumbo crash with large numbers of casualties at a major airport, the access road would immediately become congested with enthusiastic onlookers, and a multiplicity of emergency vehicles. This, he revealed, could be bypassed by the use of the larger type of helicopter carrying inflatable operating theatres, treatment units, holding wards, etc.

We, in this country, are used to the role of the helicopter in air sea rescue, mountain rescue, and to a lesser extent in interhospital travel, but certainly we are far less used to the more enthusiastic use of the machine in an urban situation and in large distance travel.

This, as was pointed out, may be due to the extreme expense to the National Health Service, or more probably to the extremely efficient Ambulance Service in a smaller area with less arduous terrain.

Useful discussion followed all the presentations and a more general debate wound up the session on a lively level.

Care of the Acutely Ill and Injured
Edited by D. H. Wilson and A. K. Marsden
© 1982, John Wiley & Sons Ltd.

THE ROLE OF THE HELICOPTER IN THE S.A.M.U. 94
DEPARTMENT, 1975-1980

Hrouda P. Simon D. and Abbeys J.M.

SAMU 94. Departement d'Anesthesie-Reanimation.
Hospital Henri Mondor. 94 010-F Creteil, France.

ABSTRACT

During the five years 1975-1980, the SAMU of the Val de Marne (94)
carried out 733 helicopter flights.   The district served is a
suburb of Paris covering 245 sq.km. and housing 1,500,000
inhabitants.   Two types of helicopter flights are described, those
in which the helicopter flew to the location of the ill or injured
patient and those in which it was used for an inter-hospital
transfer.   The age and diagnoses of the patints, the mobilisation
time of the medical team and the distances covered by the flights
are discussed.

INTRODUCTION

The area for which the Val de Marne S.A.M.U. provides medical first
aid is traversed by important motorways, numerous railways and two
large rivers.   It contains the Orly International Airport, a
university and many factories for the manufacturing industry.

Emergency medical treatment is assured day and night by four main
hospitals, two of them being university hospitals.   They can
provide the necessary care for most patients but cases requiring
specialist treatment for multiple injuries, neurosurgery, thoracic
or cardiac surgery can be transported to appropriate hospitals
anywhere in the Paris area.

Specialised medical transport, called S.M.U.R., provides some
6,000 journeys a year in the SAMU 94 district, this is mostly by
ambulances fully equipped for resuscitation but when necessary a
helicopter is used.

THE ROLE OF THE HELICOPTER

An Alouette III helicopter has been employed for this work.   It
can accommodate a pilot, a mechanic, an emergency physician and a
nurse together with their medical equipment and, of course, the
patient lying on a stretcher.   The take-off time is about three
minutes and during the five years under review there has been an
increasing use of the Alouette III.   In 1980 215 out of 5,985,
or 3.5% of all medical journeys, were made by helicopter.

Advantages: The first advantage of using a helicopter is in saving

125

time, especially over long distances. While an ambulance has
travelled 30 km. a helicopter will have covered 100 km. The
helicopter is not subject to traffic conditions, especially
traffic jams. The medical team not only reaches the patient more
quickly but less of their total time is spent travelling and they
are more readily available for other emergencies. This advantage
is also valid for the transport of the patient: for instance if a
patient requiring neurosurgery were to be transported from the south
to the north of Paris at 6.00 p.m. the journey would take more than
an hour by ambulance but it can be accomplished in six minutes by
helicopter. The patient also has a more comfortable ride by
helicopter, the amplitude of acceleration and deceleration stress
is less than it is in an ambulance.

Disadvantages: The disadvantages of helicopter transport are, first
of all, its dependence on favourable meteorological conditions.
Adverse weather can make flights impossible and night time helicopter
flights over Paris have been banned since 1973. The number of
flights is much less in winter than in summer. The level of noise
in the helicopter is a further inconvenience. In the Alouette III
the crew, the medical staff and the patient have to wear ear
protectors; the problem is less severe in the more recent Dauphin
or Ecureuil models. Finally some hospitals still do not have a
correctly beaconed landing zone.

DIAGNOSIS OF PATIENTS TRANSPORTED BY HELICOPTER

Most of the patients transported by helicopter had neurological,
neorusurgical or cardiosurgical diagnoses. Only 18% of patients
had a trauma diagnosis. Several patients, who had been in
intensive care units, were transported by helicopter back to their
base hospital or to a convalescent home. This is because they were
still in a weak condition and helicopter transport is more rapid and
more comfortable.

AGE DISTRIBUTION OF PATIENTS

Certain diagnoses among these patients have a characteristic peak
incidence. From 0-15 years neonatology problems and serious
childhood neurological problems predominate. Patients in the
15-25 years group are mainly surgical. Cardiac patients were most
common in patients aged between 45 and 55 years. Very few patients
over 75 years of age were transported by helicopter.

DISTANCES TRAVELLED BY HELICOPTERS

Primary missions to the site of the acutely ill or injured patient
were usually less than 50 km. corresponding to a flight time of
16 minutes or less. Secondary missions, taking patients between
hospitals, were sometimes up to 160 km. Beyond this distance the
Alouette III helicopter begins to lose its efficiency.

CONCLUSIONS

In our opinion there are very precise indications for transporting
a patient by helicopter. The cost, when using an Alouette III

helicopter, is quite reasonable - about 30 French francs per km.
compared with 42 French francs for some emergency ambulance
journeys.   The reason why, at the present time, only 3.5% of our
patients are transported by helicopter is because the French public
authorities have not yet realised all the advantages.

In a recent study we showed that, based on German and Swiss
experience, 10 Dauphin and 30 Ecureuil helicopters under S.A.M.U.
control would be sufficient to give a quick response to all medical
and surgical distress calls for the whole of France.

REFERENCES

A.D.A.C. 1977. Der Luftrettungsdienst in der Bundesrepublik
  Deutschland.   Document A.D.A.C.

Huguenard P. et al. 1975. Les helicopteres et les SAMU: la
  position du SAMU 94.   Ann.Ane.Fra.   16.   453-463.

Johnson A. Jr. et al. 1976.   Five years of emergency aeronotical
  evacuations in the U.S.   Avi.Spa.env.med.   47.   662-666.

Mackensie C.F. et al. 1979.   Two years of mortality in 760 patients
  transported by helicopter directly from the road accident scene.
  Am.Surg. 45.   101-108.

Metrot J.   1974.   Accelerations et vibrations en transport routier
  et aerien.   Etude physique.   Ann.Ane.Fra. 15.9M.

Sonsino G. 1979.   Realisation d'un batiment et d'une helistation
  a l'usage du SAMU et du SMUR a l'Hopital Henri Mondor.
  These med. CHU H.Mondor.Creteil.

Care of the Acutely Ill and Injured
Edited by D. H. Wilson and A. K. Marsden
© 1982, John Wiley & Sons Ltd.

THE ROLE OF THE HELICOPTER IN A RURAL
EMERGENCY MEDICAL SERVICE SYSTEM

Albert Cram, M.D.

Associate Professor of Surgery
University of Iowa Medical College
Iowa City, Iowa

ABSTRACT

The University of Iowa Hospital is an 1100-bed teaching institution
which instituted a hospital-based helicopter ambulance system in
April, 1979. Experience with the system reveals that flights to an
accident scene are relatively infrequent while transfer of critical
patients from small rural hospitals to the tertiary care center com-
prise the bulk of the flights. Rapid delivery of the patient to the
tertiary care center was found to be less important to patient outcome than the rapid delivery of experienced personnel to the rural
hospital.

INTRODUCTION

Rapid delivery of a severely injured patient to a facility capable
of managing all injuries sustained is assumed to increase survival
and decrease morbidity. The rural physician often has inadequate
experience and lacks necessary equipment for managing the multiple
injury patient. Transportation of such patients to a trauma center
is usually carried out in ground ambulances with the patient attended by poorly equipped and inexperienced paramedical personnel. The
University of Iowa Hospitals began a helicopter ambulance service on
the premise that decreased transportation time to the trauma center
would improve survival. After two years of service we reviewed the
charts of severe trauma patients transported by helicopter to evaluate the effectiveness of the program.

METHODS

A total of 366 patients' charts were reviewed in detail. Four experienced trauma surgeons reviewed each chart and categorized helicopter transport as: essential, beneficial, or not a factor in patient outcome.

RESULTS

Helicopter transport was judged essential to patient outcome in 24%
and beneficial in 11%. The remaining patients appeared to derive
no benefit from rapid helicopter transport. No cases were found in
which helicopter transport was judged detrimental to patient outcome. Endotracheal intubation, chest tube insertion, or institution
of massive fluid replacement at the rural hospital by the flight
nurse was the most common finding when helicopter transport was
judged essential or beneficial to patient outcome.

DISCUSSION

Lack of experience in dealing with the multiple trauma patient often
results in delayed recognition and inadequate stabilization by rural
physicians. The rapid delivery of well trained and highly experienced personnel to the rural hospital often results in the institution of live-saving measures which make delivery of a salvageable
patient to a distant trauma center possible. Helicopter transport
plays an important role in the rural emergency medical service system.

Care of the Acutely Ill and Injured
Edited by D. H. Wilson and A. K. Marsden
© 1982, John Wiley & Sons Ltd.

LONG DISTANCE TRANSPORT OF CRITICALLY ILL PATIENTS

Bordone G. Graziina A. Scarani F. Sganzerla E.
Rossi G.P. Vesconi S. Fairhorst J.

Institute of Anaesthesiology - University of Milan.
European Assistance Institution, Milan, Italy.

ABSTRACT

The training of specialised medical staff and the availability of
miniaturised, battery charged medical equipment has made the
transport of high risk patients possible, even over long distances.
Now that treatment can be given at the site of the accident and
during transport there are very few situations in which a patient
must be regarded as "untransportable".

The transport of a high risk patient from Pakistan to Italy is
described as an example of what can be achieved.

INTRODUCTION

Countries which have a high standard of health care have a growing
interest in the problems of medical transport. This may involve
the provision of specialised personnel and equipment at the site
of an accident or the transfer of critically ill patients from one
hospital to another or from one country to another either by land
or by air. Two of the factors which have led to an increasing
demand for such services are:

1) the rapid development of new medical technology and the
    centralisation of medical skills in a few highly specialised
    centres.

2) the frequent need to transfer patients from countries where
    the local health services are inadequate to a specialised
    centre which can give a high level of care.

The long distance transport of patients whose condition is already
stabilised does not usually cause any serious problem and it is
now widely practised. However the transport of "high risk
patients" with an unstable condition which requires constant
monitoring is seldom effected. To transfer such a patient it is
essential not only to monitor their condition but also to be able
to correct any changes which occur in their vital functions
during the journey.

We therefore deemed it interesting to refer to our experience in
the long distance transport of 191 patients which we have carried
out with the help of a company which specialises in this work.

METHODS

The medical staff involved in this work are all physicians working in the Policlinico Hospital of Milan. The role of the company is to give the necessary organisation and support to the activity and to process all the relevant information. Most of the work involves "high risk patients" who require intensive care and continuous monitoring of their vital functions during the journey. Some patients, who were thought to be in a stable condition before the journey began, developed unexpected major complications during transport. Until recently many of the patients in this series would have been considered "untransportable" but attitudes are changing because of the success obtained by specialised medical teams, with the necessary equipment, using appropriate means of transport. None of our patients suffered a deterioration of their general condition as a consequence of the transport itself and, at the end of the journey, they were in a centre which offered them much better care in terms of expertise and equipment.

GENERAL MEDICINE	40.3%
ACUTE MYOCARDIAL INFARCTION	10.4%
ACUTE RESPIRATORY FAILURE	0.5%
PSYCHIATRIC	5.7%
POST OPERATED PATIENTS	5.2%
POLYTRAUMA	27.7%
SPINAL CORD INJURY	5.2%
BURNED PATIENTS	4.7%

Figure 1

Different pathologies transported in the period 1978-1980 referring to a total of 191 patients.

Figure 1 shows the diagnoses of 191 patients transported during a three year period. On a final assessment 60% of them fulfilled the description of "high risk patients" transported over long distances. Figure 2 indicates the type of transport used and in 52.4% of these journeys the medical staff accompanying the patient consisted of two doctors and a nurse.

MEDICAL PLANE	55%
AIR LINER WITH STRETCHER	11%
NORMAL FLIGHT	15.2%
AMBULANCE	16.2%
TRAIN	2.6%

Figure 2

Means of transport used.

The geographical distribution of our activity is shown in Figure 3.
During the past three years we have received an increasing number of
requests for the transport of patients from countries where the
emergency health care is inadequate when compared with European
standards.

	1978/79	1980
EUROPE	60%	39.3%
MEDITERRANEAN COUNTRIES	19%	24.2%
ITALY	11.4%	19.6%
MIDDLE EAST	4.8%	6.1%
OTHER COUNTRIES	4.8%	10.8%

Figure 3

Geographical distribution of requests for medical
transport

CASE REPORT

A 49 year old Italian employed by an Italian firm in Pakistan
suffered a myocardial infarction when working 200 kilometres from
Sukkur.   We received a telex on 13th December indicating that he
was diabetic and had been suffering from hypertension.   The local
doctor had diagnosed an anterior inferior infarction and reported
that the patient was in considerable pain and developing left
ventricular insufficiency.   He was being cared for at a first aid
post where there were no facilities for monitoring his condition
nor even for intravenous therapy.

We suggested the immediate evacuation of the patient by an air
ambulance despite the long distance and the opposition of the local
doctors.

A cardiologist, an anaesthesiologist trained in intensive care and
an intensive care nurse left Milan in an air ambulance on
14th December.   To save time spent on beaurocratic matters,
arrangements for visas and customs regulations were obtained during
the flight.   On arrival it was noted that there were no local
facilities for cardiovascular monitoring and that continuous medical
care or intravenous therapy were not available and were never carried
out.

The patient was immediately connected to a cardiac monitor, an ECG
confirmed the recent inferior infarction with anterior extension.
A catheter was introduced to monitor central venous pressure and
this confirmed a state of dehydration due to hyperglycaemia and
glycosuria which were demonstrated with reactive stripe.

After being placed on the stretcher an intravenous infusion was
started.   The helicopter flight to Sukkur airport took 1½ hours

and there the patient was transferred to the medical plane for a
14 hour flight to Rome.   During the journey the standard of care
was such as would have been given in an intensive care unit.
Isotonic saline was given intravenously to correct the dehydration,
vasodilators were used to improve his haemodynamic condition and
short acting insulin injections maintained his blood sugar within
the normal range.

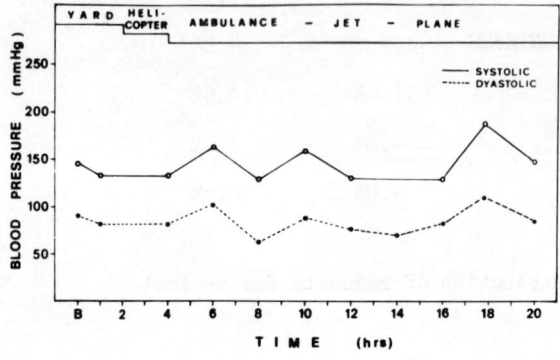

Figure 4
Arterial pressure
during transport

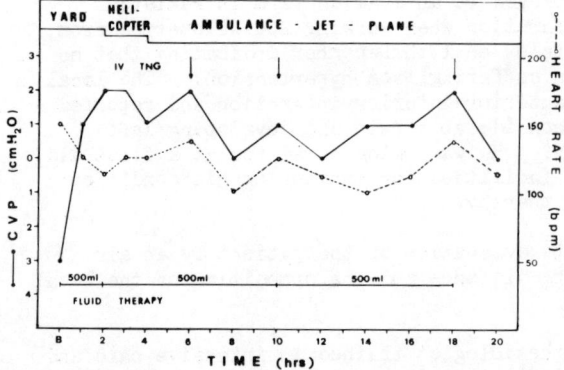

Figure 5
CVP and pulse rate
during transport

Figures 4 and 5 show the course of the principal clinical parameters.
The general condition of the patient was considerably improved on
arrival in Italy.   From Rome airport he was immediately referred to
a coronary care unit and from there he was transferred to a general
ward 5 days later.

CONCLUSION

We consider that when a patient is severely ill as a result of an
injury or acute illness and the local treatment facilities are not
adequate then the patient should be transferred as quickly as
possible.   If the team go to the patient a specialist assessment
and appropriate treatment can be started immediately and during the
journey the patient is managed just as if he were already in an

intensive care unit.

REFERENCES

Ivanoff S. Hurtaud J.P. and De Courly A. 1979. Les transports aeriens medicalises de longue duree. La Nouvelle Presse Medicale 8. 1359.

Durner P. Sehati-Chafai G.M. and Fagerlund B. 1980. Prerequisite repatriation flights, in Types and events of disaster. Organisation in various disaster situations. (Ed.Frey and Spring-Verlag) pp.302. Berlin, Heidelberg, New York.

Care of the Acutely Ill and Injured
Edited by D. H. Wilson and A. K. Marsden
© 1982, John Wiley & Sons Ltd.

HELICOPTER SEARCH AND RESCUE;
THE RAF EXPERIENCE

A J Merrifield

RAF Hospital Ely
Cambs England

ABSTRACT

The use cf RAF helicopters is outlined. The training of the
winchmen and the medical equipment used is described. Problems of
airway control, hypothermia and monitoring are discussed.

RAF Search and Rescue helicopters are tasked with picking up
aircrew who have ejected from aircraft usually over the sea, though
sometimes in remote inland areas. The search and rescue organisation
is now fairlyextensive and it would be underused if it were not
integrated into the general rescue services of the UK.

The Air Force and the Navy work closely together — the Navy cover
the South and South West at Lee—on—Solent and Culdrose — they have a
back—up facility at Prestwick. The RAF have flights at Lossiemouth,
Leuchars, Boulmer, Leconfield, Coltishall, Manston, Chivenor, Brawdy
and Valley. Close liaison is maintained with the Police and
Coastguard and RNLI; a flight can be activated by a phone call from
these organisations but all incidents are reported to the Rescue
Co—ordination Centres at Petrevie and Plymouth, so in a major
incident the aircraft may be re—directed or the operation modified.
These Co—ordination Centres also handle the long range searches of
the Nimrod aircraft for incidents out of helicopter range, though
they not infrequently work together.

The injuries and medical emergencies that are encountered can be of
any kind; fractures, burns, head and chest trauma, and all these
may be aggravated by hypothermia and exposure. Many are near
drowned victims who may develop secondary drowning before arrival
in hospital. More often than not the priority is to get the victim
out of his hazardous situation quickly, however badly injured he
may be, as on site treatment may be impossible.

Sea search can be done by fixed wing aircraft as well as helicopters, but the latter are used for virtually all rescue operations. The "hover" capability of the helicopter which is so easily taken for granted, is a major factor in the safe rescue of victims at sites where access could be impossible by conventional means, and at sea the facility for stationing the helicopter over a damaged craft can be important when the alongside position of a lifeboat becomes difficult to maintain, highly skilled though these crews are. The helicopter is less suitable for large numbers of victims but where a lifeboat has salvaged perhaps five or six seamen rapid aircraft transfer of the more seriously ill or injured from the boat to hospital can be life saving.

The aircraft used are the Wessex, Puma, Lynx and Gazelle. These last three are operational aircraft but they can and are used for carrying patients. Now we have the Westland HA3 Sea King — with a crew of four, an endurance of six hours with a top speed of 125 knots, which carrys three stretcher patients and twelve sitting. It has complete all weather navigational equipment and superb stabilisation facility — the automatic hover. With two pilots there can be a look out on both sides which helps when rotor blades are a few feet from a rock face. There is a big down wash which can blow a survivor off a cliff face — hence the need for a long line, which in the Sea King is 75 metres. Finally we have the Chinook with capacity for 12 stretchers which makes it highly suitable for multiple victims.

There are still difficulties in radio—location of marine craft because of differences in radio frequencies. SAR aircraft carry marine frequency radios, but survivors who have left the main vessel need an electronic locator similar to that carried by aircrew; and these can be small, automatic, and will facilitate precision location of a small life raft. Both the locator and the homer are being developed for British Merchant Ships as an extension of the military aircraft system.

Winching and the training of the winchman is vital. The equipment used includes the essential rescue loop which goes around the chest of the victim, and a stretcher shackle if it is not possible to use the loop. Training is done in gulleys and crevasses so that close manoeuvring to rock faces is practised, and experience is gained by winching victims up from marine craft and life boats. But for the winch line the helicopter would lose most of its value. Stretchers used in conjunction with the line include the Neil Robertson and the Stokes litter.

One advance is the use of pneumatic supports in flight to reduce vibration of the victim who has to remain on the stretcher. The stretcher can be winched from virtually anywhere that the winchman can be positioned: sometimes the most hazardous places.

High line transfer winching is very important with the Sea King —
with a long line the placement of the winchman can be very difficult.
He uses this line by throwing it to the ships, crew or other
survivors and by using it as a stay he can be steadied when going
down or up with a victim. Clearly, snagging of this line might
jeopardise the aircraft so it has a built in 90 kilogram breaking
strain shackle. The winch operator — the man at the top end can use
a little joy stick and virtually fly the aircraft within prescribed
limits in order to position the winchman precisely.

General first aid equipment is carried in a back pack so that the
winchman can be lowered with his hands unencumbered. This kit
contains all the standard items for injury treatment including
parenteral analgesics. Entonox is also carried and is most
valuable if a victim with severe pain has to be moved quickly.
Splints of various kinds are used including the Hare but a simple
webbing strip with "velcro" is effective and can be applied with
gloved hands; an important consideration in conditions of extreme
cold. Where a doctor is able to go with the aircraft and the need
for respiratory assistance is anticipated a custom kit is taken
containing everything required for endotracheal intubation. Oxygen
is carried in 325 litre standard cylinders with a modified domestic
regulator, mounted in a fibreglass suitcase. For artificial
ventilation the Pneupac portable ventilator is used; in general
mechanical ventilation is preferred to hand ventilation particularly
in difficult cabin conditions, but the lightness and simplicity of
the self inflating bag make it a most useful back up item. Adequate
suction equipment is obviously essential, and in the Sea King the
Laerdal electric sucker is employed.

The cold wet near-drowned human being presents considerable problems
in a casualty department, in an aircraft cabin with limited
facilities very little comprehensive treatment can be carried out.
Where the transit time to hospital is short simple supportive
measures and passive insulation are used. Once the cabin door is
closed the ambient temperature rises so that some rewarming will
occur in any event. Temperature measurement is not easy in these
conditions and inhibitions about the precipitation of ventricular
fibrillation through movement and techniques such as oral suction,
are usually outweighed by the need to give artificial ventilation
and get the victim to hospital.

Work has been done on attempting to provide some rewarming by the
inspiration of warm moist air. The heat and humidity are generated
by the discharge of carbon dioxide into anaesthetic soda lime.
Rewarming by this method is extremely slow but respiratory heat loss
is cancelled and it is possible that at critical levels the incident
of ventricular fibrillation may be lessened. Further work is
required to justify the use of this equipment routinely, but research
done so far has been valuable to many workers concerned about the

treatment of accidental hypothermia. Future development may involve
a type of water blanket with both the energy for the circulation
pump and the water temperature rise provided by the same portable
heat source.

Where the flight may be of several hours duration some form of
monitoring has been considered and small portable electrocardiographs
are being evaluated. A reasonable signal is difficult to obtain
unless a "nutmeg grater" type of electrode is used and these can be
applied on the wrists; where heavy clothing or sailing wet suits are
worn other points of access to skin areas are limited. Also the use
of oesophageal electrodes in conjunction with the oesophageal
obturator airway or with the Vygon "oesocaths" has been considered,
and a reasonable monitoring trace has been obtained.

The medical training of the rear crewmen, that is the winchman who
is suspended on the winch cable and the winch operator who controls
his descent and ascent, is extensive and continuous, with a
comprehensive first aid component. Apart from standard techniques,
such as expired air resuscitation and the more important aspects of
handling injured victims, the winchman learn to give effective
ventilation with oropharyngeal airways and a self inflating bag.
This is done in operating theatres where the crewman is presented
with an anaesthetised apnoeic patient prior to intubation, and he is
instructed in artificial ventilation with the equipment mentioned
later. Oxygen is added so that the manoeuvre is no different from
that practised in routine anaesthetic induction, and it gives the
crewman greatly increased confidence in this technique. At present
intubation is not taught. This constraint is based on the problem
of endotracheal intubation under extremely adverse conditions in a
small aircraft cabin, and the difficulties that would be encountered
in the maintenance of constant practice. With inadequate experience
technical skill may be less important than the judgement needed to
stop trying and to revert to the simple bag and mask method. With
this system good ventilation can be obtained, and when it is
considered that these crewmen are primarily aviators and not
paramedical personnel their success record with artificial
ventilation is of a high order.

We are interested in an alternative to endotracheal intubation — the
oesophageal obturator airway. This device occludes the oesophagus
and allows ventilation to occur around the obturator. It has its
snags, but there are occasions when it might be useful and it is
still being evaluated.

The hazards of this work are obvious, and the courage and skill of
the crewmen who take great risks to save lives, cannot be too
highly commended.

Care of the Acutely Ill and Injured
Edited by D. H. Wilson and A. K. Marsden
© 1982, John Wiley & Sons Ltd.

A STUDY OF THE ORGANIZATION OF AN AEROMEDICAL
RESCUE AND TRANSPORT SERVICE IN A DEFINED
GEOGRAPHICAL AREA

O. Chiara, G. Bordone, G.P. Rossi

Clinica Chirurgica I - Istituto di Anestesia e
Rianimazione, Universita degli Studi di Milano, Italy.

In Italy, and particularly in our own region of Lombardy, an
organization specifically for the purpose of aeromedical assistance
does not exist.   Only occasionally and in cases of extreme emergency is this function carried out by various military institutions,
whose aircraft are not specifically equipped, and personnel not
adequately trained, to deal with medical problems.   Moreover, these
institutions carry out rescue missions only subordinately to their
military function.   For these reasons, we would like to see an
aeromedical assistance organization set up, capable of operating over
the whole region, utilizing helicopters which follow a direct call
from anyone needing emergency help.   Geographically, our region is
composed of a mountainous zone at the North, with a flat area at the
South.   Milan, the town where we operate, is located in the middle
of the flat area, about 30 miles from the mountains.   The
requisite characteristics of such a service would be:-

  1. An around the clock service, operating even in
      bad weather conditions.

  2. A range of operation of 120 square miles, both on flat
      country and on mountains.

  3. An ability to move into action in under fifteen minutes.

  4. The presence on board of medical facilities and
      qualified medical personnel able to give first aid
      and emergency therapy throughout the mission.

  5) The setting up of an operations room in Milan which
      receives and evaluates the emergency calls, co-ordinates
      the missions and directs the patients to the appropriate
      hospital centre.

  6) The construction in every regional hospital of helicopter
      take-off and landing pads.

The best helicopters for this purpose are the AB212 and the A109.
The AB212 is considered an aircraft able to reach mountainous areas
and other places inaccessible by land.   The A109 is proposed for its

speed; this helicopter is particularly useful for operation in flat
country.   The type of mission we consider possible is as follows:-

1.   Search and rescue.

2.   Search and rescue of traumatized or severely ill patients
     in places difficult to reach by land.

3.   Transport of emergency cases from one hospital to
     another.

4.   Transport of medical personnel and supplies to inaccess-
     ible places, where transport by land would result in
     serious delay.

5.   Transport of medical and paramedical personnel, drugs
     and equipment to districts where natural calamities
     have brought about a breakdown of communications.

6.   Finally we consider that the helicopter could be used
     for other purposes when not engaged in emergency opera-
     tions, for example, fire control, pollution control etc.

Last year 50 operations were carried out in Lombardy using Air Force
helicopters:

a.   Transport of a premature baby;

b.   Transport of seven seriously ill patients to hospital;

c.   Twenty rescue operations to find people lost in the
     mountains;

d.   Twenty-two rescue missions to traumatized patients
     in places impossible to reach by land.

In all these cases the use of the helicopter was the determinant
factor in the success of the operation.   In view of these results,
we consider necessary the institution of a specific aeromedical
assistance service in our region and throughout out country,
modelled on those which exist in many other parts of Europe.

SECTION THREE

CARDIOPULMONARY RESUSCITATION

Care of the Acutely Ill and Injured
Edited by D. H. Wilson and A. K. Marsden
© 1982, John Wiley & Sons Ltd.

CARDIOPULMONARY RESUSCITATION

Editorial Overview

Andrew K. Marsden

Recent years have seen an insidious change in the role
of the Emergency Department from coping almost exclusively with
traumatic emergencies to having to provide an increasing service
to urgent medical problems.   Not least amongst these pure medical
emergencies is collapse from coronary artery disease and its
sequelae.

Resuscitation from cardio-respiratory arrest, rightly, earned
itself a place of importance in the Congress programme.   We heard
how innovations in organisation, communications and technology are
affecting the results of treatment of acute heart attack.   The role
of the paramedic in a CPR programme in   the USA was highlighted
by Handal - and, in France, the real costs analysed by Piganiol.
Vincent outlined the concept of a public education scheme in
Resuscitation successfully practised in the conference town of
Brighton.

From Salford, UK came reports of a novel approach to ventricular
asystole. The abandonment of the time-honoured drugs adrenaline
and calcium chloride in favour of intracardiac atropine followed,
if required, by early ventricular pacing is already showing
promise of a significant reduction in mortality from this
condition in the Emergency Room.

Care of the Acutely Ill and Injured
Edited by D. H. Wilson and A. K. Marsden
© 1982, John Wiley & Sons Ltd.

RESUSCITATION —
THE STATE OF THE ART

Kathleen A. Handal, M.D.

Long Island Jewish-Hillside Medical Center
New Hyde Park, New York, U.S.A.

With the realization of wall to wall Emergency Medical Service (EMS) Systems to its population, patients are more rapidly being delivered to Emergency Departments (E.D.) with an ever increasing likelihood for successful resuscitation.

The organization of an EMS into regions throughout the country has formed standards for training, operations and care. These activities are licensed and protected by legislation. All this has enabled physicians to start their therapy at the scene. The advanced life support (ALS) units of this system, in the form of Paramedics trained in Basic Life Support (BLS), the use of adjunctive equipment, cardiac monitoring, defibrillation, venous access, drug therapy have enabled stabilization and transport to hospital. With the paramedics as their hands and eyes medical care is communicated over radio waves and telemetry bands from the designated control hospital emergency physician. Standing protocols written by a Medical Advisory Committee exists as a guarantee. EMS is involved in setting of standards and auditing E.D.s that can receive the critically ill. These standards include minimum staffing, equipment and educational requirements. Hospitals are designated horizontally and also vertically as trauma, burn, spinal and re-implantation centers. Thus enabling stabilization and rapid transport to a definitive care center.

Paralleling the growth of EMS, was the formalization of resuscitation as a field. The National Conference on Cardiopulmonary Resuscitation and Emergency Cardiac Care in 1974 and again 1980, published standards and guidelines for resuscitation. Pediatric and Adult BLS and ALS measures, medication, indications, doses, along with adjunct methods and maneuvers were specified. Also included were recommendations for certification training and medico-legal considerations. The American Heart Association became the formal body providing certification through the teaching and testing of these standards.[1] Courses were designed for instructors and providers. The provider course being given in minimum of sixteen (16) hours with continuing education credits awarded for successful completion. The curriculum includes didactic lectures and skill practice sessions. Course content includes: adjuncts for airway, ventilation, artificial circulation, monitoring and dysrhythmia recognition, defibrillation, synchronized cardioversion, intravenous techniques (including central line placement), essential and useful drugs in emergency cardiac care, acid-base balance, stabilization and transport to definitive care institution.

Progress in this area owes much to the coming of age of a new medical specialty. Emergency Medicine, in September of 1979, became the 23rd medical specialty in the United States. This new specialist is trained in the critical aspects of all branches of medicine. These physicians have assumed the primary leadership roles in EMS.

Kathleen A. Handal, M.D.

Trauma is the leading cause of death in the first three (3) decades of life in the United States. As with most ciritical illness the initial observation and therapy influence the ultimate outcome. To address this problem EMS in Nebraska began in 1979 to develop with Lincoln Medical Education Foundation, a course curriculum for resuscitation of the traumatized patient. In 1979 the American College of Surgeons (ACS), Committee on Trauma, adopted the program nationwide. The ATLS course is a minimum of sixteen (16) hours, designed to train physicians in advanced concepts, skills and techniques. ATLS content includes upper airway management, shock, thoracic, abdominal, spinal cord and extremity trauma and burns. These topics are integrated with appropriate manual skills required, as is interpretation of radiographs.

Communities with large numbers of lay persons trained in BLS and with a rapid response system of well trained Paramedics, have demonstrated that more than 40% of patients with documented ventricular fibrillation out of hospital, can be successfully resuscitated if CRP is provided promptly and followed by ACLS.[2] Successful resuscitation in selected subgroups of patients with documented cardiac arrests has been accomplished in 60-80% of cases.[3] Discharge rates as high as 23% have been reported for patients with out of hospital cardiac arrests due to ventricular fibrillation.[4] Based on these and other statistics, it has been estimated that 100,000-200,000 deaths from cardiac disease could be saved each year in the United States with early and aggressive BLS and ACLS.[1]

This is but the beginning of a new field, the formalization and aggressive interest has provided a new impetus for research. In November, 1980 the 2nd Wolfcreek Conference on Resuscitation heard forty-five (45) papers on current research topics.[5] Data was presented that would have us seriously question the 'basics', for example, in one man rescue the ratio of 15 heart compressions to 2 ventilations is not as effective as 15 to 1. Investigation from John Hopkins showed that increased intrathoracic pressure provides much, if not all, of the force that moves blood into the circulation with external compressions and not the fixed sternum and vertebral column. The endotracheal route is now an accepted means of drug administration and is advised in standards for ACLS over intra-cardiac. Epinephrine and Naloxone have been found to achieve therapeutic levels via this route.

Pharmacological developments, example: Bretylium Tosylate, for refractory ventricular fibrillation, further aided the physician in maintaining an aggressive posture with the extremus patients.

Perhaps this is the birth of a new field — Critical Care Medicine!

[1] Standards for Cardiopulmonary Resuscitation and Emergency Cardiac Care. JAMA 244 (Supplement): 453-509, 1980.

[2] Eisenberg, M.S., Bergner, L., Hallstrom, A.: Cardiac Resuscitation in Community. JAMA 241: 1905-1907, 1979.

[3] Lund, I., Skulberg, A.: Cardiopulmonary Resuscitation by Lay People. Lancet 2:702-704, 1976.

[4] Cobb, L.A., Baum, R.S., Alvarez, H. et al: Resuscitation from Out-of-hospital Ventricular Fibrillation. Circulation 51, 223-228, 1975.

[5] Critical Care Medicine: 2nd Wolfcreek Conference on C.P.R. Critical Care Medicine, Volume 9, 5, 1981.

Care of the Acutely Ill and Injured
Edited by D. H. Wilson and A. K. Marsden
© 1982, John Wiley & Sons Ltd.

EPIDEMIOLOGY AND PROGNOSIS OF CARDIO-RESPIRATORY ARREST
BASED ON 73 CASES TREATED IN AN EMERGENCY DEPARTMENT

G. Piganiol, B. Blettery, J. Saugeot and C. Virot

Service de Reanimation Medicale et Medecine d'Urgence
Hopital General, 3,rue du FaubourgRaines - 21033 Dijon Cedex,
France.

The authors have reviewed the case records of 73 patients treated
for cardiac arrest in the Emergency Department of the General
Hospital at Dijon Cedex during a two year period, 1978-79.   The
average age of patients was 57 years and six months, with a range
from 6 to 86 years.   The male/female ratio was 48 men to 25 women
which corresponds to the sex ratio for all patients attending the
Emergency Department.

Patients who regained temporary, but satisfactory, haemodynamic
activity were regarded as having a good short-term prognosis even
though they subsequently died in hospital.   Patients who were able
to leave hospital were considered as having a good long-term prognosis.

Although the short-term results appear to be fairly satisfactory,
31.8% recovery, the long-term results are only mediocre, only 3
patients out of 73 left hospital alive, i.e. 4.1%.   The results are
independent of age and sex.   Patients under 60 years of age and
female patients appeared to have a better prognosis but in neither
was the difference statistically significant.

Conversely,the results were significantly better for patients in
whom the cardiac arrest was due to ventricular fibrillation, 18.8%
had a good result, whereas no patient who arrived in asystole had a
long-term recovery.   Moreover it must be noted that, for the three
patients who left hospital, in each case treatment was started within
less than 3 minutes of the onset of the arrest.

We have tried to evaluate the financial cost of treating a cardiac
arrest.   The calculation is based on the cost to "la Securite Sociale"
of each cardiac arrest.   It is a fairly gross estimate which doesn't
take account of the cost of maintaining a medical and paramedical
team, with their highly specialised equipment, in constant readiness
for 24 hours a day.   The figure works out at 2570 French francs for
each patient having a cardiac arrest.   As only three patients left
hospital alive, the total financial outlay to achieve these good
results is 62,537 French francs per patient with a good long-term
prognosis.

Even though a human life is without price, doctors should be mindful of the expenditure they create. It seems to us essential to weigh the indications for cardio-respiratory resuscitation. Even though age and sex may not be relevant factors, the type of cardiac arrest and the speed with which resuscitation is started are important prognostic indicators of the probable outcome of the treatment and are relevant when deciding how long to continue the attempt at resuscitation.

Care of the Acutely Ill and Injured
Edited by D. H. Wilson and A. K. Marsden
© 1982, John Wiley & Sons Ltd.

COMMUNITY TRAINING
IN CARDIOPULMONARY RESUSCITATION

R.Vincent, B.Martin, and D.A.Chamberlain

Royal Sussex County Hospital,
Brighton, Sussex, U.K.

ABSTRACT

To augment the work of the existing Coronary Ambulance
Service, community training in cardiopulmonary
resuscitation was introduced into the Brighton Health
District in 1978.   By June 1981, 12912 members of the
lay public had attended the 2-hour instruction sessions.
Twenty-seven incidents have been reported involving
trainees of the scheme and we believe that, as a result,
at least four lives have been saved.   The scheme is
likely to bring benefits in addition to successful
resuscitation although these may be difficult to
quantify.   Its effect in the community is likely to
become more apparent as the number trained approaches the
target of 50000.

INTRODUCTION

The attrition rate from myocardial infarction is at its
highest in the immediate few hours following the onset
of symptoms.   Armstrong and his colleagues (1972) found
that in a group of patients dying within 4 weeks of their
attack 50% had perished within two hours.   Often such
deaths result from potentially reversible arrhythmias
rather than from serious myocardial damage.   And yet in
many cases a successful outcome is precluded by the long
delay before skilled help can be given, help which
usually follows admission to hospital.   Conventional
referral procedures result in a median time for hospital
admission of about six hours - long exceeding the period
of greatest risk.

In 1971, recognising the vulnerable and unattended
period following myocardial infarction, the Brighton
Health District introduced resuscitation ambulances for
the urgent management of the collapsed patient.   The

ambulances carry no medical personnel but a crew of
specially trained ambulance staff who are proficient in
the interpretation of arrhythmias and in defibrillation,
as well as in the usual techniques for cardiopulmonary
resuscitation.   A small number of ambulance personnel
is also able to perform tracheal intubation and to give
drugs intravenously (Briggs et al.,1976).

The introduction of this service, with an increased
awareness of the value of early skilled help after
myocardial infarction, has lessened the median admission
time to the Cardiac Care Unit in this District to
approximately two hours.   Moreover, out-of-hospital
resuscitation has undoubtedly enabled the survival to
good health of a small but important number of patients
each year.   More than ten such cases have been recorded
in the first five months of this year (1981) including
a 20 year old man suffering from an acute myocarditis
who required 27 minutes of out-of-hospital resuscitation
prior to his transfer to ITU. (He has now been discharged home in good health.)

But even with an efficient coronary ambulance service
there remains an endangered interval following a
coronary attack in which most patients will be remote
from skilled help.   In an attempt to increase the
salvage of victims of sudden coronary death, attention
has been directed to providing cardiopulmonary support
until the arrival of professional help.   We have
considered that this would best be achieved by training
a proportion of the general public in heart/lung
resuscitation aiming at a total of 50,000 people trained
before full evaluation of the scheme.   We report here a
preliminary assessment of the first three years of our
work in this area.

THE TRAINING SCHEME

A training scheme for the community in cardiopulmonary
resuscitation (CPR) was commenced early in 1978 and was
aimed initially at personnel sponsored by commercial
organisations in the Brighton area, and by public
service groups such as the police, GPO, and fire brigade.
Later that year a publicity campaign was introduced to
attract members of the public throughout Brighton and
Hove to become students of "public" classes.   Publicity
was achieved through leaflets, local radio and press,
and by displays at community functions.

Class attenders have been trained at an average rate of

325 per month reaching a total of 12,912 by the end of
May this year.   Classes are held on two evenings every
week with a usual attendance of eight to ten per class.
In addition, private classes have been arranged as
requested by many different organisations in the
community at an average rate of seven per month.
Training is provided in a single two-hour session in
which the students are divided into groups of six to
eight.   Each group receives teaching from a certified
instructor following an agreed outline.   The
instructors are drawn from a pool of 45 more intensely
trained lay personnel and 23 supervisory instructors who
mostly are members of the Ambulance Service.   The scheme
has a single co-ordinator, the only full-time salaried
member of the training team.

Training is given in airway protection, mouth-to-mouth
ventilation, and external cardiac massage.   The
techniques are carefully explained and demonstrated, and
adequate time is given for supervised practice with
teaching models.   At the end of the training session
each student receives a certificate of attendance and a
pamphlet reiterating the essential points of cardiopulmonary resuscitation covered during the evening's
tuition.   The training has been well received and, we
believe, has encouraged an increasing community   interest
in CPR.

RESULTS

Twenty-seven incidents have been reported in which
trainees of the scheme have implemented resuscitation
techniques learned on the course.   The outcome of these
cases is illustrated in Figure 1.   Ten patients were
dead on arrival at hospital or died shortly after their
admission to the Casualty area.   The outcome of two
incidents was unknown (a total of three of the 27
incidents occurred abroad).   Fifteen patients attended by
trainees of the CPR scheme were alive on admission and
eight survived to be discharged from hospital.   Those
leaving hospital alive had the following diagnoses.

1.   Asystole from facial injury

2.   Myocardial infarction

3.   Concussion

4.   Hypoglycaemia

5.   Transient arrhythmia

6.   Unknown

7.   Drowning

8.   Grand mal epilepsy

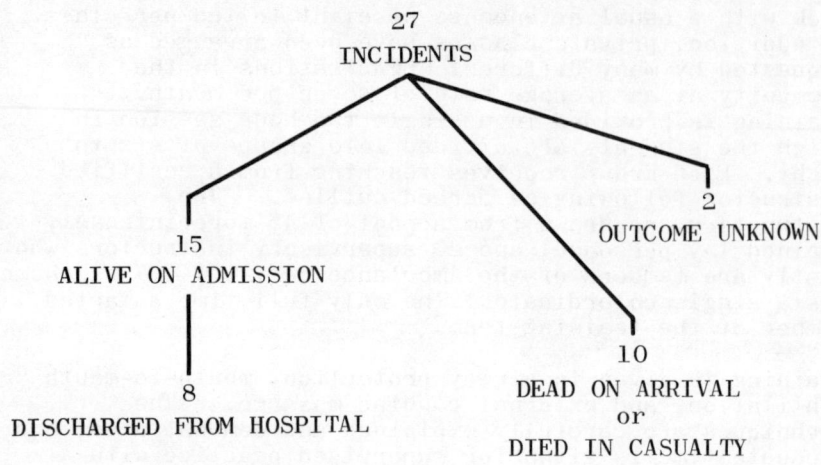

Fig.1.   Outcome of 27 incidents attended by
trainees of the scheme.

Although a number of conditions listed above were self-
limiting it seems likely that cardiopulmonary
resuscitation - including airway protection - afforded
benefit to the patients treated.   Moreover, in at least
four cases urgent treatment given by bystanders who had
received CPR training undeniably sustained life prior
to transfer to hospital.

DISCUSSION

The potential rewards of immediate resuscitation are
little understood by the community.   Indeed even those
professionally involved in health care may be unaware
that a disorder may be rapidly fatal but potentially
short-lived or reversible if temporary life-support can
be given.   Educating the community in the benefits of
CPR and in the simple techniques involved relies heavily
on the vision, enthusiasm, and activity of a small core
group.   This has been especially true in Brighton where
there is only one full-time member of staff to advance
the scheme.   Nevertheless close to 13,000 members of the
lay public have received instruction in CPR and we are
beginning to see practical results of this training.

Lives threatened by acute ischaemic heart disease – and by other conditions – have been protected by community application of CPR.

The benefits of the scheme, however, are difficult to quantify.   A simple count of the number of lives saved directly by trainees of the scheme draws attention to the most rewarding and dramatic result of CPR training.   But increased community awareness of the need for urgent attention to a collapsed patient, better understanding of the early symptoms of coronary attack, and reduced fear of becoming involved in the face of catastrophic illness may seen as additional benefits from this instruction.

A community training scheme for CPR will be effective only if backed by professional support for the secondary management of the resuscitated patient.   Indeed training of the community has usually followed the appropriate organisation of rescue services, both here and in America.

CONCLUSION

We conclude that to train members of the community in cardiopulmonary resuscitation appears feasible and need not be unduly expensive.   There is potential for aiding recovery from circulatory arrest due to trauma accompanied by excessive autonomic discharge, to electro-cution, or to drowning as well as from the fatal arrhythmias of ischaemic heart disease.   The number of lives saved so far as the result of this scheme is small. Other benefits from CPR training are likely, but are difficult to quantify. The influence of the CPR programme should increase as further students are trained and it will be of interest to analyse the effect of the scheme when the target number of trainees has been reached.

REFERENCES

Armstrong, A., Duncan, B., Oliver, M.E., Julian, D.G., Donald, K.W., Fulton, M., Lutz, W., and Morrison, S.L., 1972.   Natural history of acute coronary heart attacks: A community study. British Heart Journal, 34, 67.
Briggs, R.S., Brown, P.M., Crabb, M.E., Cox, T.J., Ead, H.W., Hawkes, R.A., Jequier, P.W., Southall, D.P., Grainger, R., Williams, J.H., and Chamberlain, D.A., 1976. The Brighton resuscitation ambulance: A continuing experiment in prehospital care by ambulance staff. British Medical Journal, 2, 1161.

Care of the Acutely Ill and Injured
Edited by D. H. Wilson and A. K. Marsden
© 1982, John Wiley & Sons Ltd.

CARDIAC ARREST   -   A NEW CONCEPT

Gordon Laing and Anthony Redmond

Department of Accident & Emergency Medicine
Hope Hospital, Salford.

University of Manchester School of Medicine. U.K.

ABSTRACT

It is known that cardiac arrest is the result of either ventricular
fibrillation or ventricular asystole. The treatment of ventricular
fibrillation by D.C. cardioversion has greatly improved the
survival.   However, when cardiac arrest is the result of asystole
the survival rate remains appallingly low. It is our belief that
the treatment of asystole can be improved. The heart may only be
held captive in asystole by excessive parasympathetic stimulation.
If this parasympathetic stranglehold can be broken then the heart
is free to respond to resuscitative measures. We would recommend
that the management of the asystolic patient commences with an
intracardiac infusion of Atropine.

INTRODUCTION

The rationale for giving Atropine is based on the assumption that
when asystole is reversible the condition must be the result of
parasympathetic stimulation. There is good evidence to support this.
The presence of receptors in the ventricles affecting the
circulatory system was discovered over 100 years ago (Bezold 1867)
and the finding that injections of veratrum alkaloids resulted in
hypotension and bradycardia. Reflex slowing of the heart following
a pressure rise in the left ventricle was thought to be due to
stimulation of these receptors. (Daly 1927). The presence of these
receptors was clearly demonstrated (Jarisch 1939) and the conclusion
was that they were responsible for triggering the Bezold Jarisch
reflex. It has also been shown that this reflex may be produced by
acute coronary obstruction by tying a coronary artery in animals
(Constantin 1963) (Ascanio 1965). This work was later confirmed
(Thoren 1972). The mechanism was thought to be important in the
hypotension associated with acute myocardial infarction. (Gunner
& Loeb 1973). Further experiments in animals have shown that the
receptors are activated by distension of the ventricle producing
this reflex (Thoren 1972). These receptors can also be stimulated
by infusion of Adrenaline (Thoren 1972) and which may account for
the poor response to Adrenaline in cardiac arrest. In fact
Adrenaline may provoke ventricular fibrillation, but should asystole
ensue after Adrenaline then in our experience the asystole becomes
irreversible.

Circulatory collapse in asphyxia in man was thought to be due to
receptor stimulation (Benzinger 1942) and vaso vagal syncope was
considered to be similarly induced (Sharpey Shafer 1956)
Carotid body chemo receptor stimulation from hypoxia causes a
profound bradycardia due to increased vagal activity contributing
to the arrest state (De Burgh Daly, Angell-James, Elsner 1979)

DISCUSSION

All the above evidence provides good physiological support for the
concept that following an episode of asystole a return to sinus
rhythm may be prevented by parasympathetic overactivity.
It would seem logical therefore to administer Atropine to the
asystolic patient in the hope that the episode of Asystole is
of this nature.

Furthermore, in the asystolic patient if a drug is to be
administered the purpose of which is to block a reflex to the heart
then it can only be administered directly into the heart.   A
peripheral infusion in a patient with no circulation serves no
physiological function

CONCLUSION

It is our recommendation therefore, that the initial management
of the asystolic patient should commence with an intracardiac
injection of Atropine.

REFERENCES

Benzinger T.H. Doring H, and Hornberger W. Wissenschaftliche
    Grundlagen der Prufung auf Hohenfestigkeit Mittelst Atmung
    definierter Gasgemische. Luft fahrtsmedizin. 1942. 6. 234-253.

Bezold A. Von and Hirt L. Uber die physiologischen Wirkungen des
    essigsauren Veratrins. Unters. Physiol. Lab. Wurtzburg.
    1867. 1. 75-156.

Constantin L. Extracardiac factors contributing to hypotension
    during coronary occlusion. Amer. J. Cardiol. 1963. 11. 205-217.

De Burgh Daly, ML. Angell-James, J.E. (1979) "Role of carotid-body
    chemoreceptors and their reflex interactions in bradycardia and
    cardiac arrest" LANCET April 7 764-767.

Gunnar, R.M. and Loeb H.S. Use of drugs in cardiogenic shock due to
    acute myocardial infarction. Circulation 1972. 45 1111-1124.

Jarisch and Zotterman (1948) "Depressor reflexes from the heart"
    Acta. Physiol. Scand. 16. 31-51.

Jarisch A. and Richter H. Die Kreislaufwirkung des Veratrins. Arch.
    exp. Path. Pharmak. 1939 a 193 347-354.

Thoren P. Left ventricular receptors activated by severe asphyxia
and by coronary artery occlusion. Acta. physiol. scand. 1972 a
85 455-463.

Thoren P. Reflex bradycardia elecited from left ventricular
receptors during acute severe hypoxia in cats. Acta. physiol.
Scand. 1972 b.

Thoren P. Evidence for a depressor reflex elecited from left
ventricular receptors during occlusion of one coronary artery in
the cat. Acta. physiol. Scand. 1972 C.

Care of the Acutely Ill and Injured
Edited by D. H. Wilson and A. K. Marsden
© 1982, John Wiley & Sons Ltd.

EMERGENCY TRANSVENOUS PACING FOR THE TREATMENT OF
ASYSTOLE — A NEW TECHNIQUE

A. D. REDMOND

HOPE HOSPITAL, SALFORD, U.K.

ABSTRACT

A new technique for the treatment of asystole is described by which
simultaneous intracardiac infusion, transvenous pacing and central
venous pressure measurement can be carried out through the one
catheter.

INTRODUCTION

The present treatment for asystole is the application of standard
cardiopulmonary resuscitation; the administration of cardioactive
drugs, and the insertion of a pacemaker.   The drugs are usually
given by intracardiac injection (Davison et al 1980) and the pacing
wire inserted via a short subclavian cannula, (Bartecchi 1979).
It is possible to give an intracardiac infusion of drugs without
recourse to cardiac puncture by the insertion of a suitable catheter
into the subclavian vein.   Through the same catheter a pacing
wire can also be passed and the central venous pressure can be
measured.

METHOD

Immediately the diagnosis of asystole has been made the subclavian
vein is cannulated with an 18 cm long, 3 mm wide catheter.   This is
long enough to reach the right atrium and therefore an intracardiac
infusion can be administered through it.   A vygon haemostatic valve
with side outlet is then attached.   A pacing wire can then be
inserted through the valve and catheter into the right ventricle.
The 3 mm bore of the catheter provides a space between the pacing
wire and the catheter.   This space, plus the provision of terminal
side outlets, allows an intracardiac infusion to be given while
pacing continues.   It also enables the catheter to be used for the
measurement of central venous pressure.

DISCUSSION

At the present time, the only method available for cannulation of
the subclavian vein with such a catheter is to use a vygon emergency

haemodialysis catheter.   This involves the use of a steel
introducer and guide wire.   A combination catheter is then
thread over the guide wire and into the subclavian vein.   The
guide wire and inner catheter are then removed.   This leaves an
18 cm long, 3 mm wide catheter in the subclavian vein.   However,
this technique can be improved.   A prototype 18 cm long, 3 mm
wide "over-needle" catheter has been developed.   This reduces the
insertion technique to a one-stage procedure and thereby reduces
the time interval from diagnosis of asystole to the establishment
of effective treatment.

REFERENCES

BARTECCHI, C. E. 1979 "Emergency Transvenous (subclavian)
   Cardiac Pacing in Elderly Patients". J. Am. Geriatric Soc.
   27, 5, 208 - 11.
DAVISON, R et al 1980 "Intracardiac Infusions During Cardiopulmonary Resuscitation". J. A. M.A. 244, 10, 1110 - 11.

SECTION FOUR

ASPECTS OF MAJOR TRAUMA

Care of the Acutely Ill and Injured
Edited by D. H. Wilson and A. K. Marsden
© 1982, John Wiley & Sons Ltd.

ASPECTS OF MAJOR TRAUMA

Editorial Overview

Andrew K. Marsden

Trauma, the leading cause of death under forty years of age, is the topic which has commanded most of the attention of the Congress. Correspondingly it occupies the bulk share of these Proceedings.

One cannot help but be impressed at the wide range of interests in and the diversity of practice of trauma care. On the one hand the Western experience of high technology,strictly formalised medicine (as represented by Dove's operating room resuscitation facility and Mayer's sophisticated autotransfusion apparatus) contrasts, on the other, with the struggles of the developing countries in gaining suitable staff and facilities to provide a safe, basic service (witness Adeleye's account of an emergency trauma service in Nigeria with its inherent problems).

All major trauma services rely on good quality educational input - the Advanced Trauma Life Support programme of the American College of Surgeons is a realistic attempt to cover the major points in trauma resuscitology. It is however frustrating to be reminded that the errors in trauma management invariably result from failure to heed basic surgical principles. Prof.Glinz's paper on the problems of assessing blunt chest injuries should be read by all traumatologists in search of a humbling experience.

The diagnosis of intraperitoneal trauma has been advanced by the use of special investigations such as diagnostic imaging techniques including ultrasound and angiography and procedures like peritoneal lavage. Several papers, practical training workshops and free discussion concentrated on some of these techniques. Finally the surgical approach to trauma was extensively reviewed at the Congress and numerous topics from the care of penetrating wounds of the heart to conservative management of the ruptured spleen received wide consideration.

Care of the Acutely Ill and Injured
Edited by D. H. Wilson and A. K. Marsden
© 1982, John Wiley & Sons Ltd.

ASSESSMENT AND MANAGEMENT OF THE SEVERELY INJURED
PATIENT: "A NIGERIAN EXPERIENCE".

Dr. E.A. Adeleye, MB, ChB. (Glasgow)

Principal Medical Officer, Accident & Emergency Centre,
Lagos University Teaching Hospital, Lagos, Nigeria.

INTRODUCTION

An accident surgeon must keep to a routine and observe basic principles when caring for injured patients. Speed and decisiveness are
necessary but a thorough examination of all the body systems is
essential if preventable fatalities are to be avoided. A peripheral
fracture must not be allowed to divert attention from a life-threatening injury to a viscus such as a ruptured spleen or liver. An
unconscious patient cannot complain of abdominal pain but a four
quadrant tap or peritoneal lavage may reveal a haemoperitoneum
requiring an urgent laparotomy. Trauma to the bowel can be slow to
present symptoms, and if the patient is anaesthetised for the treatment of a peripheral injury, peritonitis may develop before they are
sufficiently recovered to call attention to the abdomen.

Maintaining this routine of basic observations is even more important
when dealing with large numbers of patients from a mass accident. Two
such mass accidents have been handled in this centre since its
inception.

MANAGEMENT OF THE INJURED PATIENT

The clinical picture presented by the severely injured patient is not
the arithmetic sum of the several injuries. It must be realised that
the effect of one injury may enhance, diminish, or obliterate the
effect of another, and perhaps more important, different injuries
may have common clinical expression. This fact is more relevant in
the unconscious patient. An unconscious patient cannot complain of
pain, and may not show signs of other injuries that would be recognis-
able if he were conscious. Moreover a restless unconscious patient
may move injured limbs in such a way as to divert suspicion from them.
Thus with such complex and confusing possibilities, it is essential
to have a clear idea of priorities of treatment.

The first is to save life, which is most often threatened by defective breathing and defective circulation.

In the Care of the Airway: Correct positioning of the patient on the
resuscitation trolley is essential. The recovery position mitigates

against common causes of asphyxia such as falling back of the flaccid tongue to obstruct the air passage, inhalation of vomitus or secretions of the mouth. Toilet and suction of the airway to evacuate any obstructing aspirate, and in the unconscious patient, a cuffed endotracheal tube may be used to facilitate evacuation of clots or other material in the air passages.

The Care of the Circulation: Involves the prevention of shock by fluid replacement. First it is necessary to undress the patient or cut off the clothing, then to obtain baseline information of pulse, B.P., respiration, temperature and level of consciousness. Shock should be regarded as a composite picture of a cold, anxious, pale, sweating patient with rapid shallow respiration, the pulse rate raised and pulse volume reduced. The blood pressure is low and the peripheral veins are collapsed. The situation demands immediate transfusion of warmed blood under pressure possibly at multiple sites. To avoid overtransfusion, a central venous pressure (C.V.P.) monitor is a useful guide in gauging the rate and volume of transfusion.

Having dealt with the immediate treatable menaces to life, there is now time to survey the situation carefully and plan the treatment that will best ensure recovery.

General Assessment: Should involve a detailed history, careful examination of wounds, fractures and dislocations, and a comprehensive systemic examination of the thorax and abdomen. Special investigations such as X-rays, laboratory investigations and E.C.G. can then be carried out.

Planning and Execution: of an effective treatment falls under two main priorities. First is to secure and consolidate the injured persons grip on life by assuring adequate respiration and restoring an adequate circulation. To achieve this may require a craniotomy, a thoracotomy or a laparotomy. The surgeon can then repair injured tissue and take steps to combat infection.

CONCLUSION

The accident and emergency centre of the Lagos University Teaching Hospital has proved successful in the alleviation of suffering, in providing effective and specialist care of the acutely ill and injured, and in the overall reduction in the usually high mortality rate prevalent in such cases. There is varied and exciting material for research, particularly in the fields of fracture healing in Africans, and trauma metabolism, in general. I admit that there is still scope for improvement, particularly in the field of safe-transportation of patients to the hospital. Presently there is no National Ambulance Service, manned by well trained staff. Such a service would be a major contributory factor to the increased survival rate in the care of the acutely ill or injured. I do hope that this modern concept for the care and management of the severely injured will in no distant future be spread throughout the country, as a whole, as well as other countries in Africa.

Acknowledgement:

My sincere appreciation goes to Professor M.O.A. Jaja FRCS, Professor
and Head of Department of Surgery, College of Medicine, University
of Lagos, for his assistance in the preparation of this paper, and
Mrs. M.O. Akinboyewa for secretarial assistance.

Care of the Acutely Ill and Injured
Edited by D. H. Wilson and A. K. Marsden
© 1982, John Wiley & Sons Ltd.

USE OF AN EMERGENCY ROOM OPERATING ROOM FOR RESUSCITATION
AND IMMEDIATE OPERATIVE INTERVENTION OF ACUTELY INJURED
PATIENTS

Dennis B. Dove, MD, Eric Munoz, MD, Gordon Cuzner, MD,
Ralph Altman, MD, Laura Cardaci, BS, William M. Stahl, MD,
FACS and Louis R.M. del Guercio, MD, FACS

Shock-Trauma Unit and Emergency Services, Metropolitan
Hospital Center and the Department of Surgery, New York
Medical College 1901 First Avenue, New York, N.Y. 10029

INTRODUCTION

The Metropolitan Hospital Center is a 600 bed acute care facility
located in New York City's East Harlem. The Emergency Service of
this hospital records 90,000 patient visits a year with an average
of 14% of these cases involving trauma. In New York City as in most
urban areas in the United States penetrating trauma as a result of
violent person to person crimes remains the most significant category of trauma.

Hospital categorization by ability to provide trauma care is soon to
be completed in New York City. Hospitals are classified as Level I,
Level II or Level III facilities with the Level I facility evidenc-
ing the greatest commitment through staffing and equipment availability. The Metropolitan Hospital Center is a designated Level I
trauma facility and boasts one of the two emergency room operating
rooms in New York City. Patients are brought to the ER by the police
EMT's, paramedics or by their own transportation. At the injury
scene paramedics differ from all other rescuers in that they provide
resuscitation following approved protocols.

PROTOCOL

The concept of ER thoracotomies for direct cardiac compression and
for shortening the circulatory tree by thoracic aortic clamping are
well accepted procedures in trauma care. However, traumatologists
the world over remain frustrated as they helplessly witness the dis-
ruptive process of patient transfer from the resuscitation area of
the ER to the operating room. It is in response to this frustration
that we developed the concept of a functioning operating room in the
ER in this hospital in 1974.

Protocols established in 1978 recognize three categories of patients
who are admitted directly to the ER-OR. 1) Patients in whom signs
of life are lost in transit to the emergency room; 2) Patients with
injuries to the base of the neck and central injuries to the thorax;
3) Patients in profound shock with or without MAST trousers. All
other patients are taken to an adjacent trauma resuscitation room.

171

Resuscitation is not performed if the patient never showed signs of life. The ER-OR is staffed exclusively by emergency department nurses with special OR training. Anesthesia and surgical staff are immediately available since they are on a 24 hour on call schedule within the hospital.

Resuscitation consists of securing an airway, breathing the patient and restoring intravascular volume via central lines and/or groin saphenous cutdowns. Fluid resuscitation begins with Ringer's lactate and utilizes no more than 2-3 liters of this solution before beginning type specific uncrossmatched blood (TSUB). A recent review of trauma deaths at our institution revealed that 25% of these patients received inadequate or inappropriate volume replacement. A more recent two year review of our use of TSUB showed 198 patients receiving 1196 units with no transfusion reaction.

TABLE I

Mechanism of Injury-174 patients

Gun shot wounds	50%	(86)
Stab wounds	37%	(64)
Blunt trauma	13%	(24)

TABLE II

Operative Procedures-174 patients

Laparotomies	56%	(98)
Thoracotomy/stenotomy	56%	(98)
Neck Explorations	9%	(15)
Peripheral Vascular	6%	(11)
Craniotomies	1%	(2)

RESULTS

Gross data from 1974 to December 1980 is shown in Tables I-III. Utilization of the facility remained constant throughout the study period averaging 25 cases per year with peak use occurring during the summer months and in December. Of the 174 patients operated upon in this facility 42% (73 patients) survived. There was no statistical difference in survival data or in injury severity when the period 1974 to 1977 was compared with 1978 to 1980. Of note however, is that trained paramedic teams began operating out of this hospital in 1978 and have significantly influenced the probability of a severely injured patient arriving "alive" in the ER.

CONCLUSION

Survival of the severely traumatized patient can be significantly improved by early vigorous resuscitation followed by prompt surgical intervention. In our experience, this survival, may be further enhanced when these functions are performed simultaneously in an ER-OR facility.

TABLE III

Patient Outcome-174 patients

Survived	42%	(73)
Deaths	58%	(101)
ER-OR	46%	(80)
<24 hr.	9%	(15)
>24 hr.	3%	(6)

Care of the Acutely Ill and Injured
Edited by D. H. Wilson and A. K. Marsden
© 1982, John Wiley & Sons Ltd.

OVERVIEW, ADVANCED TRAUMA LIFE SUPPORT COURSE

A. Mansoory, M.D., F.A.C.S. and R. Campbell, R.N.

Wilmington Medical Center
Wilmington, Delaware   U.S.A.

Trauma is the leading cause of death for people thirty years and younger in the United States and the third cause of death in all age groups. More importantly, the mortality from trauma related catastrophies is increasing every year. Trauma strikes suddenly and often times leaves in its wake years of heartbreak either through mortality or morbidity (much of which can be decreased by effective intervention during the first one hour of assessment and treatment).

Nebraska physicians in conjunction with the Lincoln Medical Education Foundation developed a prototype Advanced Trauma Life Support Course, the first of which was field tested in Nebraska in 1978. The American College of Surgeons, Committee on Trauma, adopted the course in 1979. The course is designed to train physicians advanced concepts, skills and techniques in trauma care. There is a 2 day provider and a 2½ day instructor course.

Evaluating the victim with a systemic approach in mind facilitates the initial assessment procedure and prevents the primary physician from compounding already existing injuries, implanting the theory, "DO NO MORE HARM", through lectures as well as "hands on" experiences utilizing emergency equipment, animal labs, and live moulaged "victims".

The treatment priorities are as follows:

Airway maintenance
Breathing (control c-spine)
Circulation - control and dysrhythmias
Control hemorrhage
Treat shock
Splint fractures
Evaluate further injuries
Continuous monitoring

Imparting this information is covered in the following manner:

174

A. Mansoory, M.D., F.A.C.S. and R. Campbell, R.N.

<u>Initial</u> <u>Assessment</u> <u>and</u> <u>Management</u> <u>Priorities</u>: The objectives are to:

A) Identify the priorities of emergency medical care
B) Explain management techniques used in initial assessment
C) Conduct an initial assessment and explain management techniques
   on simulated, multiple injured patients using the ABC priority
   plan.

The student is given the opportunity to analyze the physical
findings while being critiqued by an instructor and aided by a
nurse who often times is more of a hindrance than a help. The end
result of a successful initial assessment should be the transfer of
a viable patient to a facility equipped to handle multiple trauma
victims. The victims are true to life, sometimes combative and
have been known to fall to the floor when left unattended.

<u>Upper</u> <u>Airway</u> <u>Management</u>: This includes describing the unique
anatomy of the upper airway and demonstrating the maintenance of
upper airway patency by both manual and mechanical adjunctive
methods, as well as indications for cricothyroidotomy. The
practical performance is accomplished by procedures on both an
intubation manikin as well as needle and surgical cricothyroidotomy
on anesthetized dogs.

<u>Shock</u>: The student should be able to define shock and the
classifications of hemorrhage as well as explain the basic
principles of shock treatment, fluid therapy and monitoring
principles. The clinical shock syndrome should be identified.
Clinical performance includes demonstrating central I.V. insertion
and the application of anti-shock trousers.

<u>Thoracic</u> <u>Trauma</u>: The physician will be able to identify 12 types
of thoracic trauma including the most life-threatening six.
Interestingly and sadly enough, 1 out of 4 trauma deaths are
because of chest injuries and 2 out of 3 occur after the victim
arrives in the emergency department. (85% of the surgical
procedures necessary to save a life are simple procedures!)
Students perform pleural decompression with needle thoracentesis,
chest tube insertion, and pericardiocentesis on anesthetized dogs.

<u>Abdominal</u> <u>Trauma</u>: The emphasis in this chapter is in identifying
the types of abdominal trauma, explaining principles of management
as well as outlining the diagnostic and therapeutic maneuvers.
Identifying specific organ injuries and defining complications
are also covered. Peritoneal lavages are performed on anesthetized
animals with positive tap being simulated by blood placed in the
peritoneal cavity.

<u>Head</u> <u>Trauma</u>: A review of basic anatomy and physiology is covered
as well as the principles of scalp wound management. The art
of a "mini" neuro exam and management techniques outlining
priorities is reviewed.

The student must demonstrate his assessment techniques on "Mr. Hurt" who has 8 separate head and maxillo-facial injuries, as well as reach appropriate diagnoses from interpreting accompanying x-ray films.

Spine & Spinal Cord Trauma: Evaluating and suspecting spine injuries early in the assessment can eliminate much of the morbidity caused by trauma. In this area, the principles of evaluation, types of injuries and treatment rationale are covered. Immobilization techniques are practiced on a simulated patient. Gardner-Wells tongs, used for cervical immobilization, are applied to coconuts which simulate a human skull rather nicely.

Extremity Trauma: Identifying types and management techniques of extremity trauma as well as prioritizing these injuries is reviewed. Immobilization techniques are covered utilizing Hare traction and air splints on a live volunteer.

Burns: In this chapter, extent and depth as well as stabilization, treatment, and transfer criteria are discussed.

Stabilization and Transportation: Specific conditions and general principles are applied to insure the delivery of a salvageable victim to a receiving trauma center. General guidelines must be followed including medical-legal aspects which necessitate accurate documentation and transporting procedures, always keeping in mind the primary principle, "DO NO MORE HARM" utilizing skilled personnel and adequate equipment.

In summary, the primary objectives of trauma management must be the rapid and accurate assessment of the patient's condition, the provision of stabilization and transportation on a priority basis and the assurance that each step of the way, optimum care is provided.

REFERENCES

Advanced Trauma Life Support Course Manuals
     Committee on Trauma, American College of Surgeons, 1981

Care of the Acutely Ill and Injured
Edited by D. H. Wilson and A. K. Marsden
© 1982, John Wiley & Sons Ltd.

DIAGNOSTIC DIFFICULTIES ENCOUNTERED IN THE EARLY
MANAGEMENT OF ROAD CRASH CASUALTIES

Gordon W. Trinca, OBE

Senior Surgeon, Preston & Northcote Community Hospital
National Chairman, Road Trauma Committee,
Royal Australasian College of Surgeons

ABSTRACT

Significant delays in diagnosis in the early hospital management of
road crash casualties occur because of the complex nature of road
trauma, inexperience of the first treating doctor and lack of
organisation. The teaching of road trauma as a distinct disease
entity to undergraduates and the restriction of road crash casualty
care to those hospitals capable of providing major emergency services
would overcome many of the delays and errors in diagnosis.

INTRODUCTION

Early commencement of adequate resuscitative procedures, determination and priorities of definitive care and mobilization of an
appropriate treating team in the management of road crash injuries
can be hampered if the diagnosis is delayed, incomplete or incorrect.

The clinical complexity of road trauma, inexperience amd lack of
organisation are the main contributing factors.   The extent of
the failure to detect injuries early has been studied, reasons
discussed and remedies suggested.

METHODS

Special road traffic accident forms available since 1970 for recording clinical details of all road crash casualties attending Preston
& Northcote Community Hospital, Melbourne have been reviewed.   More
than 2,000 road crash casualties are treated per year.   Initially
some 15% were admitted but this has fallen to between 8-10% in the
past 3 years.

1430 cases admitted as in-patients have been studied in detail to
determine the extent of delay in diagnosis.   The road traffic
accident forms completed in Casualty have been compared with the
in-patient medical histories and a comparison made between the
initial diagnosis on admission and the final diagnosis on discharge.

During this period emergency department services were adequate, there
was a reasonably effective triage system and although in the main,
interns and junior resident medical officers were doctors of first
contact, more senior doctors were readily available if notified.

RESULTS

88% of cases admitted sustained major or minor injury to more than
one body region.   In 298 (20.8%) of the 1430 cases, injuries 2 or
more on the Abbreviated Injury Scale (A.I.S.80) were not detected
initially.   All cases were reviewed radiologically in the Casualty
Department.   In 10% there was no record in the Casualty notes.
In 50% of the remainder, the findings were not documented.   Injuries
to the abdomen, thorax and spine had the highest incidence of non-
detection and the limbs the least. (Table 1)

TABLE 1

	UNDETECTED INJURIES PER BODY REGION (AIS 2 or ⩾)	
	No. of Injuries	Percentage Undetected
Head & Neck [1]	288	17
Facial Bones	97	19.6
Thorax	417	23.7
Abdomen	116	33
Pelvic Bones	184	18.5
Upper Limb & Shoulder Girdle	269	23
Lower Limb	518	8.3
Thoracic & Lumbar Spine	48	29

[1] Lacerations not included

DISCUSSION

Patterns of injury surveys indicate the clinical complexity of road
trauma.   Important factors to be considered are:

- High incidence of multiple body region involvement with many
  injuries hidden.
- Unsuspected progression of underlying pathology (head, thorax
  and abdomen)
- Varying clinical presentation depending on category of road user,
  degree of protection in a crash and nature, direction and
  degree of the injuring force.

Delays and errors in diagnosis result from excessive work load, lack
of triage and inexperience of doctor of first contact.   Errors
follow acting on false information provided, incorrect interpretation
of signs and inadequate clinical exmaination.   Diagnostic errors
and failure to detect injuries can be avoided by the application of
sound clinical principles rather than dependence in the first
instance on sophisticated investigations and the inevitable delay
attendant on them.

It is suggested that increased clinical awareness of road trauma
would occur if the subject was included as a distinct disease
entity in the undergraduate curriculum and taught by those experienced in trauma management irrespective of their surgical discipline.
It is also suggested that hospitals should be graded as to the level
of emergency services they can provide and that road crash
casualties be taken to those hospitals capable of providing
continuous major emergency services which commence in the Casualty
Department.

Care of the Acutely Ill and Injured
Edited by D. H. Wilson and A. K. Marsden
© 1982, John Wiley & Sons Ltd.

CARE OF THE INJURED PATIENT'S EMOTIONAL TRAUMA

V. Morkovin, M.D.
Emergency Medicine
Illinois Masonic Medical Center, 836 Wellington Avenue,
Chicago, Illinois 60657, USA.

Emergency physicians and trauma surgeons are aware that
seriously injured patients suffer profound emotional as well as physical trauma, although there is a paucity of data about this in the
literature. It is hoped that this discussion will provoke further
interest in the subject and stimulate future investigation.

We have been particularly interested in the immediate and late psychological effects of human violence when it is the case of physical
trauma. In this category are those patients who are beaten, raped,
shot, or stabbed by either strangers, parents, spouses, or lovers.
In other words, it includes the "violence syndromes", such as child
abuse, incest, sexual assault, the battered wife syndrome, and abuse
of the elderly. These have been extensively studied in recent years.
We have now come to believe that criminal assaults by strangers, such
as muggings, kidnappings, and robbery cause similar emotional trauma.
Attempted suicides, whose psychological implications are better understood, may also be included in this group, since they also are
victims of violence, directed against themselves.

To some degree, almost all victims pass through certain stages of reactions. During the first shock, at the time of the assault or soon
afterwards, there is denial; "This can't be happening to me." Then
fear takes over. During and immediately after the attack, there is
fear for one's life, and later, fear of another attack. Anger that
such a thing could have happened is the healthiest sequel, but the
anger stage may frequently be repressed because of guilt, resulting
in a period of apathy when victims appear indifferent to their fate.
Finally, resolution should occur although this stage is not always
reached. The duration of these stages can vary tremendously. Families and close associates of victims often experience a similar
sequence.

There is a common group of delayed phenomena which are almost universal for victims of violence or of major trauma. These include frequent flash backs, inability to concentrate, nightmares, sleep disturbances, and a variety of psychosomatic symptoms. Such manifestations of anxiety may be severe enough to change the victims lifestyle
dramatically. Frequently victims move from their homes or change
jobs; their distrust of people may result in isolation from family
and friends. Depression, with the associated inability to function,

179

may even lead to suicide. This sequence of events, well described in
Burgess and Holstrom's study of the rape victim, is also characteristic of post-traumatic depression.

It has now been shown that the attitude of the first responder to a
victim can significantly modify the severity of these delayed symptoms. Thus it is important to train physicians, nurses, and prehospital personnel to be aware of these psychological processess, and
to behave in ways which will minimize them and assist victims toward
emotional as well as physical recovery.

One reaction peculiarly common to victims of violence is the sense of
guilt. This is a projection of society's attitude which holds victims responsible for their misfortunes. Martin Symonds postulates
that the need to blame the victim is a very primitive and powerful
instinct, which serves the purpose of protecting ourselves from feeling vulnerable. If we can believe that the victim somehow was the
cause of his disaster, we can sustain the confidence that it could
not happen to us. When people can be made to think that unfortunates
such as slaves or victims of a holocaust, are somehow inferior and
deserve their fate, they can justify being complacent and accepting
these horrors. It has been experimentally demonstrated that subjects
devalue those victims whose injuries they are unable to prevent.
Victims themselves, inculcated with these same societal attitudes,
often blame themselves for their misfortunes. They feel especially
guilty if they have cooperated with criminals, even when such com-
pliance was absolutely necessary to save their lives. This phenomena
has been rocorded in prisoners of war and people who have been kid-
napped.

Families of victims are similarly affected, often being rejected by
persons who would otherwise offer sympathy. It is as if mere contact
with unfortunate people could be contagious. Fear of contamination
by mere contact with misfortune has been shown to be a basic instinct
in observing small children and even animals.

It is evident that all victims, at the time they are attacked or injured, suffer from two overwhelming emotions; fear of death and loss
of control. We may not realize that emergency departments and trauma
units, to many patients, also produce the same fears and sense of
helplessness. In the unfamiliar and formidable hospital environment,
the medical staff may be viewed as assailants, and medical procedures
as life threats. Imagine yourself awakening strapped to a board, intubated, and in pain, with amnesia for the accident and the events
preceeding arrival at the hospital. Overwhelmed with their helplessness under such conditions, patients tend to regress to child-like
states. They feel frightened and yet completely dependent upon their
"captors". Such regression can even be useful during the temporary
period when they must be passive and allow many things to be done to
them.

Extreme humiliation, often sensed in semi-comatose states, can be a
major cause of agitation, especially in the elderly. In confused
states, catheterization may be perceived as bed-wetting. Being dis-

robed among strangers violates the life-long ingrained sense of modesty. Psychological trauma of such magnitude can actually induce syncope. Thus when evaluating the agitated or obtunded states in the injured patient, the syncope resulting from psychological shock must be considered as one possible etiological factor, in addition to head injury, cerebral hypoxia, and other physiological disturbances. When the psychological concerns can be dealt with, it is frequently possible to minimize the use of drugs and physical restraints, and to restore the patient's ability to cooperate.

As in all other aspects of surgery, the first rule is "do no harm." Persons who appear unconscious or confused may be intermittently aware of their surroundings, despite their apparent lack of response. It is unwise to assume that any patient cannot hear; thus it becomes extremely important to avoid careless talk and grave prognoses in the trauma room.

The first essential step is to establish communication with the patient. This can best be done by one member of the trauma team who is responsible for keeping in constant touch. This person should stay close to the patient's head, speak slowly and clearly, and remain in the line of vision as much as possible. For patients who are unable to speak because of their injuries, or because of having been intubated or tracheostomized, it is important to offer a means of communication, such as "Blink if you can hear me", "Squeeze my hand once for yes; twice for no". Touch is as important as speech. Stroking the forehead, clasping the shoulder, holding the hand; these acts can penetrate through the patient's isolation, confusion, and panic.

As soon as communication can be established, the following steps are important:

1. Tell the patient where he is and what is happening. Inform him in advance about procedures to be done, such as catheterization, intravenous connulation, or thora centesis. Use short sentences and repeat the information frequently. Encourage other members of the team to be as quiet as possible, as confusion and noise aggravate the patient's panic.
2. Validate the victim's experience. When he is able to speak, ask what happened. Try to get a detailed history of events. Share his memories of what he has been through, and give him feedback to show that you understand.
3. As early as possible, allow the patient to participate in making decisions about his care. Cover him up as soon as possible after examination. Treat the patient as an adult, and begin the process of personality re-integration to counteract the initial infantile regression. This is the first step in helping him to regain control of his life.
4. As far as possible, avoid leaving trauma victims alone. When separated from their families, they tend to believe they have been abandoned by those closest to them, a perception which may reinforce their sense of unworthiness.
5. Above all, avoid feeding into the patient's own feelings of guilt or self-blame. To do this, staff members must understand

their own unconscious tendency to blame victims. The implication that the rape or battery victim "asked for it" or that the
victim of an assault must have been in the wrong place at a
particular time, or that the patient's carelessness caused his
own accident - - all these "natural" responses must be avoided.
It is particularly important for someone to explain to the family and friends, before they visit the patient, how devastating
such attitudes can be. They too need to be made aware of the
self-serving motives which make people blame victims.

While acknowledging these concepts, emergency physicians often protest that there is no time, during the stressful management of critical trauma cases, to apply these principles. Actually, two approaches can make it possible. Workshops and discussions of psychological
concepts can sensitize the entire emergency team to patients' feelings, so that all personnel will be able to avoid inadvertent errors
and can contribute to providing psychological support. If the importance of this is realized, it is usually possible to assign one
individual, either a nurse, social worker, or trained volunteer, to
maintain communication with the patient without interfering with
efficient care.

After the critical period, this individual should continue contact
with the patient and the family, at least for a short period of time.
He or she should make sure the services of a social worker or other
mental health worker are available to continue assisting with psychological recovery, if needed, during hospitalization and later.

The fact that a major accident often results in permanant personality
disturbance is commonplace knowledge. Collaboration between emergency medicine and behavioral science is essential to insure patients
the best chance for full psychological as well as physical recovery.

REFERENCES

Burges G, Holstrom LL: Rape trauma syndrome, Am J Nursing, 131: 981-
    986, 1974.
Symonds M: Victims of violence: Psychological effects and after-ef-
    fects, Am J Psychoanalysis, 35: 19-26, 1975.
Strain JJ: Psychological reactions to acute medical illness and
    critical care, Crit Care Med 6: 39-44, 1978
Schnaper N: The psychological implications of severe trauma: Emotion-
    al sequelae to unconsciousness, J Trauma, 15: 94-98, 1975.
Schnaper N, Cowley RA: Overview: Psychiatric sequelae to multiple
    trauma, Am J Psychiatry, 133: 883-889, 1976.
Titchener JL: Management and study of psychological response to
    trauma, J Trauma, 10: 974-980, 1970 (quoted in Mattsson)

Care of the Acutely Ill and Injured
Edited by D. H. Wilson and A. K. Marsden
© 1982, John Wiley & Sons Ltd.

INTRAOPERATIVE AUTOTRANSFUSION IN
EMERGENCY SURGERY

H.R. Mayer, G. Kieninger, W. Neugebauer

Chirurgische Universitätsklinik Tübingen,
Direktor: Prof. Dr. L. Koslowski
Germany

INTRODUCTION

The number of polytraumatised patients with massive hemorrhaging
into the large body cavities has increased as traffic grows more
and more dense.
When the patient is delivered, generally to the closest local county
hospital, the surgeon there is usually only able to have him referred farther to a surgical center, since there is a lack of technical equipment, personnel, and, above all, blood.
This unnecessary loss of time very often results in irreversible
shock for the patient.
Even in elective surgery with an unforeseen massive hemorrhaging,
often only the possibility of a blood bank is considered.
Loss of time, shock as well as grave coagulation disturbances
following transfusion of foreign blood and limited blood supplies
call for the greatest possible independance from blood banks.
Other methods of acute blood replacement during emergency operations are needed.

Intraoperative autotransfusion permits the immediate obtaining and
re-use of the patient's own blood by means of a technically simple,
thoroughly tested and safe procedure. This contributes decisively
to the rationalization and optimation of acute blood replacement in
a surgical emergency.
Autologous blood transfusion after the patient's own blood has been
taken preoperatively (8) and after pre-operative hemodilution (9)
can be considered only for a few elective operations.
Intraoperative autotransfusion with technically unsophisticated equipment was used more than 100 years ago in isolated instances.
Following introduction of this method of blood replacement in 1868
by Volkmann and again in 1874 by Highmore, it was employed by
Thies (Leipzig) on a large scale for ruptured extrauterine pregnancies (11).
In spite of a broadening of indications subsequently, the procedure
lapsed into oblivion in the industrial nations with the introduction

of the blood bank system.
In the so-called developing nations this technique was used as always as a result of insufficient blood supplies (4,10). The equipment was simple:
The blood was spooned out of the abdomen, filtered through gas compressors in several layers, taken up in a simple container, an ACD-stabilizer[+] (an anti-coagulant) was added, transferred to bottles and then immediately re-transfused.

We performed intraoperative autotransfusion in Abeokuta/Nigeria between 1966 and 1980 following the same procedure, without, by the way, ever observing a single complication.

Dyer (1) took up this procedure again in the U.S. in 1966.
Klebanoff and Watkins (7) created the autotransfusion machine in its present form in 1968.
The data from numerous experiments on animals as well as from clinical application (2-6) justify the use of this technique of blood replacement as a routine clinical procedure.
We have been using the Bentley ATS machine (Bentley Laboratories GmbH, Düsseldorf) since 1973.

AUTOTRANSFUSION SYSTEM AND METHOD

The autotransfusion machine consists of a roller pump with a device for regulating suction velocity and transfusion pressure.
The blood level is monitored by a photoelectric cell which gives an optical as well as acoustical alarm when the blood level falls below the allowed minimum.
The attachments are delivered as a sterile disposable set. This consists of a 2000 ml reservoir with tube and 2 conduits as well as a suction pump.
The sterile disposable set can be connected to the pump within a few minutes, making the apparatus immediately operable at all times.
The aspirated blood is filtered and defoamed in the reservoir. This is accomplished by a nylon tripodnet with a pore size of 125 u, within the net is the polymethane defoaming device. The blood is transfused immediately afterwards.
In case of only slight hemorrhaging the reservoir is emptied by force of gravity.
The pumping speed should always be at the lowest level which is sufficient for aspiration in order to avoid unnecessary traumatization of the corpuscular blood components.

[+] Biotest, Frankfurt. Composition: Sodiumcitrate 13,2 g, Citric Acid 4,4 g, Glucose monohydrate 14,7 g, destilled water added to 1000 ml.

In case of massive hemorrhaging the blood must be retransfused under pressure. The air-outlet on the side of the pump is closed with a lever. The reservoir tolerates a pressure of up to 300 mm/hg. The blood can be returned at a maximum flow of 500 - 600 ml/min if necessary. Because of the danger of air-embolism which exists only in high-pressure transfusion, the greatest attention must be paid to checking the blood level.

ANTICOAGULATION

There are 2 procedures available for preventing coagulation of the blood taken:

1) Anticoagulation in the reservoir with ACD-solution which is administered at a dose of 300 ml ACD per filling.
2) Systemic heparinization before operation and autotransfusion (in this case 200 - 300 I.U. Heparin/kg body weight is administered).

Heparinization is used for hemorrhaging during vascular surgery. For all traumatically induced hemorrhages and for all intra- and postoperative bleeding in cases of extra-uterine pregnancy, ACD-anticoagulation is used.

OWN EXPERIENCES

We have performed a total of 324 intraoperative autotransfusions in Abeokuta/Nigeria since 1966 and at the Chirurgische Klinik at the University of Tübingen since 1973.

INDICATIONS FOR AUTOTRANSFUSION

Ruptured ectopic pregnancy	131
Rupture of the spleen	50
Rupture of the liver	39
Ruptured aortic aneurism	27
Postoperative hemorrhage	21
Pelvic vein thrombosis	16
Porto-caval + spleno-renal shunt	16
Rupture of the kidney	14
Hemothorax	13
Rupture of blood vessels	9
Fracture of the pelvis	6
Rupture of the urinary bladder	4
Partial hepatectomy	4
Traumatic rupture of the aorta	3
Nephrotomy	3
Varia	12
Total number of patients (31.12.80)	324

The greatest blood volume per patient, 20 l, was transfused into a patient with a ruptured aortic aneurism; The average amount was 2,1 l. Bank blood was given if necessary.
Anti-coagulation was accomplished with 40 patients by systemic heparinization, with 284 by ACD-solution.
Total re-transfused blood volume was 660 l.

Of the 193 autotransfused surgical patients 20 were referred from other hospitals in a state of irreversible shock and could not be saved even with intensive measures.
The coagulation disturbances which occurred following autotransfusion corresponded to those which are well-known from usual blood-transfusions. Platelet and fibrinogen levels fell post-operatively, and for the following 3 days, but reached the normal range after the 6th day (5).
In the initial period of our autotransfusion experience with the Bentley machine, we had two air embolisms with fatal consequences. Other grave complications with fatal results did not occur in Nigeria, however, even with the rather primitive method already described.
Of the 131 patients operated on and autotransfused in Nigeria, a large portion would have died from a lack of blood supplies and those in Tübingen because of lacking rare blood group supplies.

These figures admit of no argument, in our opinion, against intraoperative autotransfusion.

Further, the cost to the blood bank for 660 l of retransfused blood would have been about 200.000 marks and can be contrasted the expenses of purchasing an autotransfusion machine, sterile filters and ACD-solution which would total ca. 40.000 marks.

This alone, on purely economic grounds, would recommend the use of this technique of autotransfusion.

INDICATIONS

From our own experimental data, and from that in the literature as well as from clinical experience (2 - 6), we present the indications for intraoperative autotransfusion:

1) In all traumatic hemorrhaging of the abdominal, thoracic and retro-peritoneal cavities.
2) In emergency vascular surgery, especially with aortic aneurysms and injury to the large vessels.
3) In pelvic vein-thromboses.
4) In ruptured extra-uterine pregnancies.
5) In massive hemorrhaging during elective surgery, as shunt operations, hepatic surgery etc.

6) In all cases of post-operative bleeding which necessitate a re-
   intervention.
7) In cases where blood transfusions are refused on religious
   grounds, as the Jehovah Witnesses.

Our autotransfusion machine is always in functioning condition in
surgery. The pump can be ready in less than five minutes. Should
the use of the completely prepared autotransfusion-system prove
to be unnecessary or not indicated, the reservoir with the tubing
section and the suction pump can be re-used after sterilisation
with gas.

CONTRAINDICATIONS

Definite contraindications for use of intraoperative autotransfusions
are surgery of malignant tumors, septic surgery and contamination
of the blood with large bowel contents.
In our opinion, rupture of the uterus must also be considered a
definite contraindication due to the danger of embolism in the
amniotic fluid.
An injury to the stomach or the small intestine presents a relative
contraindication. This is also essentially a quantitative problem.
If the degree of contamination is small and the defect can be effectively closed or covered, then the blood can be used if necessary.
A fissure in the biliary ducts should not be considered a contraindication. Here, it is sufficient to refer to the favourable experiences in the treatment of hepatic rupture.

Retransfusion of blood, which had been mixed with urine, after
nephrotomies and cystotomies, showed no essential hemolysis (5).
Obviously, in those cases where the patient would surely die without the autotransfusion, all contra-indications become relative.

SUMMARY

Based on our excellent experiences with intraoperative autotransfusion we are able to recommend it as a routine procedure in
emergency surgery. The main advantages are:

1) Immediate availability of blood (especially in rare blood groups)
2) Transfusion of fresh blood
3) No risk of hepatitis
4) No immunisation
5) No risk of incomatibility
6) Economic aspects

Aside from the 131 cases of ruptured ectopic pregnancies who
were predominently operated on in Nigeria, the following becomes evident: In over 60% of cases a trauma preceded surgery
and autotransfusion; 82% of traumas were the result of a traffic

accident.

We would like here to refer to our opening remarks and empha-
size that most traffic accident cases get to the Surgical Center
only after an unnecessary detour by the local county hospital.
Lack of blood supplies should not result in loss of time for treating
patients. Immediate autotransfusion which can be performed even
in the most primitive conditions - as shown here - in the African
bush country, should be introduced into every local hospital dealing
with emergency operations.
The fatal consequences of irreversible shock would be more often
avoided.
One ought not ask the number of patients who have died as a consequence of insufficient blood bank supplies and the absence of the
autotransfusion procedure.

The decisive importance of autotransfusion in disaster situation
can not be adequately judged as yet in peacetime.

REFERENCES

(1) Dyer, R.H.: Intraoperative autotransfusion. A preliminary report and new method. Amer.J.Surg. 112 (1966), 874.
(2) Hauer, J.M., H.A. Shub, W.I. Wolff: The case for autotransfusion. Resident & Staff Physician 118 (1977), 17s.
(3) Kern, E., P. Klaue, B. Homann: Die intraoperative maschi-
nelle Autotransfusion bei Massivblutungen. Dtsch.med.Wschr.
102 (1977), 188
(4) Kieninger, G., H. Junger, K. Schmidt: Die Anwendung der
intraoperativen Autotransfusion in der Gynäkologie und Chirurgie.
Anaesthesist 25 (1976), 357.
(5) Kieninger, G., L. Koslowski, W. Neugebauer, H. Junger,
R. Stunkat, W. Epting: Methodik, Indikationen und Ergebnisse der
intraoperativen Autotransfusion. Akt.Chir. 11 (1976), 351.
(6) Kieninger, G., H. Junger, K. Schmidt: Intraoperative autotransfusion. Review of its use in ill surgical and gyneologic patients.
Curr.Top.crit. Care Med. 2 (1977), 108.
(7) Klebanoff, G., D. Watkins: A disposable autotransfusion unit.
Amer.J.Surg. 116 (1968), 475.
(8) Klövekorn, W.P., H. Pichlmaier, E. Ott, H. Bauer, L. Sunder-
Plassmann, K. Meßner: Akute präoperative Hämodilution - eine
Möglichkeit zur autologen Bluttransfusion. Chirurg 45 (1974), 452.
(9) Newman, M.M., R. Hamstra, M. Block: Use of banked autologous blood in elective surgery.J.Amer.med.Ass.218(1971),861.
(10) Pathak, U.N., D.B.Stewart: Autotransfusion in ruptured ectopic pregnancy. Lancet 1970/I, 961.
(11) Thies,J.: Zur Behandlung der Extrauteringravidität.Zbl.Gynäk.
34 (1914), 1191.

Care of the Acutely Ill and Injured
Edited by D. H. Wilson and A. K. Marsden
© 1982, John Wiley & Sons Ltd.

DIAGNOSTIC DIFFICULTIES AND PROBLEMS IN ASSESSMENT OF BLUNT CHEST INJURIES

W. Glinz

Surgical Clinic B, University Hospital
Zurich, Switzerland

On site resuscitation, faster transport to the hospital and better clinical care have improved the prognosis of patients with blunt chest trauma considerably. But one of the main reasons for a fatal outcome in thoracic-injured patients, who are admitted alive is: Misdiagnosis: Misdiagnosis with one s meaning the wrong diagnosis, and with two s's: The missed diagnosis.

CLINICAL MATERIAL

Table 1 shows our clinical material of a 5 year period. An analysis of these 675 patients with severe blunt chest trauma shows that diagnosis in four thoracic injuries of considerable clinical importance may be difficult and is frequently missed or delayed: Cardiac contusion (present in 16 % of severe thoracic injuries), diaphragmatic rupture (the incidence is 4 %), aortic rupture(2 %), and bronchial rupture (0,6 %).

TABLE 1. THORACIC INJURIES IN 675 PATIENTS WITH SEVERE BLUNT CHEST TRAUMA

Hemothorax	344	51 %
Pneumothorax	121	18 %
Cardiac contusion	108	16 %
Rupture of pericardium	2	0,3 %
Pulmonary contusion	141	21 %
Rupture of diaphragm	26	4 %
Aortic rupture	15	2 %
Lesions of other thoracic vessels	6	0,9 %
Bronchial rupture	4	0,6 %
Chylothorax	1	0,15 %
Rupture of esophagus	0	–

CARDIAC CONTUSION

Every textbook describes impressive, severe cardiac
injuries: Cardiac ruptures, traumatic septal defects and
heart valve lesions. However, in clinical practice these
cases represent decided rarities.

In contrast to these rare injuries, cardiac contusion is
very frequent. The diagnosis of this injury is often not
established. The pathologic picture is not well known;
furthermore in the majority of cases the diagnosis is not
easy.   (Figure 1).

There are two situations in which cardiac injury is
overlocked:

1) In very severe thoracic trauma, the surgeon is so overwhelmed by multiple rib fractures, paradoxical respiration,
hemothorax, pneumothorax, that the heart is often not
considered.

2) The second situation is almost the opposite of the one
previously described. If there are no rib fractures, the
force of the internal impact is underestimated. In the
youthful elastic thorax the heart can be injured between
the sternum and spinal column without fracture of the ribs.
On occasion, contusion marks will then point to the
severity of the thoracic trauma. Heart injuries without
rib fractures are not at all uncommon; among our patients,
rib fractures were not present in 25 % of all heart
injuries caused by blunt force.

The ECG (table 2) may - rarely - reveal a pattern of acute
infarction. Very often there are unspecified ST-T wave
changes and findings of subepicardial damage. But the ECG
can be normal. Every possible variation of ECG can be
observed. There is no typical ECG pattern for cardiac
contusion. Furthermore, electrocardiographic patterns
change very rapidly.

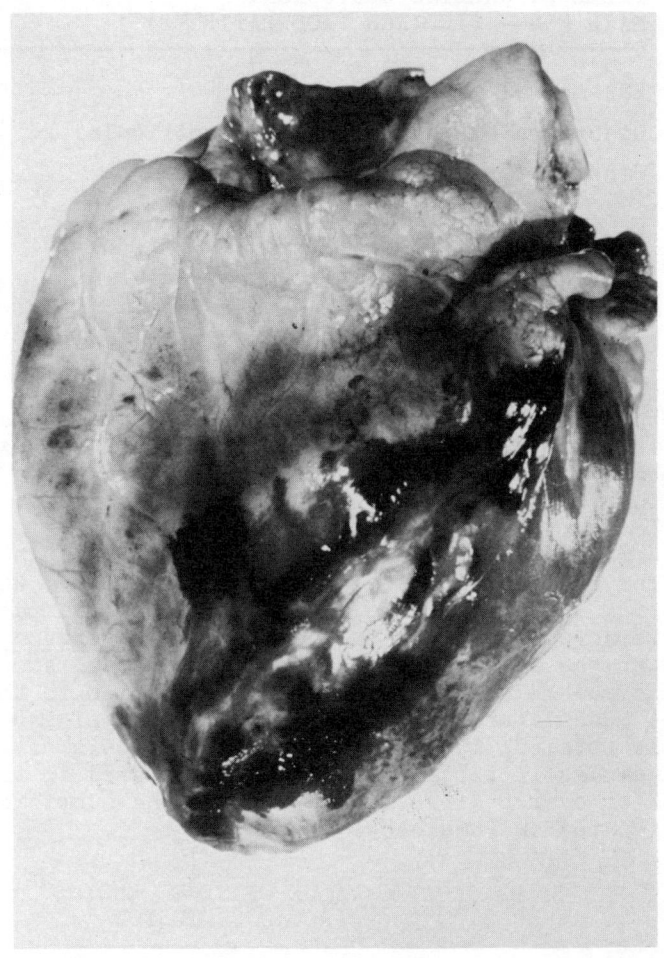

Fig. 1:   Extensive hemorrhagic involvement of the anterior wall
          of the heart in severe cardiac contusion

TABLE 2. CARDIAC CONTUSION:
MAIN ECG - FINDINGS (108 PATIENTS)

ECG normal	13
Disorders of rhythm, mainly ventricular	24 ⎤
Other arrhythmias and disturbances of conduction	35 ⎦ 59
Disturbances of repolarisation	66
"Myocardial infarction"	3

What about the diagnostic value of <u>serum enzymes</u> in
cardiac contusion ? A rise in <u>CK</u> is found in every severe
trauma victim. Values of over 3000 to 4000 IU far exceed
those observed in myocardial infarction since every injury
to peripheral musculature results in a CK increase.

The determination of the <u>CK isoenzymes</u> is more authori-
tative for the diagnosis of cardiac injury. Since we
began using this method, we have found among all patients
with cardiac contusion an increase of the <u>isoenzyme MB</u>
already on the day of the accident. Since small amounts
of isoenzymes MB are released also in injuries to the
skeletal musculature the proportional amount of isoenzymes
MB in the total CK is significant for diagnosis of myocardial damage: A percentage of CK MB compared to the
total CK of over 8 % provides a very strong suspicion of
cardiac contusion (table 3).

TABLE 3. DIAGNOSTIC VALUE OF SERUM ENZYMES IN
CARDIAC CONTUSION

Total LDH	↑	not specific
$LDH_1 + LDH_2$ isoenzymes	↑	
Total CK	↑	in all trauma patients, no diagnostic value
CK-MB isoenzymes	↑	$\dfrac{CK\ MB}{CK\ total} > 8\ \%$ strongly suggesting cardiac trauma

The same is true for the determination of Lactate-
dehydrogenase (LDH). In all patients with cardiac
contusion, we found an increase in LDH_1 and LDH_2
isoenzymes. The enzyme remained elevated for a long time,
more than one week.

It must be kept in mind that in some cases it is not
until the total findings have been evaluated that the
diagnosis of cardiac contusion can be made. A normal
ECG does not rule out the possibility of cardiac contusion. The determination of CK MB as well as the LDH_1
and LDH_2 isoenzymes is very helpful.

Why is it important, that cardiac contusion be recognized?
I can lead to threatening situations, which if promptly
recognized can usually be dealt with effectively. Of
particular importance are the disturbances in heart
rhythm. Indeed disorders of rhythm and acute cardiac
failure are encounted quite frequently (table 4).

TABLE 4. CARDIAC CONTUSION: CLINICAL COURSE

		108 patients, surviving 1st day after trauma. Therapy required:
Frequent:	Disorders of rhythm	40
	Acute cardiac failure	17
Rare:	Cardiac tamponade	2
	Secondary heart rupture	0
	Aneurysm	0

So the plea is: A patient with cardiac contusion must be
treated in an intensive care unit with cardiac monitoring.
In our series of 108 patients with cardiac contusion who
survived the first day, only two died due to heart injury.

Secondary heart rupture or aneurysm formation is rare:
We have not observed a case, but two cases of cardiac
tamponade because of post-traumatic pericarditis.

DIAPHRAGMATIC RUPTURE

Number two on our list of difficult diagnoses has been
rupture of diaphragm. The chest X-ray may imitate hemothorax. Introducing an intercostal tube the surgeon may
be very suprised to drain gastric contents from the
thorax. A stomach full of air, when dislocated into the
thorax, may give the impression of a tension pneumothorax.
(Figure 2).
Rupture of the left diagphram is by far more frequent
than of the right (85 % out of 1845 ruptures in the
literature).

The diagnosis of a right sided rupture is much more
difficult. It can be proved preoperatively by placing a
small dialysis catheter into the abdomen, as it is used
for peritoneal lavage, and insufflation of air intra-
abdominally. During spontaneous breathing, this results
in a pneumothorax if there is a diaphragmatic rupture.
If the diaphragm is intact it can be seen clearly with
this simple technique.

Associated injuries play an important role in rupture of
the diaphragm, reflecting the severe impact on thorax and
abdomen (table 5). Note the high incidence of intraabdominal injuries and the frequent association of pelvic
fractures (20 % in the literature, 5o % in our material).

TABLE 5. RUPTURE OF DIAPHRAGM: ASSOCIATED INJURIES

	655 acute ruptures of diaphragm in recent literature	Own clinical material (26 cases)
Rib fractures	297 (45.%)	19 (73 %)
Pelvic fractures	134 (20 %)	13 (50 %)
Extremity fractures		10 (38 %)
Head injuries		8 (31 %)
Vertebral fractures		3 (12 %)
Injuries to abdominal organs:		
Spleen	195 (30 %)	8 (31 %)
Liver	89 (14 %)	11 (42 %)
G I tract	95 (15 %)	5 (19 %)
Kidneys	60 (9 %)	5 (19 %)

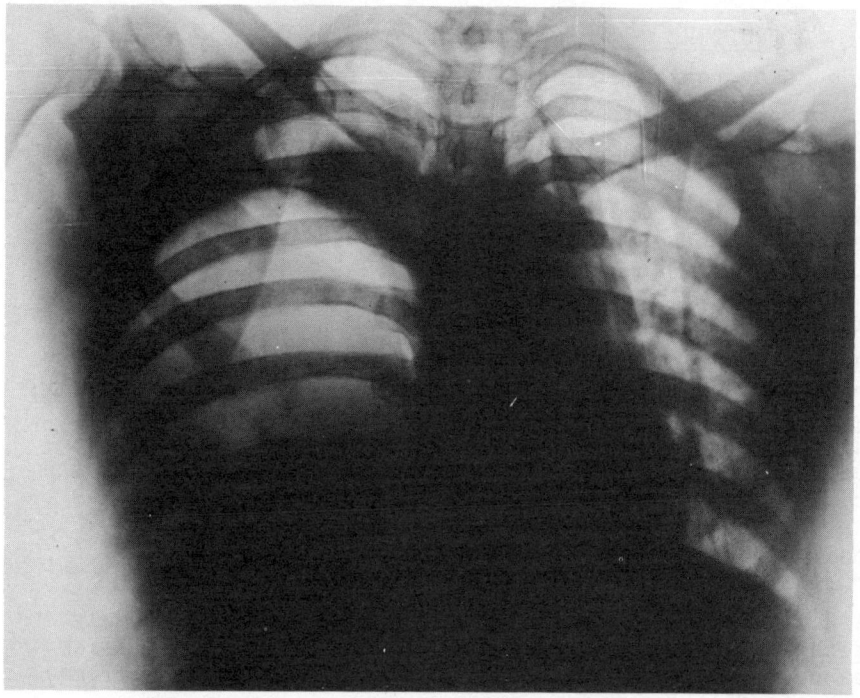

Fig. 2: The displacement of a large, air-filled magenblase into the
left thorax in a diaphragmatic rupture can result in a situation
comparable to a tension pneumothorax

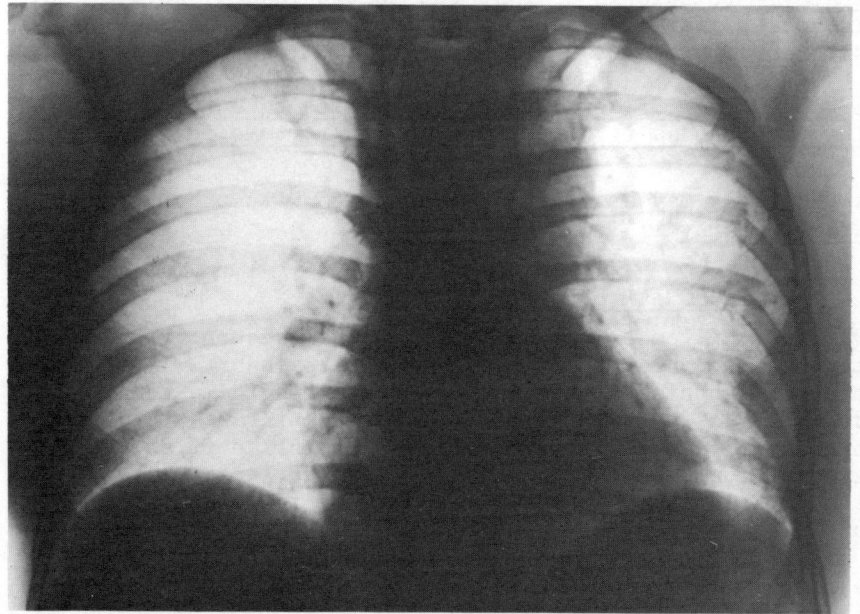

Fig. 3: Widened mediastinum in rupture of the aorta. No attention
was paid to this finding until there was a perforation
with fatal results

RUPTURE OF THE AORTA

The main problem of aortic rupture is timely diagnosis.
It must be kept in mind that many more patients die of an
overlooked rupture of the aorta than of operative
difficulties or postoperative complications.

Reviewing the recent literature we find that 93 % of
ruptures in cases who came into clinical observation are
localized at the classical site, just distal to the left
subclavian artery. Much less common are ruptures of the
ascending aorta.

There may be a variety of clinical symptoms in aortic
rupture, but the most important diagnostic sign is the
widening of the mediastinum of the chest roentgenogram.
However, even when the mediastinum is widened, the cause
can be traced to aortic rupture in only a minority of the
cases. Of 64 patients, whose first roentgenograms taken
after emergency admission showed a widened upper
mediastinum, only 11 were subsequently found to have
ruptured aortas.   (Figure 3).

A widening of the mediastinum can also occur for purely
technical reasons: The patient in supine position, X-ray
exposure anterior-posteriorly, and a small distance from
tube to film.

The presence of a widened superior mediastinum always
demands aortography - or, if available, computertomography - to rule in or rule out aortic injury. Aortography
is more reliable than explorative operation: It can even
show a rupture of the intima only.   (Figure 4).

A good number of negative aortographies have to be taken
into account as to detect one aortic rupture in time.

Aortography may and should be combined with other organ
arteriography if indicated.

BRONCHIAL RUPTURE

The fourth item on our list of lesions frequently diagnosed
late is bronchial rupture. It is a rare injury. In the
past, diagnosis of these injuries has generally been
delayed, and only 15 % (Bishop) to 25 % (Krauss) of
bronchial lesions were recognized within the first week
after trauma, and unfortunately often not until late
complications have occured (according to Burke in 68 %
of the cases).

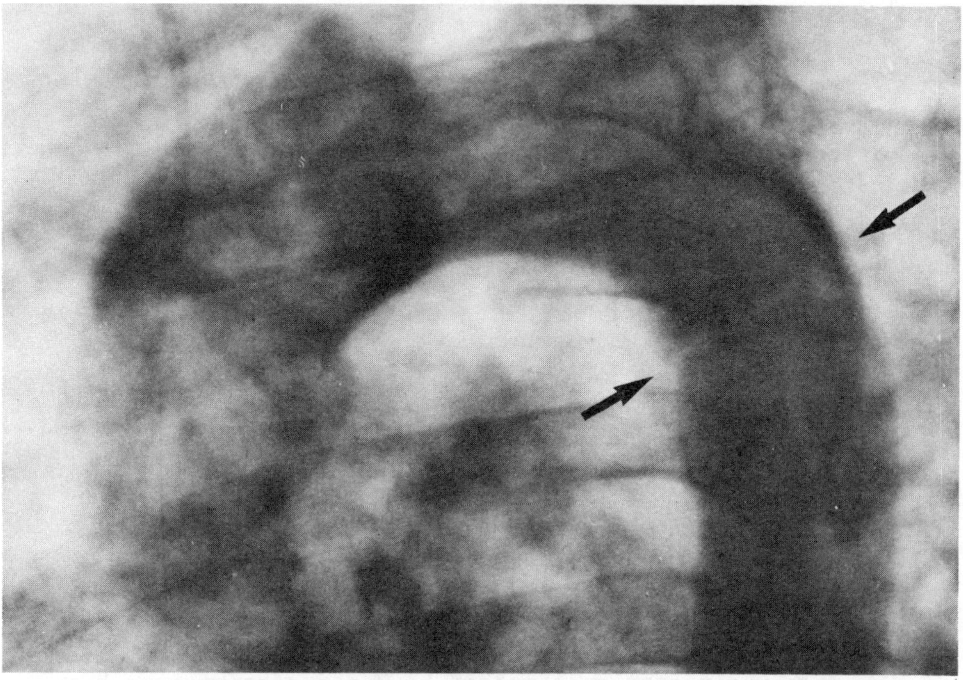

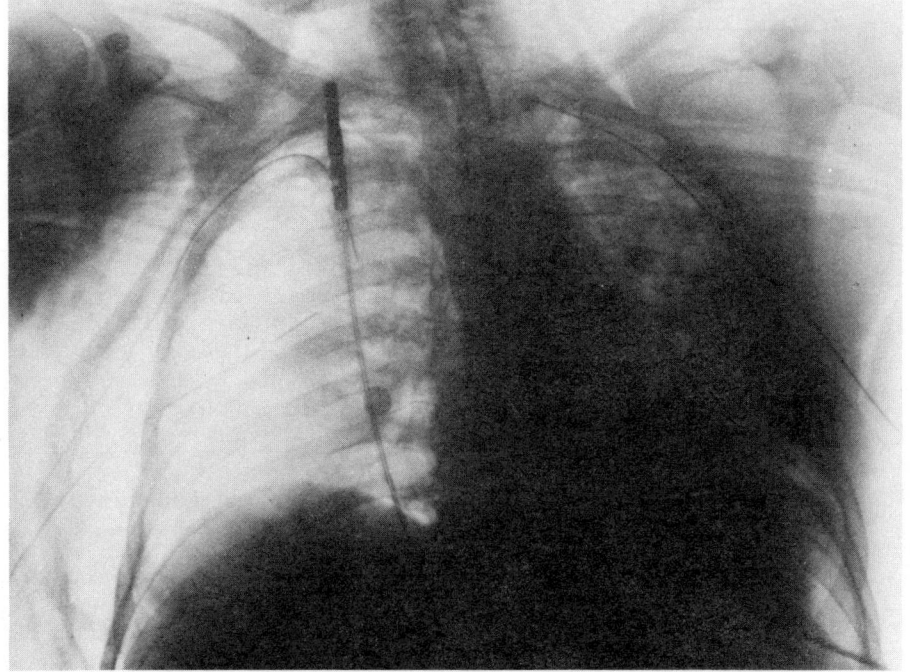

Fig. 4: Transverse intimal tear of the descending aorta at the typical site without extravasation of contrast medium during angiography, confirmed intraoperatively

Fig. 5: Despite abundant thoracic drainage, a tension pneumothorax cannot be eliminated: rupture of the bronchus of the upper lobe on the right side and injuries to the lung parenchyma

Three situations demand always further investigation:

1) Failure in expanding the lung in pneumothorax by intercostal tube drainage.   (Figure 5).

2) Marked mediastinal emphysema.

3) Atelectasis of a lung not relieved by the usual therapeutic management.

The issue is not making of the diagnosis on the basis of clinical signs. The issue is the indication for bronchoscopy.

Bronchoscopy always clears the situation. You will never regret making use of early bronchoscopic examination.

PULMONARY CONTUSION

Aortic rupture, rupture of diaphragm and bronchial rupture are not common injuries found in blunt chest trauma. Pulmonary contusion, on the other hand, was found in 21% of patients with severe thoracic injuries. This condition is generally easily diagnosed by X-ray examination; but it is often underestimated in its functional consequences. If arterial blood gas analysis demonstrates a significant intrapulmonary right-to-left shunt, immediate mechanical ventilation with PEEP has markedly improved the prognosis of this condition.

CONCLUDING REMARKS

Trauma has no respect for anatomic boundaries. This is especially true for blunt trauma. We have found more than 3/4 of our thoracic patients suffering from additional injuries to other regions of the body.

These patients belong in the care of a facility that accepts responsibility for the treatment of all of their wounds and they may not be parcelled out to a multiplicity of specialists on the basis of their injured organs.

REFERENCES:

Glinz, W. 1981. Chest Trauma; Diagnosis and Management. Springer-Verlag, Berlin-Heidelberg-New York.

Care of the Acutely Ill and Injured
Edited by D. H. Wilson and A. K. Marsden
© 1982, John Wiley & Sons Ltd.

PULMONARY FUNCTION AFTER ACCIDENTAL
INJURY AND THORACOTOMY

J. Bancewicz*, Pamela Bithell, R.A. Little, J. McBeath[+],
M. Stansfield, H.B. Stoner and D.W. Yates

Depts. of Surgery* and Anaesthesia[+] and M.R.C. Trauma
Unit, Hope Hospital (University of Manchester School of
Medicine), Salford, U.K.

INTRODUCTION

Despite increasing interest in the pulmonary complications of
trauma there have been few studies of the functional sequelae
of chest injuries. The investigations that have been done have
concentrated on the long-term effects of major chest injuries
in patients who were admitted to an intensive therapy unit (eg:
Davidson, Bargh, Cruickshank and Duthie, 1969; Hanning,
Ledingham and Ledingham, 1981). We are now studying the early
changes in pulmonary function after chest injuries that are
frequently considered to be of only minor or moderate severity,
and after a surgical thoracotomy.

METHODS

Three groups of patients have been studied: (1) Accidental
fracture of 1 - 3 ribs (n=14), (2) Thoracotomy for Nissen
fundoplication - without Epidural anaesthesia (n=9), (3)
Thoracotomy and laparotomy for oesophageal resection - with
Epidural anaesthesia (n=6). Pulmonary function was assessed
preoperatively (where appropriate), as soon after injury or
operation as possible and at intervals thereafter using a
Morgan TLC system (P.K. Morgan, Chatham, Kent), and/or a wedge
spirometer (Vitalograph Ltd., Buckingham).

RESULTS

The measurements require active cooperation from the patients
and we have been unable to obtain reliable values for pulmonary
function during the first two days following operation in the
patients without an epidural anaesthetic. However, in those
receiving an epidural (Marcain - 0·375% infusion at 5ml/h) some
measurements have been made during this period, despite the
greater degree of intra-thoracic manipulation, and the presence
of an abdominal incision in this group. FEV_1 (Table 1), and T_L
(transfer factor) were markedly reduced in both groups of
surgical patients (to 20 - 40% of predicted values) during the
first week after operation, and were still reduced three months
later. Total lung capacity (TLC) was not reduced to such an
extent (60 - 70% of predicted), and had recovered within three

J. Bancewicz et al.

TABLE 1   Forced expiratory volume (FEV_1) measured at
intervals after accidental or surgical injury (%
predicted, mean±S.E.).

	Time after injury				
	0	1-2D	3-5D	6-16D	1-3M
(1) Trauma	43±7 (10)	34±6 (6)	46±10 (6)	54±12 (6)	90±26 (3)
(2) Thoracotomy (- Epidural)	–	28±5 (2)	41±4 (8)	53±7 (7)	73±6 (4)
(3) Thoracotomy (+ Epidural)	–	25±3 (5)	37±6 (4)	44±4 (5)	68±13 (4)

months. After the accidental chest injuries FEV_1 (Table 1) and
T_L were reduced acutely to values as low as 20% of predicted
and took up to three months to recover. TLC was also reduced
after accidental injury, and following the fracture of three
ribs the reduction was greater (to 50% of predicted) than after
a major intra-thoracic operation (eg Group 3).

CONCLUSIONS

Accidental chest injuries which are not generally considered
serious may lead to a greater deficit in pulmonary function
than is commonly realized. Epidural anaesthesia may have a role
in the post-operative management of patients following
oesophageal resection.

REFERENCES

Davidson, I.A., Bargh, W., Cruickshank, A.N., and Duthie, W.H.,
1969. Crush injuries of the chest. A follow-up study of
patients treated in an artificial ventilation unit. Thorax,
24, 563-567.
Hanning, C.D., Ledingham, E., and Ledingham, I.McA., 1981. Late
respiratory sequelae of blunt chest injury: a preliminary
report. Thorax, 36, 204-207.

Care of the Acutely Ill and Injured
Edited by D. H. Wilson and A. K. Marsden
© 1982, John Wiley & Sons Ltd.

ANAESTHESIA FOR CIVILIAN WARFARE:
CHEST WOUNDS

R S J Clarke

Department of Anaesthetics, The Queen's University of
Belfast, Whitla Medical Building, 97 Lisburn Road,
Belfast BT9 7BL, Northern Ireland

I am taking my title to include the anaesthetist's role in the
management of patients with chest injuries. I am however covering
the whole intensive care management because these patients do not
always need formal anaesthetics, but for many hours and days after
their injuries they require management in an Intensive Care Unit.
The reader is also referred to surveys by Keen (1975), Coppel (1978)
and Clarke (1981).

First I would like to stress that civil disturbance provides less
than half of our acute trauma, car accidents contributing more to our
numbers and agricultural mishaps providing some of our most rewarding
problems. Having reviewed our numbers, I will therefore discuss the
routine situation of fractured ribs that we all see and return to
bomb blasts as one of the causes of Post-traumatic Pulmonary
Insufficiency.

ADMISSIONS TO THE INTENSIVE CARE UNIT

The admissions due to civil disturbance to the Royal Victoria
Hospital, Belfast have totalled 3,418 from 1971 to 1980 inclusive,
of whom 387 have come to the Intensive Care Unit. We have had
between 16 and 96 admissions to the Unit per year but rarely more
than three such patients at once in a 12-bed unit. Although the
bomb injuries are more spectacular and place a greater burden on the
Accident and Emergency staff there have been more than twice as many
gunshot wounds. The overall mortality from the two groups is
similar - 35 and 39 per cent respectively. Table 1 shows the
mortality in the Unit according to site of injury and it is notable
that chest injuries have the best prognosis, followed by those of
jaw and neck. The higher mortality from injuries of the abdomen was
usually associated with severe peritonitis, while deaths due to
severe haemorrhage would usually occur before patients reached the
Intensive Care Unit.

TABLE 1.   Outcome of injuries (1971-1980) due to civil
            disturbance in relation to site.

Site	Total number	Deaths	
		Number	Percentage
Head	120	60	50
Neck/Jaw	26	6	23
Chest	64	11	17
Abdomen	21	11	52
Chest+Abdomen	37	13	35
Multiple	119	38	32
Total	387	139	36

Our Intensive Care Unit has a closer connection than most with the
Accident and Emergency area of the hospital, because it lies just
across a corridor from it on the ground floor. It is in the same
block as the neurosurgery and fracture wards which means that we
have a close connection with these fields but the price is that we
are rather too far from the thoracic and cardiac surgical units. We
have twelve beds, six open and six in cubicles, the latter being
kept usually for post-trachaeostomy patients, those with renal
failure and burns.

The management of chest as with other injuries depends in the early
stages on the ability to get air into the chest and the arrest of
haemorrhage. Most airway problems occur in the mandible-tongue-
larynx region and early intubation, while it may be difficult, is
vital. In the chest, the acute problems interfering with respiration
are pneumothorax and haemothorax and they are essentially managed by
the thoracic surgeon. However, a chest drain should be inserted by
any competent person who is available when the need is urgent.

FRACTURED RIBS

These are by far the commonest chest problems which the anaesthetist
has to manage and should be looked for particularly in any road
casualties. Physical signs include:

1. Crepitus and/or tenderness along the ribs

2. Bruising (but this may take days to develop)

3. Paradoxical chest movements

4. Surgical emphysema

and where there is pneumothorax

5. Displacement of the apex beat

6. Hyper-resonance with shifting dullness

The patient arriving in hospital with fractured ribs will be complaining mainly of pain and if dyspnoeic, this is often secondary to the pain. One of the most useful first analgesics is Entonox, 50 per cent nitrous oxide in oxygen in one cylinder which can be given at the scene of the accident or at any stage later. Its great advantages are:

1. It is rapidly effective

2. It has little effect on cardiovascular or respiratory systems

3. It allows administration of 50 per cent oxygen

4. Its use encourages observation of the patient's respiration

5. But it can be administered by the patient on his own

6. Its effects wear off quickly so that analgesia need not be withheld until all specialists have examined the patient. This applies particularly to assessment of consciousness by the neurosurgeon.

The other regimes which have proved effective include the use of a lignocaine infusion (1.4 mg.ml^{-1}). Surprisingly, this has few side effects and does appear to produce acceptable analgesia without depression of respiration or the cough reflex. The patients are being closely observed so that early signs of central nervous system excitability would be detected.

The thoracic extradural technique is troublesome to set up and, because of the uncertainty of further chest trauma (Gibbons, James and Quail, 1973),we have not used it very often.

The use of opiate analgesics in addition is of course frequently necessary and here the intravenous route is rapid, reliable and safe, avoiding the uncertainties of giving intramuscular injections to the shocked patient. As with all trauma the dose should be tailored to the patient's needs giving adequate analgesia to the strong and healthy young man, though head and chest injuries are often less painful than those of the abdomen or limbs.

Once the pain is relieved, the patient should be able to breathe deeply and cough as required. However, he will need frequent encouragement from the physiotherapist. Sometimes the passage of a soft catheter through the nose will help to stimulate coughing and remove tenacious secretions. Some patients clearly need more active management from the beginning and certain factors militate against straightforward recovery. In particular, the patient with a flail segment or lung contusion from a severe injury may have no hope of keeping normal blood gases. If however the patient does manage to breathe, a careful watch should be kept for exhaustion, restlessness, pallor, cyanosis or redness from CO_2 accumulation, since it may require several days before sufficient sputum accumulates to produce these findings.

Age and pre-existing chronic bronchitis may also lead to early
respiratory failure. Atelectasis may lead to hypoxia which
stimulates ventilation but leads to exhaustion. The resulting low
$PaCO_2$ may then be misleading. This kind of sequence in the presence
of some of the factors mentioned should encourage early intubation
under anaesthesia as a means of proper expansion of the lungs and
aspiration of secretions. Physiotherapy may be poorly tolerated
because of pain, but the use of anaesthesia or at least N_2O/O_2 does
allow more vigorous efforts. It is rarely satisfactory to leave an
orotracheal tube in position in the conscious patient. The naso-
tracheal tube is an alternative but in general it is our practice to
carry out a trachaeostomy if the chest needs frequent inflation and
aspiration. Trachaeostomy is certainly more comfortable for the
patient than either an oral or nasal tube and does allow swallowing
and movement with less irritation of the vocal cords.

Indications that spontaneous ventilation is not going to be adequate
arise from the appearance and blood gases of the patient. However
the nature of the injuries, especially marked instability may
necessitate early ventilation. It is logical to institute
ventilation early in a patient with severe paradoxical movement of
the chest, so that the ribs may stabilise in an expanded position
rather than sinking inwards, with collapse of the underlying lung
(Shackford et al, 1976). This may be described as pneumatic
stabilisation as distinct from surgical stabilisation which is
rarely practised in our hospital. Widespread lung contusion may
likewise force one to early ventilation. However, a broncho pleural
fistula or parenchymal tear with bubbling of air from the chest
drains, is an indication to delay. Certainly a large leak is
unlikely to heal while the patient is being ventilated. Once the
decision has been made intravenous opiates can be given for sedation
without worry and we usually alternate morphine with diazepam. It
is probably best to curarise the patient in addition at least until
the fractures stabilise. Suction on the chest drain (+ 5 cm H_2O) is
often necessary to expand a collapsed lung and to keep the
pneumothorax evacuated.

Diaphragmatic rupture should always be considered if there is a
loculated air pocket or total collapse in the left lower zone on
x-ray. Once suspected, confirmation is usually by barium meal
radiography and surgical treatment is urgent.

POST-TRAUMATIC PULMONARY INSUFFICIENCY

I am using this term to include the patchy or confluent atelectasis
which develops in so many patients after injury. Principal causes
include fat embolism, oxygen toxicity, large transfusions of stored
blood, fluid overload, aspiration of gastric contents and blast lung.
All are rather vague terms and classification is largely subjective,
especially since they frequently co-exist in the same patient.

Fat embolism should be suspected in any patient with a major

fracture who becomes confused or develops any pulmonary signs. The
presence of petechiae is confirmatory but rare and measurement of
arterial oxygen tension should not be delayed until frank cyanosis
is seen.

Oxygen toxicity can be avoided by keeping the F_1O_2 as low as
arterial oxygenation permits and is much less common since the
introduction of PEEP which I will return to below.

Massive transfusion of stored blood is now a recognised cause of
pulmonary complications (Reul, Beall and Greenberg, 1974) but these
have been reduced by the use of fine-screen filtration. On the
other hand these filters are now always used when large transfusions
are being given rapidly because they certainly reduce the flow rate.

Fluid overload also should be avoided by central venous pressure
monitoring but this is often set up late in patients after major
injuries. Certainly there is a tendency for some patients to reach
the Intensive Care Unit with an excess of 2-4 litres of crystalloid
which must then be removed by diuretics over the next few days.

Aspiration of gastric contents is likely in all injured patients who
lose consciousness even for a short time. It is all the more likely
since many of these patients have had an excessive alcohol intake.
Suction of the trachea is desirable as soon as possible but many
patients have soiling of the lungs which is not suspected for many
hours after the injury.

Blast lung is a term used rather vaguely for chest problems in
patients involved in explosions but our figures indicate that it was
the diagnosis in only 9 out of 22 bomb victims with respiratory
insufficiency (1971-80). In fact it is only a diagnosis of
exclusion when the above factors do not account for the chest
problems (McCaughey, Coppel and Dundee, 1973).

Patients with primary blast injuries of the lungs present with
dyspnoea of sudden onset and haemoptysis. They may be cyanosed with
moist crepitations in both lung fields. Chest x-ray may reveal
pneumothoraces or bilateral intra-pulmonary haemorrhage and oedema.
External injuries may be extensive or relatively superficial but the
presence of flash burns indicates close proximity to the explosion.

However, having made these general points, injuries following
explosions have been very variable. Some patients have lost two
limbs with little pulmonary disturbance. Others have recovered
after some weeks on ventilation. One girl died with complete
consolidation of both lungs and yet had no external injuries beyond
superficial scratches. Much appears to depend on the way the
patient was facing and the presence of blast-reflecting surfaces.

Certain differentiation of these causes is therefore rarely possible
but fortunately the same general lines of treatment seem to be
applicable. These are:

1. Administration of humidified oxygen to maintain the PaO_2 at an acceptable level. This is sufficient for many patients with fat embolism of a minor degree.

2. Paralysis and IPPV to reduce the work of breathing.

3. Addition of PEEP up to +10 or rarely + 15 cm H_2O to improve arterial oxygenation while keeping the F_1O_2 as low as possible.

The improvement in PaO_2 with PEEP is at the cost of a fall in venous return and cardiac output (Gamble, Coppel and Dundee, 1974). However it has been shown that by ensuring that the blood volume is adequately maintained and by reducing the tidal volume these cardiovascular effects can be minimised. Certainly the introduction of PEEP has been of the greatest benefit in the management of post-traumatic pulmonary insufficiency over the past ten years.

REFERENCES

Clarke, R. S. J., 1981. The management of respiratory trauma, in *Trauma Care* (Eds. Odling-Smee and Crockard), pp 153-173. Academic Press, London.

Coppel, D. L., 1978. The management of chest injuries, in *Medical Management of the Critically Ill* (Eds. Hanson and Wright), pp 386-397. Academic Press, London.

Gamble, J. A. S., Coppel, D. L., and Dundee, J. W., 1974. The cardiorespiratory effects of positive end expiratory pressure at varying tidal volumes. *Proceedings of the First World Congress on Intensive Care*, London, June 1974. p 69.

Gibbons, J., James, O., and Quail, A., 1973. Relief of pain in chest injury. *British Journal of Anaesthesia*, 45, 1136-1138.

Keen, G., 1975. *Chest Injuries*. Wright, Bristol.

McCaughey, W., Coppel, D. L., and Dundee, J. W., 1973. Blast injuries to the lungs: a report of two cases. *Anaesthesia*, 28, 2-9.

Reul, G. J., Beall, A. C., and Greenberg, S. D., 1974. Protection of the pulmonary microvasculature by fine screen blood filtration. *Chest*, 66, 4-9.

Shackford, S. R., Smith, D. E., Zarins, C. K., Rice, C. L., and Virgilio, R. W., 1976. The management of flail chest. A comparison of ventilatory and non-ventilatory treatment. *American Journal of Surgery*, 132, 759-762.

Care of the Acutely Ill and Injured
Edited by D. H. Wilson and A. K. Marsden
© 1982, John Wiley & Sons Ltd.

EXPERIENCE IN THE SURGICAL MANAGEMENT OF TWELVE
CONSECUTIVE WOUNDS OF THE HEART

Ronzani C. and Gennari A.

Clinica Chirurgica 1°, University of Milan, Italy.

ABSTRACT

Twelve consecutive patients with cardiac wounds underwent
emergency surgery between 1970 and 1980.   The diagnosis in each
case was made on the degree of shock, the E.C.G. and the chest
X Ray.   Immediate operation is advised.   Pericardiocentesis is
employed only for diagnosis or the emergency relief of tamponade.

Between 1970 and 1980 twelve patients with wounds of the heart
were operated upon in the Department of Emergency Surgery at the
University of Milan.   Of these patients two had gunshot wounds
(16.6%), two had blunt trauma (16.6%) whilst eight had penetrating
stab wounds (66.8%).

All patients were in haemorrhagic shock on arrival - in two
there was cardiac arrest and in one irreversible cerebral damage
and coma.   Four patients exhibited signs of cardiac tamponade;
venous distension;   raised C.V.P.;   pulsus paradoxus;   muffled
heart sounds and slight enlargement of the non-pulsating cardiac
shadow on fluoroscopic screening.   A chest X Ray invariably
showed haemothorax which often masked the changes in the left
ventricular contour.

All patients showed subepicardial ischaemia on the E.C.G.

An immediate thoracotomy was performed in all patients;   in each
case there was a wound to the pericardium with haemopericardium
and haemothorax.   Cardiac injuries were located in the right
ventricle in four cases;   in the right antrium in four cases;   in
the left ventricle in three cases and in the left antrium in one
case.   One patient had an injury to the left anterior descending
coronary artery.   Six patients had associated wounds - lung,
liver, diaphragm and spleen and, in one case, both colon and
stomach.

Of the twelve patients there were three deaths - an overall
mortality of 25%.   Two patients were operated upon in cardiac
arrest with irreparable injuries to the heart and other organs.
One was in coma because of craniocerebral trauma associated with
injuries to the left atrium, diaphragmatic hernia and splenic
rupture.

TREATMENT

All patients were treated by cardiorrhaphy and the injured
coronary arteries by ligation.   The pericardium was always
incompletely sutured to allow free drainage into the drained
hemithorax.   In one patient who underwent immediate laparotomy
because of serious abdominal injury pericardiocentesis was
required to relieve a cardiac tamponade pending thoracotomy.

CONCLUSIONS

The diagnosis of cardiac trauma is not always easy, mainly because
associated injuries and shock.   Furthermore the classical signs
of cardiac tamponade are not always present.   Nevertheless a
careful observation of the patient, a chest X Ray and an electro-
cardiograph are together often sufficient for a conclusive
diagnosis.   In this way immediate exploratory thoracotomy is
always indicated.

Care of the Acutely Ill and Injured
Edited by D. H. Wilson and A. K. Marsden
© 1982, John Wiley & Sons Ltd.

DIAPHRAGMATIC TRAUMA : REPORT ON 150 CASES.

Augustin Besson FACS, Frédéric Saegesser FACS

Centre Hospitalier Universitaire Vaudois, 1011 CHUV

Lausanne, Switzerland.

Thoracoabdominal trauma is frequent and severe. Young men with a
life-expectancy of 40 years are especially at risk when violently
decelerated.

In a series of 1915 chest trauma cases, 33 % also involve the abdomen. 150 diaphragmatic injuries - open or blunt - were observed.
Type of injuries are as follow : rupture, tear or dehiscence or peripheral avulsion (91 cases), contusion (3), phrenic palsy (12),
post-traumatic relaxation (9) and open wounds (35).

Major cases included 60 left hemidiaphragm rupture (with one effort
rupture), 12 right hemidiaphragm rupture, 1 bilateral rupture, 2
central pericardodiaphragmatic rupture, 8 tear through fractured
ribs and 5 suture line dehiscence, 3 patients in this group where
suspected to suffer diaphragm rupture, but surgery was unrevealing.

Type of accidents resulting in diaphragmatic trauma were : car accidents (35 %), other road traffic accidents (15 %), fall from a
height (6 %), blast or crush-injury (14 %), homicidal or suicidal
attempt (22 %), miscellaneous (8 %).

Mortality was 27 %, but death was unrelated to diaphragm injury in
14 %. The high mortality of blunt trauma (34 %) can be explained
by (a) quick transportation of severely wounded patients, (b) high
incidence (75 %) of multiple wound patients, (c) a number of patients referred to our hospital secundarily.

Diaphragmatic trauma results in various symptoms and signs, most
often severe (or even life-threatening). It is therefore essential
to suspect or to document the diagnosis in the early phase : this
is usually easy in the face of left or right evisceration of abdominal viscera into the chest.

A. Besson and F. Saegesser

THORACIC EVISCERATION OF VISCERA IN DIAPHRAGM RUPTURE (n = 89)

Several viscera can be herniated

Left (n = 71)

Gastrothorax	- uncomplicated	17	
	- compressive	29	48 (68 %)
	- strangulated	1	
	- ruptured	1	
Colothorax	- uncomplicated	18	25 (35 %)
	- tension	7	
Splenothorax	- intact spleen	12	21 (30 %)
	- ruptured spleen	9	
Transdiaphragmatic splenic hemorrhage			5 (7 %)
Evisceration of omentum			15 (21 %)
" small bowel			12 (17 %)
No evisceration or incomplete file			10 (14 %)

Central (into pericardium) (n = 2)

Evisceration of colon and omentum	1

Right (n = 16)

Hepatothorax	- progressive	2	9 (56 %)
	- complete	7	
Transdiaphragmatic hepatic hemorrhage			2 (13 %)
Colothorax	- uncomplicated	2	3 (19 %)
	- strangulated	1	
Evisceration of omentum			1 (6 %)
" stomach			1 (6 %)
" small bowel			1 (6 %)
" kidney			1 (6 %)
No evisceration or incomplete file			4 (25 %)

Associated injuries are frequently encountered; they are helpful in diagnosis and are of prognostic significance. Surgical treatment is mandatory in most instances of diaphragmatic trauma. Indications to surgery are known. Laparotomy is often the best approach to repair the left diaphragmatic injuries as well as concomitant trauma to abdominal viscera. Thoracotomy is more appropriate for right injuries. Procedures are relatively easy to perform when diagnosis is made early; late cases require different tactical approach and more complicated surgery.

*

Complete reference on the subject can be obtained from the authors on request or in chapter 10 of : CHEST TRAUMA, a colour atlas and textbook for surgeons, radiologists, epidemiologists and the intensive care or emergency room teams. Wolfe, London, to appear in early 1982.

Care of the Acutely Ill and Injured
Edited by D. H. Wilson and A. K. Marsden
© 1982, John Wiley & Sons Ltd.

RUPTURE OF THE RIGHT HEMIDIAPHRAGM

V. Pezzangora, R. Barina, A. Saggioro,
M. Rizzo, S. Vattolo and V. Averno

Umberto I Hospital, 1st Department of Surgery
Venezia-Mestre, Italy.

ABSTRACT

Ruptures of the right diaphragm are rare conditions accounting for
only 10-13% of all post traumatic diaphragmatic rupture. Three
cases are described and diagnostic and treatment methods discussed.

INTRODUCTION

Road trauma has resulted in an increased incidence of diaphragmatic
rupture. It is, however, suprising to note how often such lesions
are misinterpreted or unrecognised. The majority of cases are of
rupture of the left hemi diaphragm (83 to 90% according to the
literature) and only rarely is the right hemi diaphragm involved.
Here the diagnostic problems are considerably more complex and
definitive diagnosis often made only in the operating theatre.

METHODS

Between 1971 and 1980 twenty three cases of ruptured diaphragm were
studied. With the exception of a patient who fell from scaffolding
all cases resulted from road accidents. Of the 23 cases 20 involved
the left diaphragm and only three the right. Associated pathology
was as follows:

	Number of pts.	%
Head Injury	7	30.4
Bony injuries	8	34.8
Rib fractures	19	82.6
Splenic rupture	3	13.0
Liver rupture	5	21.7
Other visceral rupture	3	13.0
Shock	20	85.9

There was a delay in diagnosis ranging from two hours to two days.

We used a simple diagnostic test which gave true positive results
in 95% cases and false positives in 2% : A nasogastric tube is
inserted and connected to a water manometer. The oscillations of
the liquid gauge are observed in relation to respiratory movements.
If a ruptured diaphragm exists the negative intrathoracic pressures

211

will be referred to the stomach and hence to the monometer system. The sensitivity of the test can be increased by asking the patient to take a deep breath out.

RESULTS

We treated three cases of rupture of the right hemi diaphragm with no mortality.

Diagnosis was made pre-operatively in one case only.   Peritoneal lavage proved essential in indicating emergency surgery in the other two cases.

In all three patients there were fractures of the right ribs.

There are no pathognomonic features of right hemi diaphragmatic rupture on radiological examination but some signs, if present, may point towards the diagnosis.   These include modification of the diaphragmatic profile;   convex opacity at the lung base and mediastinal displacement.

Surgery comprised repair of the diaphragmatic breach at separate points in a U-shape with sutures of nonabsorbable material.

CONCLUSIONS

Diagnosis of rupture of the right half of the diaphragm is substantially different from that of the left.   Peritoneal lavage is an important indicant of emergency laparotomy.   The surgical approach will be influenced by the presence of associated lesions but must be sufficiently adequate to allow exposure of the abdominal contents.

REFERENCES

Fontaine R. et al., 1966. Le poumon et le coeur. 22, 1-47
Harrington S. W., 1950. S. Clin. North Amer. 30, 961
State D., 1949. Surgery. 25, 461
Thibault J. C. G., These strasbourlt. 1964. IV, 11

Care of the Acutely Ill and Injured
Edited by D. H. Wilson and A. K. Marsden
© 1982, John Wiley & Sons Ltd.

THE THERAPEUTIC APPROACH TO THORACO-ABDOMINAL INJURIES

I.Suteu, M.Soare and Gh.Popovici

IInd Surgical Clinic, Emergency Clinical Hospital
Bucharest, Romania.

ABSTRACT

During the period 1972-1979, 139 patients with thoraco-abdominal
injuries were admitted to this Clinic.   Of these 89 (65.9%)had
closed thoraco-abdominal trauma and 50 (34%) open chest and
abdominal wounds.

INTRODUCTION

Patients with thoraco-abdominal injuries exhibit complex lesions
of viscera and bodily systems - frequently the diaphragm is
involved.   Numerous authors (e.g. Oancea 1975, Lazar 1973) have
emphasised the gravity of this condition but have only described
a small number of cases.

METHODS

We retrospectively examined the records of 139 patients with
thoraco-abdominal wounding, investigating the type of injury;
age;   causation;   accident to admission to surgery time;   type
and number of concomitant injuries and surgical techniques.

RESULTS

Road accidents were the cause of 61 cases of wounding (43.9%) and
firearms of 42 cases (30.2%).   Most patients were aged between
21 and 50 years.   Sixty eight patients were admitted three hours
after the accident.

Depending upon the degree of shock patients were received in the
reception unit, the resuscitation/intensive care service or
directly in the operating theatre.   98 patients (70.5%) were
operated upon within the first three hours after admission.

Multiple, complex and associated lesions were found on clinical
or radiological examination.   There were multiple rib fractures
in 78 cases '56%);   haemopneumothorax in 108 cases (77.7%); splenic
injuries in 65 cases (43.9%);   liver injuries in 42 cases (30.2%)
and diaphragmatic tears in 48 cases (34.5%).   All patients had
more than one organ injuried, some as many as six.   71 cases
(50%) had three organs involved.

The severity of injuries increased with the number of associated lesions - a mortality rate of 80% was seen when six organs were injuried.   The overall mortality was 15.1% - twenty one of the 139 patients.

The surgical approach depended upon the site and disposition of the injuries.   We performed minimal pleurotomy and laparotomy in 69 cases (50%);   laparotomy alone in 43 cases (31%).   In 19 cases thoracotomy followed by immediate laparotomy was required and in 4 cases thoracoabdominal laparotomy dividing the diaphragm.

DISCUSSION

Patients with thoracoabdominal injuries present complex lesions involving two or more organs requiring emergency surgery.   The approaches of thoracotomy, laparotomy or thoracophrenolaparotomy were dictated by the clinical picture established preoperatively.

REFERENCES

Lazar C. et al., 1973.   Experienta Clinicii I chirurgicale lasi in politraumatismele cu predominanta toracica si abdominala, Al Xlll-lea Congres national de chirurgie, Bucuresti. 194-195.

Oancea Tr. et al. 1975. Traumatismele toracelui, Edit. militara, Bucuresti. 441-462. 472-477.

Care of the Acutely Ill and Injured
Edited by D. H. Wilson and A. K. Marsden
© 1982, John Wiley & Sons Ltd.

PROBLEMS IN THE MANAGEMENT OF LIVER
TRAUMA

R.Grundmann

Chirurgische Universitätsklinik Köln-
Lindenthal, Joseph-Stelzmann-Str. 9,
D-5000 Köln 41, Germany

In the last ten years we treated 66 patients with liver
trauma. 55 of these patients had blunt and 11 patients
penetrating liver wounds. The penetrating wounds were
caused by knifing or gun shots, whereas the blunt liver
injury was mainly due to road traffic accidents. The extent of injuries and the concomitant injuries are given
in table 1.

TABLE 1

	penetrating injuries (n=11)		blunt injuries (n=55)	
	number n	lethal (n)	number n	lethal (n)
Extent of injury				
- superficial lacerations	8	(0)	9	(2)
- deep rupture	3	(0)	32	(19)
- serious disruption	0	(0)	14	(12)
Concomitant injuries				
0	6	(0)	4	(3)
1	5	(0)	15	(8)
$\leqq$ 2	0	(0)	36	(22)
Therapy				
- suture and drainage	11	(0)	36	(18)
- resection of liver lobe	-	-	7	(4)
- tamponade and coagulation	-	-	4	(3)
- lig. a. hepatica	-	-	2	(2)
- no	-	-	6	(6)

RESULTS

The results are summarized in table 1. The main causes of
death were shock and its sequelae in 25 patients. 10 of
these patients died due to uncontrollable liver bleeding
and 8 patients due to other uncontrollable hemorrhage.
The mortality rate depended on the number of concomitant
injuries, the mortality rate increased from 40 to 100% if

4 additional injuries instead of 1 were present. A clear
correlation between the mortality rate and the degree of
blood loss (given as the number of the perioperatively
transfused units of stored blood) could be detected: the
mortality rate increased from 29 to 72% if 4 or more
units of blood instead of 1 had to be given. Finally a
significant correlation between the age of the patients
and the mortality rate could be demonstrated.

POSTOPERATIVE COMPLICATIONS

25 of 46 patients surviving more than 1 day developed
postoperative complications. Pneumonia occured most
commonly (n=11) and 4 patients consequently died. Wound
infections were relatively rare (n=6), as were also peri-
hepatic abscesses (n=4). Liver abscesse or liver failure
were not postoperatively observed.

DISCUSSION

The prognosis of liver trauma depends most decisively on
the type of injury. In our patients all penetrating
wounds were survived whereas the mortality rate of blunt
injury was about 60%. This means that statistics compiled
on the mortality rate of liver trauma in general are misleading, the proportion of blunt and penetrating liver
wounds must be indicated. The high mortality rate of our
patients with serious liver disruption can be referred
back to the concomitant injuries that unfavourably affected the outcome. Besides this the prognosis depended on
the age of the patients, older patients do not possess
sufficient energy reserves to compensate hemorrhagic
shock and its sequelae. Nevertheless these two factors
are not the only cause of the high mortality rate, on the
contrary, it must be admitted that in 10 of 55 patients
with blunt liver injury a rapid control of bleeding did
not succeed and consequently in these cases uncontrollable liver bleeding was the main cause of death. This
brings to discussion the therapeutic procedure in the
case of serious blunt liver injury: the rapid control of
bleeding has to be the center of all efforts. Different
techniques have been described for this. If additional
intraabdominal injuries are present and the operative
field is unclear, subdiaphragmatic clamping of the aorta
is recommended for control of bleeding. However, by this
step renal blood flow is also cut off. Therefore the
clamping of the liver hilus, Pringle's maneuver, should
be preferred in all cases where bleeding is mainly due to
liver injury. The ischemic tolerance of the human liver
is excellent and therefore one has 30 mins to 1 hr to
carry out the final treatment of the liver wound. Before
clamping the liver hilus we administer to the patient 1 g
of methyl-prednisolone since it was possible in rat experiments to improve the hepatic ischemic tolerance in

this way (Wienand, Grundmann, Wahl and Pichlmaier, 1980).

Another possibility of rapid control of bleeding consists
in hepatic compression which can be performed either bi-
manually or with tourniquets.

The definite treatment of the liver wound has to be performed according to the extent of the trauma. Several
procedures are available: the suture of the liver wound -
the more or less extensive removal of the crushed tissue
(the debridement) - the complete resection of the destroyed liver lobe (hepatic lobectomy) - finally hepatic
artery ligation or embolisation, resp..

What type of procedure should be performed in a particular
case?
The final treatment of the liver wound has to be as spa-
ring as possible and therefore suture and drainage should
be preferred to all other procedures. If the bleeding does
not end after suture, a pedicled omentum flap which serves
as tamponade can be sewn on the liver wound. The extensive
removal of the crushed tissue (debridement) is only indicated in those cases where multiple lacerations of the
liver exist. In these cases the removal of the devital-
ized tissue is thought to lower the risk of infection and
abscess formation. On the other hand the risk of liver abscess must not be overemphasized, particulary, since these
abscesses can be drained relatively easily in a second
operation. It should also be remarked that we did not find
any abscess formation which made a second operation necessary.

As regards hepatic lobectomy it has to be emphasized that
this procedure is seldom necessary in cases of liver
trauma. Liver resection is apparently an ideal operation,
allowing a rapid control of bleeding and preventing later
complications such as abscess formation. The circumstances during liver resection for trauma are however fundamentally different from those during liver resection for
tumor or hydatid disease. In many patients there are
numerous concomitant injuries, and hemorrhagic shock and
its sequelae aggravate the initial situation of the patient. The prognosis of liver resection due to trauma
is therefore serious and this procedure can be recommended for selected cases only. We would perform liver resection in those cases where multiple lacerations of one
liver lobe exist, especially lacerations of the right
liver lobe with bleeding of the retrohepatic vena cava.
In this situation we were able to control the bleeding in
3 patients by right hepatic lobectomy. These patients had
no postoperative complications.

In a few isolated cases, when both liver lobes are injured
the ligation of the hepatic artery can be used for both
control of the bleeding and as final therapy. Aaron (1975)
and Flint (1977) recommend this procedure in those cases

where suture and tamponade failed to control the hemorrhage. We were also able to use this procedure successfully in two patients. In man the risk of liver failure
due to hepatic artery ligation is relatively low, after
ligation of the artery the utilization of the portal
vein oxygen concentration increases. Consequently, after
hepatic artery ligation only a short-term rise of the
serum-transaminase concentration is seen. Nevertheless,
the mortality rate after ligation of the hepatic artery
was relatively high in the cases reported so far, but
this was mainly caused by the concomitant injuries in
these patients. Therefore, we intend to argue against hepatic artery ligation not because of the risk of this
procedure, but on account of its effect: In the case that
the liver lobe lacerations are so extensive that they can
not be treated successfully with suture and tamponade,
the effect of hepatic artery ligation is also restricted.
This is based on the fact that in most of these cases the
hepatic veins are also injured, and the bleeding of the
veins can not be treated by artery ligation.

CONCLUSIONS

The final treatment of a liver wound is determined by the
extent of the trauma. The therapy has to be as conservative as possible. In the case that suture and drainage
of the wound are not successful, clamping of the hepatic
artery should be tried. If the bleeding stops, hepatic
artery ligation can be consequently performed. If this
procedure also fails liver lobe resection is indicated.

REFERENCES

Aaron,S., Fulton,R.L.,and Mays,E.T., 1975. Selevtive li-
    gation of the hepatic artery for trauma of the liver.
    Surg. Gynecol. Obstet., 141, 187 - 189.
Flint,L.M., Mays,E.T., Aaron,W.S., Fulton,R.L.,and Polk,
    H.C., 1977. Selectivity in the management of hepatic
    trauma. Ann. Surg., 185, 613 - 618.
Wienand,R., Grundmann,R., Wahl,K., and Pichlmaier,H.,1980
    Die Steroidschutzwirkung auf die ischämische Ratten-
    leber, in Experimentelle und Klinische Hepatologie
    (Eds. Zelder, Fischer, Eckert and Bode), pp 175 - 180.
    Georg Thieme Verlag Stuttgart·New York.

Care of the Acutely Ill and Injured
Edited by D. H. Wilson and A. K. Marsden
© 1982, John Wiley & Sons Ltd.

STUDY OF 520 ACUTE THORACO-ABDOMINAL INJURIES WITH LIVER AND BILIARY TRAUMA

P.Blidaru, M.Ciuta, R.Dop and A.Blidaru

IInd Surgical Clinic, Emergency Clinical Hospital Bucharest, Romania

ABSTRACT

The present paper, based on ample experimentation in swine is a retrospective clinico-statistical study of 520 cases of thoraco-abdominal injuries with hepato-biliary involvement. Classical and modern therapeutical procedures were applied and, in a restricted number of cases, 2 techniques used in experimental surgery.

INTRODUCTION

The increased incidence of liver injuries in multiple trauma and the high mortality rate of 10-80% in terms of the associated lesions, demand careful study of the morphofunctional alterations and therapeutical principles.

METHODS

In 4 animal lots, total or partial clamping of the liver pedicles was permanently or intermittently performed in hypothermia and hypobarism. Under protection of THAM and hypertonic glucose solutions clamping was prolonged up to 57-58 minutes without microscopically detectable hepatic lesions. Wounds of various extent and depth were produced then covered by pedicled diaphragmatic flaps (wounds of the convex aspect of the liver) thus realizing a haemostatic phrenohepatorraphy (Blidaru technique, figs. 1,2,3). Wounds on the inferior aspect of the liver were covered with free split skin grafts for compaction, contention, haemostasis and biliostasis, hence using autogenous, heterotopic, homovital grafts (figs. 4,5).

RESULTS

Phrenohepatorraphy gave very good results. The skin grafts were fixed with absorbable suture or simple application on the damaged liver;

the grafts readily "took" and realized spontaneous haemostasis and biliostasis. It is suggested that richness of the dermal collagen and hepatic fibrinogen contributed to this host-graft complex.Macroscopic and microscopic control by second look or by sacrificing the animals at 24 and 48 hours, and 7, 30 and 60 days after grafting, revealed perfect adherence of the dermal connective tissue to the liver parenchyma. By extrapolation of the two procedures to human traumatology satisfactory compaction, haemostasis and biliostasis were obtained (fig.6: microscopic image 60 days after grafting showing perfect coalescence between the skin graft and liver host).

DISCUSSION

Swine liver is increasingly used for hepatic clearance and transplantations. The original therapeutical procedures experimented by the first author in swine and extrapolated to the human clinic with good results, lend further support to this study,

REFERENCES

Blidaru, P., 1977. Contributions au traitment des traumatismes hépatiques par hématophrenoraphie et autogreffes cutanées, III Congrès Intern.de Chirurgie d'Urgence, Paris, 105.

Blidaru, P., 1974. Traumatismele complexe hepatice.   Doctor'thesis.

Blidaru, P., 1975. Le traitement des hémorragies hépatiques au moyen d'un transplant de peaux (derm), Journées Médicales Balkaniques, V-ème Session Athenes.

Blidaru,P., 1977. Traumatismele hepatice, Ed.Acad.RSR.

Blidaru,P., Cherchez, E. and Dop R., 1978. Appréciations thérapeutiques sur les traumatismes hépatiques complexes. Congresso nazionale Societa Italiana di Chirurgia d'urgenza, Milano,25-28 July.

Blidaru.P., Popescu,I. and Blidaru A., 1981. Particularita diagnostiche e terapeutice dei traumi epatobiliary chiusi. Incontri Internationali di Chirurgie, Milano, 10-13 Maggio.

Suteu, I. and Blidaru, P. 1977. Appréciations clinico-thérapéutiques sur 395 traumatismes hépato-biliaires, III Congrès Intern. de Chirurgie d'Urgence, Paris, Juin.

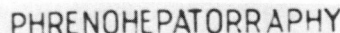

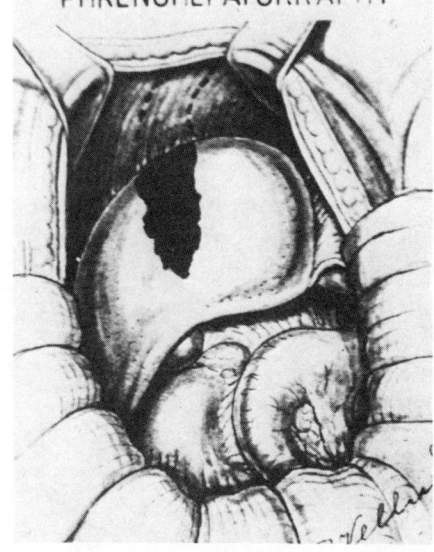

Figure 1
Wound on Upper Aspect of Liver

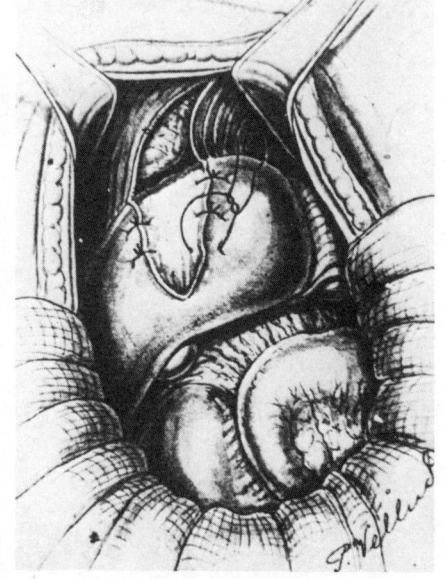

Figure 2
Grafting of Diaphragmatic Flap

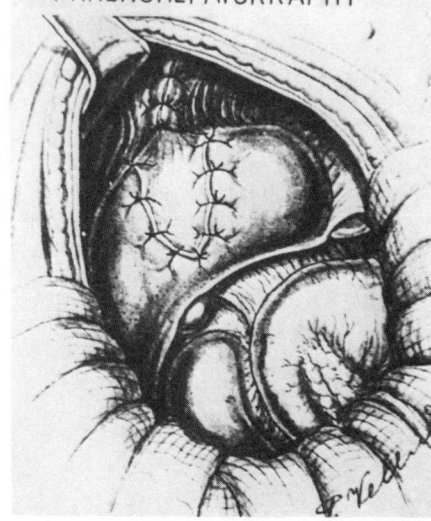

Figure 3
Completion of Phrenohepatorraphy
and Suture of Diaphragm

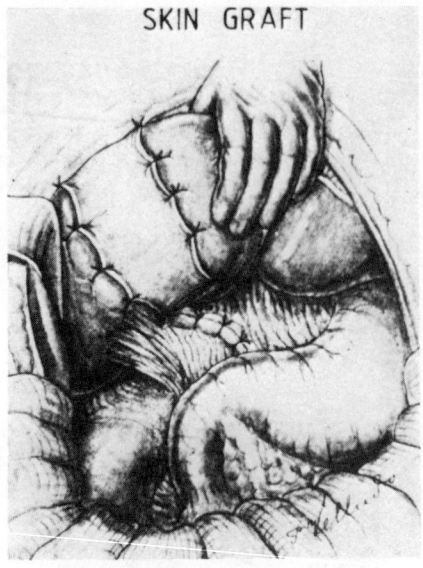

Figure 4
Suturing of Skin Graft Hemostasis
and Biliostasis

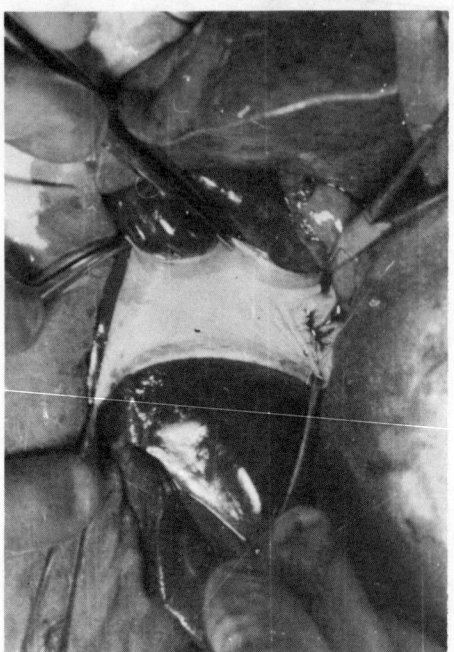

Figure 5
Skin Graft - Blidaru Technique

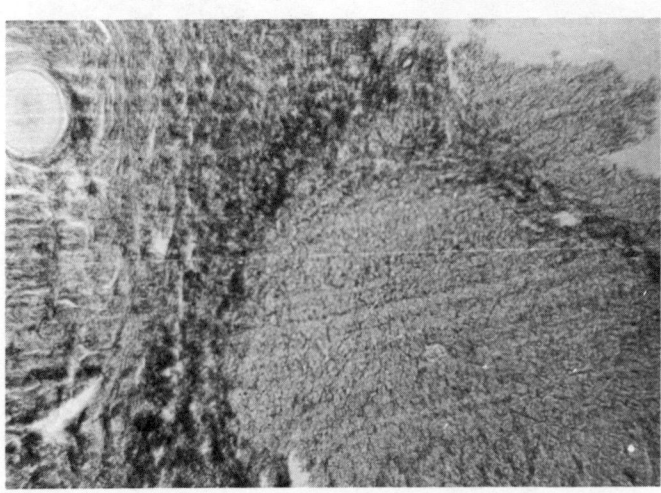

Figure 6
Histology 60
days after
grafting

Care of the Acutely Ill and Injured
Edited by D. H. Wilson and A. K. Marsden
© 1982, John Wiley & Sons Ltd.

CONSERVATIVE TREATMENT OF THE RUPTURED SPLEEN

H. Green

University of the Witwatersrand,
Johannesburg Hospital, Johannesburg, South Africa

Splenectomy has been performed for 350 years with apparently satisfactory results.

The preventive role of the spleen was demonstrated by King and Shummaker in 1952, and its relevance to splenectomy for trauma since 1957. Today the condition of Post Splenectomy Fulminant Infection (P.S.F.I.) is accepted.

To put it into its correct perspective P.S.F.I. :-

1.   Is a relatively uncommon condition.

2.   It occurs more frequently after splenectomy for haematological conditions.

3.   It occurs mainly in the young and the incidence decreases with time.

Nevertheless P.S.F.I. can occur 20 years or more after splenectomy and the incidence never reaches zero.

It is imperative to administer pneumococcal vaccine. However there is some evidence to suggest that the vaccine is less effective after splenectomy. The patient is thus still exposed to some pneumococci and other organisms involved in P.S.F.I.

One can conclude that the spleen should, where possible, be preserved partially or completely in the young. When practicable and safe, it should also be preserved in whole or part in the adult.

NON-OPERATIVE TREATMENT.

It has been shown that in the paediatric patient, splenic lacerations can be treated conservatively. Is this applicable to the adult?

a)   Often, on operating for splenic injury the bleeding has stopped.

b)   It is probable that the spleen is injured - not diagnosed - and so treated conservatively.

c)   The spleen is occasionally damaged during upper abdominal
            procedures and bleeding frequently stops.

We thus adopted a policy of non-operative treatment in patients in
whom we have diagnosed splenic injury - confirmed by scan and/or
arteriography, provided that:-

1.   The spleen is the only organ injured.

2.   The patient is haemodynamically stable and does not
            deteriorate.

3.   Frequent clinical reassessment is satisfactory.

4.   Bowel sounds do not disappear.

5.   Lavage fluid does not contain bile, amylase, organisms or
            faecal debris.

6.   X-ray does not show free gas.

Seven cases have so far been treated non-operatively, and without
complications.

CONSERVATIVE SURGERY.

This implies leaving the whole spleen, or as much as possible in
situ. The splenic artery usually divides into two branches and then
segmental arteries supply its own segment. These are end arteries.

Experiments on post mortem spleen and in clinical situations, have
shown that segmental artery ligation will stop the bleeding in that
segment. Using this procedure, we have been able to save, in whole
or part about 50% of spleens submitted to laparotomy.

By further extension one can ligate the main branches or even the
main splenic artery. This can be done with relative impunity.

Thereafter, but usually not necessary, the injuries can be sutured
or resection carried out in an avascular or relatively avascular
area.

The procedure is safe, rapid and does not need splenic mobilization.

A plea is made for consideration of non-operative treatment in
selected individuals, and a conservative approach when the damaged
spleen is found at operation.

Care of the Acutely Ill and Injured
Edited by D. H. Wilson and A. K. Marsden
© 1982, John Wiley & Sons Ltd.

PANCREATIC TRAUMA

C. A. Giani, Chief - Emergency Department

Santojanni Hospital
Pilar 950
1408 Buenos Aires, Argentina

ABSTRACT

The surgical approach and postoperative results in 26 patients
presenting Pancreatic Trauma (PT) are discussed. Major complications arose in 13 patients of whom 5 subsequently died. In 19 cases
PT was associated with visceral, vascular or parietal injuries.
Traumatic agents included blunt trauma (8) and penetrating wounds
(18). Of the latter, 4 were iatrogenic trauma , 6 were bullet wounds
and 8 were stab wounds. 8 were caudal, 5 corporal, 1 cephalic and
caudal, 9 duodeno-cephalic and 3 cephalic localised.

INTRODUCTION

In emergency surgery, a broad tactical approach is essential in view
of the unpredictable nature of the patients' condition. Patients
presenting with accidental or criminal injuries require the surgeon
to use his imagination, to improvise and to be creative. PT is one
of the most severe consequences of accidental or criminal injury.
This paper demonstrates the value of a schematic approach to surgery
involving this class of patient and discusses the relevance of such
an approach in a wide range of conditions.

MATERIALS AND METHODS

The cases described consisted of 26 individuals all of whom were
receiving medical treatment prior to pre-operative investigation.
Each patient was maintained and monitored in an intensive care unit.
The body fluids obtained as a result of abdominal paracentesis were
used to reinforce decisions on early laparotomy. Where PT was
observed during surgery, whether as a disruption or a haematoma, the
postoperative medication was administered according to the normal
routine for patients with acute pancreatitis.

RESULTS

Table 1 shows the outcome of the 8 different surgical procedures
used to treat PT, in 26 cases. In 10 cases one additional operation
was required and in two cases a third intervention was necessary
(* in the Table).

TABLE 1.   Relation between surgical method, morbidity and mortality

Operation	Cases	Major Complic.	Deaths
Duodenopancreatectomy*	2	2	2
Corporocaudal pancreatectomy or pancreatosplenectomy (Walton 1923)	4	2	1
Caudopancreatectomy with splenectomy	8	3	1
Cephalic Duodenopancreatectomy	1	0	0
Cholecistectomy, choledocus drainage with T tube and Wirsung drainage (Doubilet and Mulholland 1959)	2	1	1
Duodenal suture, antrectomy, precolic gastrojejunal anastomose and vagotomy plus cholecistectomy and T drainage of the bile duct	4	2	0
Duodenal diverticulisation	4	2	0
Splenectomy, hepatic and gastric suture, and pancreatic lodge drainage	1	1	0
Total	26	13	5

DISCUSSION

The study shows a 19% mortality rate in PT surgery which is within
the limits found at other centres throughout the world (Bach and
Frey, 1971). Half of the patients suffered major complications
including 6 individuals who developed post-traumatic acute pancreatitis. Three patients in this latter group died. Of 12 patients
who underwent distal pancreatectomies, only 2 died. Implant of
distal remaining pancreas in the jejunum was performed once, with
success. Late total duodenopancreatectomy failed in 2 cases of
second reoperation, demonstrating that an earlier aggressive tactic
may have been necessary. The Table emphasizes the range of surgical
resources which must be available to a surgeon dealing with cases of
PT.

REFERENCES

Bach, R. D. and Frey, C. F. 1971. Diagnosis and treatment of
    pancreatic trauma. American Journal of Surgery 121, pp 20.
Doubilet, H. and Mulholland, J. H. 1963. Some observations on the
    treatment of trauma to the pancreas. American Journal of Surgery
    105, pp 741.
Walton, J. J. 1923. A textbook of surgical dyspepsias. London,
    Edward Arnold and Co.

Care of the Acutely Ill and Injured
Edited by D. H. Wilson and A. K. Marsden
© 1982, John Wiley & Sons Ltd.

BLUNT TRAUMA OF THE PANCREAS

J.E.Murat, J.L.Bernard, J.L. Vaur, N.Huten and
L.Debbiche

Emergency Department University of Tours School of
Medicine, F 37044 Tours cedex

ABSTRACT

The results of two groups of patients with blunt trauma of the
pancreas operated by the same team from 1969 to 1974 and 1975
to 1981 allow observations of changes occurring in the management
and re-evaluation of treatment of pancreatic trauma.

INTRODUCTION

Previous work of Graham and Jordan (1) and us (2) has demonstrated
the uncertainty of diagnosis and sometimes initial treatment.

METHODS

32 consecutive patients from 17 years old up to 75 were studied.
There was neither difference in the frequency of incidence of
blunt injuries between the two periods nor in associated lesions
(spleen, duodenum, kidney ahead of major vascular division).
Anatomical classification has been performed and computed against
treatments and results as shown in Table 1.

RESULTS

Excepting injuries to the portal vein or the vessels around the
head, early surgery for the injured pancreas carries a better
prognosis than the delayed case when pancreatitis may have
developed.   Two cases which were not operated on until 4 or 5
days after injury succumbed to necrotising pancreatitis.

Distal pancreatectomy is a safe and simple procedure for injuries
of the body and tail - either as a primary procedure (10 cases)
or after failure of drainage procedures in presumed superficial
pancreatic contusion (7 cases).

Whipple's procedure is reserved for severe vascular and duodenal
laceration of the head of pancreas (1 case).

Subtotal left to right pancreatico-jejunostomies performed
elsewhere for pancreatic trauma gave poor results and had to be
secondarily revised.

227

228   J.E. Murat et al

Cystojejunostomy was used once as a secondary procedure.

Total or sub-total pancreatectomy for lesions with secondary total pancreatitis may be excessive - instead laparostomy (abdominal open-wound technique) should be contemplated for the repeated removal of necrosis (one case was able to be re-opened four times).

Complications (the major being pancreatitis fistulae) led to reoperation in eight cases (one third of the series). There were seven deaths mainly resulting from necrotic pancreatitis or from severe haemorrhage from associated lesions.

TABLE I. Results of 32 pancreatic blunt trauma.

LESIONS (right/left)	PRIMARY TREATMENT				PRIMARY RESULTS	SECONDARY TREATMENT	SECONDARY RESULTS
Contusion R 6	6				2 cyst.⎱ 2 D. ⎰	1 anast.	
L 3	2		1		2 pancr.	2 left P.	1 D.
Tears R 7	7				2 fail.⎱ 2 D. ⎰	1 left P.	1 fail.
L 3	3				2 fail.	2 left P.	1 fail.
Rupture R 0 / L 9		2	7		2 cyst.	2 left P.	1 D.
Laceration R 2	1			1	1 pancr.	1 open-wound	1 D.
L 2			2				
TOTAL : 32	19	2	10	1	4 D. 8 fail.	1 anast. 7 left P.	3 D. 2 fail.

TOTAL | 23 good results (no pain - no cyst)
2 failures
7 deaths

REFERENCES

Graham J.M., Mattox K.L. and Jordan G.L. Traumatic Injuries of the pancreas. Am.J.Surg. 136. 744-748. 1978.
Murat J.E., Crassas Y. and Debbiche L. Les contusions du pancreas. Evolution therapeutique d'aspres 17 cas personnels. Rev.Fr. Gastro-entero. 101. 5-18. 1974.

Care of the Acutely Ill and Injured
Edited by D. H. Wilson and A. K. Marsden
© 1982, John Wiley & Sons Ltd.

TRAUMATIC INJURY TO THE PANCREAS :
ANGIOGRAPHIC DIAGNOSIS

L.Bresadola and G.Pompa

Clinica chirurgica d'Urgenza e di Pronto Soccorso
Universita degli Studi di Roma

ABSTRACT

During the past three years we have employed angiography in the
diagnosis of nine cases of pancreatic trauma.   Six were emergency
cases and the other three used the technique for the late
investigation of post traumatic abdominal complications.

INTRODUCTION

The emergence in recent years of new investigative tools has
raised the diagnosed incidence of pancreatic lesions in abdominal
trauma from 2-4% to 12-19%.   Early diagnosis permits selective
surgical treatment which reduces the risk of serious complications.

METHOD AND RESULTS

At our centre we have performed emergency angiography in 84 patients
with blunt abdominal trauma : in 71 cases we were able to
diagnose the lesion, of which six cases (8.5%) were pancreatic.
Three cases of pancreatic trauma were identified by angiography
in investigating late complications.

DISCUSSION

The angiographic patterns of pancreatic lesions depend upon the
anatomical arrangements of vascular and canalicular channels.
These are differently distorted in recent or late trauma and
relate to the nature of the distorting force (contusion,laceration,
rupture and crushing) and the side of the pancreas affected.

Features of recent trauma

a) Massive extravasation of contrast medium as "puddles".
b) Limited extravasation as "little spots" near the major arteries.
c) Compression and/or interruption of vessels.
d) Kinking of vessels.

Features of late complications

a) In oedematous pancreatitis there may be perivascularisation,
    enlargement of vessels and indirect signs of compression.
b) In late necrotising haemorrhagic pancreatitis the arteries are

229

few and irregular or can produce an extravasation of contrast
medium as "puddles".

c) In chronic pancreatitis there may be parietal and/or luminal
irregularities with diffuse opacities - these changes though
are unlike those seen in generalised neoplasia.

d) In Pseudocysts the angiographic patterns are represented by
vessels stretching around a totally avascular mass.   There may
be arterial irregularity : compression and/or apparent
obstruction of the splenic vein.   The most interesting signs
to be occasionally seen are of associated lesions to the
pseudocysts - these include pseudoaneurysm, carcinomata,
cystoadenomata and extra-hepatic portal hypertension.

CONCLUSION

The present study shows the importance of angiography in the
diagnosis of pancreatic trauma - it should be used more routinely
in patients with suspected abdominal lesions.

Care of the Acutely Ill and Injured
Edited by D. H. Wilson and A. K. Marsden
© 1982, John Wiley & Sons Ltd.

A PROSPECTIVE TRIAL OF BLOOD CELL COUNTS
AND AMYLASE ESTIMATION IN BLOOD AND
PERITONEAL LAVAGE AFTER BLUNT TRAUMA

J. G. Mosley and C. R. Pascall

Department of Surgery,
Norfolk and Norwich Hospital,
Norwich, Norfolk, UK

INTRODUCTION

The clinical diagnosis of intraperitoneal injury after blunt
abdominal trauma is difficult. It is often complicated by the
presence of a head injury and multiple fractures. Several retrospective studies of blood counts and amylase in blood and peritoneal
lavage have been reported (Berman 1957, Steele 1975, Donovan 1972)
although the results lack consistency. We therefore designed a
simple prospective trial to elucidate any correlation between injury
to spleen and liver, haemoperitoneum, blood loss and white cell
count; and also to evaluate the relationship between serum and
peritoneal lavage amylase and pancreatic injury.

METHODS

We used the following groups: 1. Patients with suspected intraperitoneal injury. 2. Patients admitted acutely after a haematemesis
and/or melaena and who required transfusion. 3. Patients admitted
with a ruptured ectopic pregnancy who required transfusion. After
taking a history and examining the patients, a full blood count and
serum amylase were estimated. In the trauma group, peritoneal lavage
was performed (Root 1965). An aliquot of recovered fluid was sent
for full blood count and amylase estimation. The total blood
replacement was recorded and the patients were followed up to
discharge or post mortem to record a final diagnosis. The results
were analysed statistically by students 't' test, significance taken
to be p 0.05.

RESULTS

Table 1 shows that the average white cell count in the trauma group
with intraperitoneal bleeding was significantly higher than in any of
the other groups. The white cell count elevation in the trauma group
with intraperitoneal bleeding was not related to the amount of blood
lost, but was more consistently elevated in patients who had lost
least blood. The control groups do not show a marked increase in
white cell count which suggests that the stimulus for the elevated
white count is not simply blood loss and not simply free blood in the
peritoneal cavity.

J. G. Mosley and C. R. Pascall

Table 2 shows that the average serum and peritoneal lavage amylase in patients with a ruptured pancreas was significantly higher than in patients with an intact pancreas after trauma.

TABLE 1. Serum white and red cell counts on admission

	R.C.C.	W.C.C.
Trauma with I.P. bleeding n = 12	4.55 ∓ 0.25	17.75 ∓ 1.63
Trauma without I.P. bleeding n = 9	5.1 ∓ 0.3	13.72 ∓ 1.21
G.I. bleeding n = 11	3.2 ∓ 0.3	10.5 ∓ 1.0
Ruptured ectopic pregnancies n = 8	4.95 ∓ 0.15	13.7 ∓ 1.1

Values = mean $\mp$ standard error

TABLE 2. Serum and peritoneal lavage amylase

	Serum Amylase	Peritoneal Lavage Amylase
Trauma with ruptured pancreas n = 5	590 ∓ 370	95 ∓ 30
Trauma with intact pancreas n = 16	75 ∓ 15	15 ∓ 8

Values = mean $\mp$ standard error

CONCLUSION

We feel that a white cell count more than $16,000/mm^3$ after possible abdominal trauma may well indicate intraperitoneal injury and that if laparotomy is not already indicated, peritoneal lavage should be carried out.

A raised serum amylase or peritoneal lavage amylase is highly suggestive of a pancreatic injury.

REFERENCES

Berman, J. K., et al. Blood studies as an aid in differential diagnosis of abdominal trauma. J.A.M.A., (1957), 165, p.1537 - 1541.
Donovan, A. J., et al. Surgical Clinics in North America 1972, 52, p.649 - 665.
Root, H. D., et al. Diagnostic peritoneal lavage. Surgery, (1965), 57, p.633 - 638.
Steele, M. and Lim, R. C. Advances in management of splenic injuries. Am. J. Surg, (1975), 130, p.159 - 165.

Care of the Acutely Ill and Injured
Edited by D. H. Wilson and A. K. Marsden
© 1982, John Wiley & Sons Ltd.

EMERGENCY TREATMENT IN INJURIES OF THE PANCREAS

I.Suteu, M.Ciurel, P.Blidaru, A.Bucur, R.Florescu
and D.Culică

IInd Surgical Clinic, Emergency Clinical Hospital
Bucharest, Romania

ABSTRACT

The present study refers to 49 cases of injuries of the pancreas
caused by abdominal trauma, admitted and treated in the Clinic
between 1960 and 1979; 89% of the cases presented multiple associated
lesions, which increased the gravity of the cases producing concmi-
tant traumatic shock and acute hypovolemia.

INTRODUCTION

The frequency of abdominal injuries with affection of the pancreas is
small (1-3%) in comparison to the total number of multiple injuries
with an abdominal component, but increase the mortality rate to a
great extent. This prompted the interest of the Clinic in the pathophysiology, clinical aspects, diagnosis and treatment of injuries of
the pancreas.

METHODS

Road accidents were foremost among the causes of the injuries (52%),
followed by labour accidents (20%), sports or home accidents (19%)
and aggressions (9%). Most of the lesions affected the isthmus region
(72%), more seldom the tail of the pancreas (24%) and exceptionally
the head of the pancreas (4%). The latter lesions also involved the
duodenum, increasing the gravity of the prognosis. The clinical picture of traumas with a pancreatic component was dominated by violent
epigastric pain (90%), early postprandial vomiting (35%), oscillating
fever not in keeping with the pulse and leukocytosis (80%), paralytic
ileum (65%), abdominal contraction predominant in the epigastric region (70%). History of the case established the presumptive diagnosis
correctly in most cases. The diagnosis of certainty was established

233

I.Suteu, M.Ciurel, P.Blidaru, A.Bucur, R.Florescu, D.Culică

intraoperatively. The surgical procedure was adapted to each case in terms of the type and location of the lesion. Local and contact drainage was performed in 15 cases (3 deaths - 20%),pancreatorraphy in 20 cases (20 deaths - 9.5%), Wirsung catheterization in 2 cases (0 deaths), cephalic duodenopancreatectomy in 1 case (0 deaths), cysto-gastroanastomosis in 1 case (0 deaths) (figs. 1-5).

RESULTS

In the postoperative evolution of the 49 cases operated for acute traumatic pancreatitis the following complications developed: 6 pancreatic fistulas, 2 pseudocysts, 1 abscess, 1 duodenal fistula. The mortality rate after the primary surgical interventions, reinterventions and complications was 14.3%.

DISCUSSION

Traumatic lesions of the pancreas result in immediate acute pancreatitis, associated as a rule with lesions of the neighbouring organs. The relatively low frequency and inconclusive symptomatology of pancreatic injuries and the high mortality rate impose an early diagnosis and complex medicosurgical treatment.

REFERENCES

Petrescu, C. and Blidaru, P., 1971. Wirsung Drainage in Emergency
        Surgery, in Congress of Ass.Amer.Gastroenterology Surgery.
Turai,D., Borş, I. and Coban, P., 1964. Splenopancreatectomie în
        Chirurgia (Buc.), 12, 3,445.
Cojocaru Tr., 1972. Tratamentul chirurgical al pancreatitei acute.
        Dissertation thesis.
Turai,D. and Ciurel,M., 1970. Chirurgia pancreasului. Cercetări
        clinice si experimentale, Ed.Acad.RSR, Buc.
Culică,D., 1980, Pancreatita acută traumatică. Dissertation thesis.

Care of the Acutely Ill and Injured
Edited by D. H. Wilson and A. K. Marsden
© 1982, John Wiley & Sons Ltd.

INFERIOR VENA CAVA AND PORTAL VEIN INJURIES IN ABDOMINAL TRAUMA

E.Cerchez, R.Dop, F.Mergea and Luigia Ispas

IInd Surgical Clinic,Emergency Clinical Hospital
Bucharest, Romania

ABSTRACT

The present paper reports on the experience of the Clinic
in 2 cases of portal vein and 7 cases of inferior vena cava injuries in the course of abdominal trauma, with or
without other multiple injuries.

INTRODUCTION

Among the 2847 abdominal injuries, alone or in cases of
multiple trauma, admitted during the 1960-1980 period
there were 2 cases of portal vein injuries and 7 of the
inferior cava, with 3 postoperative deaths (1 after portal vein and 2 after vena cava lesions).

MATERIAL

There were 7 men and 2 women, 6 cases between the ages of
15-25 and 3 between 35 and 40 years. The causes were: labour accidents 4 cases, road accidents 1 case, aggression
4 cases, with 4 closed abdominal injuries and 5 open injuries. In closed abdominal trauma with wounding of the infe
rior vena cava other organs were also affected: liver and
gallbladder in 1 case with a satisfactory postoperative re
covery, liver and suprahepatic veins in 1 case with post-
operative death. In 2 cases of closed abdominal injuries
with multiple trauma and wounding of the portal vein, 1
case presented total rupture of the pylorus and pancreas,
massive haemoperitoneum, haemothorax, and died postoperatively; the other, rupture of the liver besides wounding
of the portal vein, but with a good evolution. In open abdominal injuries, 2 patients had only lesion of the inferior vena cava, and 3 also injuries of other abdominal organs. All the cases presented massive haemoperitoneum and
retroperitoneal haematoma, and were admitted in severe
shock with peripheral collapse. On principle, all the patients were brought directly to the operation theatre; after rapid, complex resuscitation, routine abdominal puncture, current analyses, emergency surgery was performed.
In 5 cases wounds of the inferior vena cava were found on
the anterior aspect and in 2 cases on the right lateral
aspect (in 4 of these cases immediately subhepatic).There

were 2 lesions of the portal vein, one lateral and the o-
ther on the right hepatic branch. The size of the linear
wounds ranged between 0.3 and 2.5 cm; there was a single
irregular lesion.

METHODS

Broad explorative laparotomy for control of the abdominal
organs often required difficult maneouvres. Provisional
haemostasis by manual compression in order to detect lesions of the abdominal organs, and rapid aspiration of the
blood from the peritoneum were of great help. After major
definitive haemostasis of the cava and portal vein, the
lesions of the other intraabdominal and retroperitoneal
organs were dealt with as follows: suture inf.vena cava +
duodenorraphy + enterectomy 1 case - died; suture inf.vena
cava + atypical hepatectomy + cholecystectomy 1 case; suture inf.vena cava 2 cases; suture inf.vena cava + hepatorrhaphy 1 case; suture inf.vena cava + atypical hepatectomy + ligature of suprahepatic veins 1 case - died; suture
inf.vena cava + hepatorrhaphy + right nephrectomy + cholecystectomy 1 case; suture right branch of portal vein 1
case; suture of portal vein + duodenorraphy + suture haemostasis of pancreas 1 case - died.

RESULTS

The greater was the number of abdominal organs affected
the longer did the intervention last, with accentuation
of shock and very few final chances for the patient. The
discharged patients followed up for some time presented
no abdominal disturbances, not even vascular, although ca-
vography indicated narrowing of the cava calibre at the
level of the sutured wound.

DISCUSSION

These cases of closed or open acute abdominal injuries
with wounds of the inferior vena cava and portal veins
are extremely difficult to solve and from the moment in
which the abdomen is opened and the diagnosis established,
surgery must be performed under emergency conditions. Experience has shown that only the concerted effort of a
team of skilled surgeons and competent anaesthetists-re-
suscitators may solve the complexity of such cases success
fully.

REFERENCES

        Cerchez Eugen, Turai I. -Pe marginea a 1000 cazuri
de traumatisme abdominale. Rev.Chirurgia,nr.11-1968,
pag.995-1017.Bucharest - Romania.

Care of the Acutely Ill and Injured
Edited by D. H. Wilson and A. K. Marsden
© 1982, John Wiley & Sons Ltd.

SUBCUTANEOUS EMPHYSEMA OF THE THIGH AS A SIGN OF RETROPERITONEAL PERFORATION

J.Waninger and D.Waldmann

Chirurgische Universitätsklinik
Hugstetterstr.55, D-78 Freiburg

Abstract

Subcutaneous emphysema of the thigh is a late sign of retroperitoneal perforation. The perforation starts insidiously. Abscess formation follows and tracks in most cases along the psoas sheath and the femoral canal down to
the thigh. 38 such cases have been reported in the lita-
rature. One patient who was treated at the Chirurgische
Universitätsklinik Freiburg had subcutaneous emphysema
due to a retroperitoneal perforation of a cecal carcinoma.

Introduction

Free colonic perforation starts with acute abdominal pain
and is one of the common causes of the acute abdomen. 10%
of gastrointestinal perforations are located in the colon
(Zühlke et al,1978). In contrast to the sudden onset of
free perforation, retroperitoneal perforation and perforation with local abscess formation start insidiously
with pain extending into the flank, hip, groin, thigh and
knee. Fever, chills, psoas spasm, abdominal pain, nausea
and vomiting will be present. 38 cases with subcutaneous
emphysema following retroperitoneal perforation have been
reported in the literature (Mair et al,1977; Robbins et
al,1977).

Pathology

Abeille (1853) was the first to describe subcutaneous gas
following colonic perforation. Retroperitoneal perforation requires a weakness of the bowel wall. Inflammation,
trauma or carcinoma may damage the bowel wall and lead to
a perforation with free access of intestinal contents to
the retroperitoneal space. Abscess formation will follow,
causing pain in the flank, hip and thigh. The most common route is either the psoas sheath or the femoral canal.
This route was reported 23 times. Other points of anato-

mical weakness such as the sciatic notch, obturator fora-
men, ischio-rectal fossa and the subcutaneous passage
from abdominal wall to thigh are less frequently involved.
The subcutaneous gas is produced by gas-forming organisms
such as E.coli, Cl.Welchii and Enterococcus. Intestinal
gas may spread directly to the thigh.

Diagnosis

It is difficult to diagnose retroperitonel perforation in
a patient presenting with hip or flank pain only. The
presence of subcutaneous gas may lead to the right diagnosis. However, the site and origin of perforation will
remain unknown until further investigations are carried
out. If the abscess is drained, contrast studies of the
abscess cavity may establish the site of perforation.
Barium enema, endoscopy, i.v. pyelogram, ultrasound and
computertomography will give further information.

Treatment

Incision and drainage of the abscess will be the first
emergency procedure. A diverting colostomy for perforations of the descending colon and sigmoid will reduce the
danger of further infection . Final treatment with resection of the involved bowel may be required when the patient is in a better condition. The high mortality rate
of 42 % in the first 24 hrs of hospital admission indicates that retroperitoneal perforation is a very dangerous complication. A 59-year-old patient with a retroperitoneal perforation due to a carcinoma of the cecum
was treated at the Chirurgische Universitätsklinik Freiburg with incision and drainage of the abscess and subsequent resection of the cecum. The course was complicated
by leakage of the anastomosis and local recurrence. The
patient died three years later from metastases.

References

Abeille,M.,1853.Perforations intestinales consécutives
      à une phlegmasie circonscrite. Péritonite générale
      ultime. Gazette des Hopitaux,105,422.
Mair,W.S.,McAdam,W.A.,Lee,P.W.,Jepson,K.,and Goligher,J.C.
      1977. Carcinoma of the large bowel presenting as a
      subcutaneous abscess of the thigh: a report of 4
      cases. Br.J.Surg,64,205.
Robbins,P.L.,Sutherland,D.E.,Najaria,J.S.and Bernstein
      W.C.,1977.Emphysema of the leg as a presenting sign
      of large intestinal perforation.Report of two cases.
      Dis.Col.Rect,2o,144.
Zühlke,V.,Siewert,R.und Peiper,H.-J.,1978.Akutes Abdomen;
      in Chirurgie der Gegenwart (Eds.Zenker, Deucher und
      Schink),Bd,2/25, Urban und Schwarzenberg,München.

SECTION FIVE

ASPECTS OF WOUNDING

Care of the Acutely Ill and Injured
Edited by D. H. Wilson and A. K. Marsden
© 1982, John Wiley & Sons Ltd.

MISSILE AND STAB INJURIES

M. S. OWEN-SMITH, MS, FRCS

Consultant Surgeon
Huntingdon County Hospital

This session on missile and stab wounds was planned two years ago.
The attacks by low velocity bullets on the chest of President Reagan
and the abdomen of the Pope have created world-wide media interest
in bullet wounds. We could not wish for a more opportune time to
utilise this interest to encourage the teaching of all medical
personnel - and in particular surgeons - the correct management
of such wounds.

When wounds are inflicted by low velocity hand-gun bullets, knives
or other penetrating weapons they can commonly be managed by
conventional surgical methods without too much harm. If these
same procedures are used in high velocity wounds from rifle
bullets or explosive blast fragments then the results can be
disastrous. Surgeons and their patients have had to learn the
hard way that these injuries require a different form of treatment.
The correct treatment has been known since World War I and the
principles have changed little from the highly developed practice
of World War II about 40 years ago.

MECHANISM OF INJURY

When a bullet strikes the body, damage is inflicted which depends
on the size, shape, stability and - above all - the velocity of the
missile, and the structures with which it comes into contact.
Bullets are divided into two groups, low velocity fired from hand
guns and high velocity from rifles. Hand guns may be revolvers
or automatics, but they all fire a fairly heavy bullet at relatively
low velocities of 200-300 m.p.s. (700-1,000 f.p.s.). A typical
military or hunting rifle fires a bullet of about 10G at over
800 m.p.s. (2,600 f.p.s.). Rifles of this type are not new as they
have been in existence for over 100 years.

Present and future developments in military rifles are towards
smaller bullets fixed at even higher velocity. For example, the
Colt Armalite rifle of calibre 5.56 mm fires a very small bullet
weighing 3.5G at a velocity of about 1,000 m.p.s. (3,250 f.p.s.)
and the Russian AK74 now in use in Afghanistan is very similar.

Pistol bullets have a relatively low amount of energy available
to cause damage and in general this only occurs at fairly close
ranges below 100 metres; they simply core out a hole through the
body and, like a knife, they only damage those tissues that they
actually touch.   There is no hidden damage.   On the contrary,
all rifle bullets have an incredible amount of energy to cause
severe wounding even at ranges of 500-1,000 metres.   They
transfer this energy by the process of "cavitation" and shock waves
that happen so quickly that ultra high speed cinephotography is
required to record it.

The external appearance of a bullet wound can be very deceptive,
because the skin is so elastic that there may well be tiny
entrance and exit holes which hide extremely severe wounds.   In
a rifle bullet wound there may be a volume of tissue destroyed
equal to the size of your fist.   This large amount of dead tissue,
uniformly and grossly contaminated with bacteria, clostridial
spores, clothing and debris from the surface is the pathological
entity of the high velocity missile wound and it does not occur
with any other wound.

TREATMENT

The majority of such wounds are of soft tissue and the treatment
is a 2-stage procedure.

Stage 1. The first operation is excision of the wound followed
4-5 days later by the second operation.

Stage 2. Delayed primary closure of the wound.

Wound Excision is the process whereby grossly contaminated, dead
and damaged tissue is thoroughly excised ("debridement").   This
leaves an area of healthy tissue with a good blood supply,
capable of combating residual surface infection provided that
the wound is not closed.

All wounds should be left open without suture of skin or deep
fascia except for the head, and the pleura and peritoneum must
be closed with sufficient muscle to make them air and water tight.

Delayed Primary Closure should be done on the 4th or 5th day
using fine sutures and, if necessary, skin grafts.

If you do not use these methods for high velocity wounds there
is a risk of gas gangrene.

LIMB WOUNDS

Limb wounds should be excised, major blood vessels repaired using
saphenous vein graft and no internal fixation should be done in
these grossly contaminated wounds.   External fixation devices are
recommended, but traction on splints or plaster slabs usually

suffice.   Delayed repair to damaged tendons and nerve should be
performed 3-6 weeks later once full skin cover has been obtained.

CHESTS

The main principles of management of penetrating chest wounds is
the early insertion of a wide bore intercostal drain to evacuate
the haemopneumothorax and to re-expand the lung.   Thoracotomy is
reserved for specific indications, usually blood loss of more than
1 litre rapidly (President Reagan), major air leak, suspected
mediastinal damage and, of course, in low velocity or stab wounds -
haemopericardium.

ABDOMEN

Penetrating missile wounds of the abdomen require urgent treatment
and the appearance of the wound may be deceptive.   A tiny wound
from a high velocity bullet may conceal enormous damage.   There
may be a place for diagnostic peritoneal lavage in stab wounds,
but not for bullet wounds.

Perforations of small bowel and stomach may be managed by suture
or resection in the surgeon's usual fashion and give little trouble.

The main problems are injuries to colon, liver and pancreas, as
well as haemorrhage from blood vessels.   The colon should be
treated with the greatest respect and by the following principles
according to the severity of the damage.

Repair by suture - with or without proximal colostomy - for minor,
low velocity stab wounds.

Resection - with proximal colostomy in most cases (as in the Pope) -
sometimes NOT on right side - proximal colostomy + mucus fistula
in severe cases.

Exteriorisation of damaged loop - on the left side only - not
right.   Thorough drainage is most important as is closure using
unabsorbable material.

LIVER

Injuries should be treated by excision of damaged tissue, or
segmental resection, haemostasis and thorough drainage.

PANCREAS

Pancreatic damage requires repair and thorough drainage if minor
or involving the head; whereas severe injuries of the body or
tail may require resection and drainage.

MORTALITY

Mortality from missile wounds is high, but it is 4-5 times as high for high velocity than for low velocity bullets and stab wounds.

The important factors that influence mortality and morbidity rates are:-

1.   The type of missile - whether high or low velocity.

2.   The part of the body that is hit.

3.   The organs that are damaged.

4.   The delay until surgery.

All these variables MUST be clearly separated and defined before any comparison of various series of gunshot wounds is made.

Care of the Acutely Ill and Injured
Edited by D. H. Wilson and A. K. Marsden
© 1982, John Wiley & Sons Ltd.

MILITARY RIFLE BULLET WOUNDS

F B Mayes and R Scott

Royal Army Medical College,
London, UK

INTRODUCTION

The development of small lightweight military rifles with repeat
or automatic capability firing lightweight bullets at high velocity
has been described in a recent book published by the Stockholm
International Peace Research Institute. (SIPRI 1978). Dudley and
his colleagues and Dimond and Rich described injuries caused by
bullets fired from the American M-16 rifle in Vietnam. (Dudley et
al. 1968, Dimond and Rich 1967). The injuries resulting in
anaesthetic pigs struck by rifle bullets at various ranges have
been described by Berlin and his colleagues, they also described
the use of blocks of soft soap to demonstrate the terminal effect
of military rifle bullets, and suggest that such tissue simulants
can be used to demonstrate the wounding potential of bullets.
(Berlin et al. 1976).

INCIDENT ANALYSIS

During the period 1969-79 there were almost 15,000 attacks on
security forces in Northern Ireland by small arms of which 114
were proved to have involved 5.56mm ammunition. 67 soldiers were
injured, 14 died almost immediately or on the way to hospital and
of the 53 who were alive on reaching hospital 8 subsequently died
after treatment.

Penetrating brain wounds carried a high mortality, all 8 soldiers
dying. Of the 29 soldiers who received penetrating trunk wounds,
7 were dead on arrival at hospital, 7 died subsequently after
treatment and 15 survived. 6 soldiers with face and neck wounds
and 24 with upper and lower limb wounds also survived.

ILLUSTRATIVE CASES

Head wound - A small stellate entrance wound 5mm diameter on the
left side of the forehead on the upper margin of the left eyebrow.
A gaping eliptical exit wound 7cms x 2cms vertical on the back of
the head to the left of the mid-line with bone defect and
protruding brain. Fatal immediately.

Chest wound - Bullet penetrated vehicle and then into right lower
chest of soldier traversing liver, diaphragm and lung. The lung
and liver lacerations were sutured and diaphragm repaired through
a right thoracotomy. Recovery was uneventful.

Abdominal wound - Small entry wound anterior left abdomen. Larger
exit wound left loin. Free blood and faeces in abdominal cavity.
Large ragged holes in transverse colon, splenic flexure and
descending colon and one hole in jejunum. Small bowel sutured,
splenic flexure resected and ends brought out at colostomy and
mucuous fistula. Convalescence was uneventful and colostomy closed
six weeks later.

Thigh wound - Small entry wound left buttock, small exit anteriorly.
Lateral popliteal nerve contusion in buttock, femoral vein severed.
Uneventful convalescence after femoral vein suture.

Arm wound - Small entry wound left anterior shoulder. No exit
wound. Comminuted fracture of upper shaft of left humerus with
metallic foreign bodies present laterally in soft tissue. Bullet
removed at operation and wound exised. Delayed primary suture at
5 days. Uneventful convalescence.

DISCUSSION

In an analysis of the first 2000 military casualties in Northern
Ireland during the recent disturbances Owen-Smith reported that
413 soldiers were wounded by high velocity rifle bullets. Of the
wounded 115 died either immediately or subsequently in hospital.
Low velocity sub-machine gun or pistol bullets were responsible for
465 casualties of whom 35 died (Owen-Smith 1981).

The mean projected area of the head and neck is 12% of total body
area (Oughterson et al 1962). Head and neck wounds were found in
14 of the 67 soldiers in this series (21%) and many of these were
undoubtedly the result of aimed fire. In a World War II analysis
Oughterson found that 29% of total hits for rifle resulted in head
wounds. He considered that exposure is one of the chief factors
in accounting for this high incidence of head wounds but
marksmanship played a small but important part.

The gelatine energy methodology used for comparisons of bullet
lethality by ammunition designers (Kokinakis et al 1979) makes the
assumption that single hits will be at random and may, therefore,
underestimate the lethality of injury due to rifle bullets.
Comparisons of the severity of wounds in experimental animals due
to rifle bullets (Berlin et al 1976) are usually made on hind limb
injuries of anaesthetised pigs. With rapid evacuation and modern
methods of surgical treatment such wounds in soldiers are seldom
fatal (Scott 1981) nevertheless, standardised experimental wounds
can give to the surgeon an indication of the degree of the
severity of injury to be expected and provide a rational basis for
the employment of new methods of treatment.

This analysis of the outcome for 67 British soldiers injured by
5.56mm bullets in Northern Ireland shows that such injury carries
a high mortality. Identification of all the responsible factors
is beyond the scope of this paper but most of them are outside
the control of the surgical team.

REFERENCES

Berlin R., Gelin L. E., Janzon B., Lewis D. H., Rybeck B.,
   Sandegard J. and Seeman T. (1976). Local effects of Assault
   rifle bullets in live tissues. Acta. Chir. Scand. Supp 459.
Dimond F. C. and Rich N. M. (1967). M-16 rifle wounds in Vietnam.
   Journal of Trauma 7 619-625.
Dudley H. A. F., Knight R. J., McNeur J. C. and Rosengarten D. S
   (1968). Civilian Battle Casualties in South Vietnam. British
   Journal of Surgery 55, 332-340.
Kokinakis W., Neades D., Piddington M. and Roecker E. (1979).
   A gelatin energy methodology for estimating vulnerability of
   personnel to military rifle systems. Acta Chirurgica
   Scandinavica Supp 489. 35-55.
Oughterson A. W., Hull H. C., Sutherland F. A. and Greiner D. J.
   (1962). Study on wound ballistics - Bougainville Campaign. in
   'Wound Ballistics' published by Office of the Surgeon General
   Department of the Army, Washington D.C.
Owen-Smith M. S. (1981). Hunterian Lecture 1980. A computerised
   Retrieval System for the Wounds of War. The Northern Ireland
   Casualties. J. R. Army Med. Corps 127. 31-54.
Scott R. (1981). High Velocity Missile Injuries in 'Topical
   Reviews in Accident Surgery - 2' ed. P. S. London and N. Tubbs.
              J. Wright and Sons Ltd Bristol.
Sipri (1978). Anti-personnel weapons. Taylor and Francis Ltd
   London.

Care of the Acutely Ill and Injured
Edited by D. H. Wilson and A. K. Marsden
© 1982, John Wiley & Sons Ltd.

SAMU 94 EXPERIENCE OF .22 LONG RIFLE HIGH VELOCITY
BULLETS AND SHOTGUN WOUNDS DURING THE LAST FEW YEARS

J.M.Abbeys, N.Dufeu and A.Margenet

SAMU 94. Departement d'Anesthesie Reanimation.
Hospital Henri Mondor. F-94 010 Creteil.

ABSTRACT

A high proportion of firearm woundings are due to the .22 rifle
and shotguns. We review the technical and ballistic characteristics
of these weapons.

INTRODUCTION

In our district in the past five years 254 cases of firearm wounding
were managed by the SAMU 94 service. This averages as one per
week. The .22 rifle was involved in 41% of cases and the shotgun
in 20% of cases - a sufficiently high proportion to cause us to
examine the specific properties of these wounding agents.

THE .22 RIFLE

.22 rifle ammunition: Uncontrolled availability of .22 long rifle
carbines and long barrelled pistols explains the high incidence of
wounding from these weapons. Since the end of the last century
these weapons have kept pace with firearms technology and are now
offering a significant wounding capability.

The .22 rifle bullet is made of raw lead and weighs about 40 grains
- it has a cylindrical pointed design, can be copper plated and
hollow pointed.

Table 1 shows the ballistics effects - muzzle velocity from a pistol
reaches 1150 f.p.s. and from the long barrel of a carbine 1350 f.p.s.
The muzzle energy from the carbine is calculated at 212 foot pound
- of more impact than the .38 special revolver bullet. The
penetrating capacity is important - three deal boards each of one
inch thickness can be traversed at a range of eleven yards.

Effects of .22 rifle bullets: The special effects noticed during
experimental work on these bullets are suprising:

- High speed photographs of a 20% gelatine block (reproducing the
density of normal tissue) traversed by a .22 rifle bullet reveal a
temporary cavity approaching half a litre in volume. This
cavitation is caused by a compression wave.

TABLE 1.   .22 long-rifle ballistics

	Cartridge	Bullet weight (grains)	Type	Muzzle vel. (feet/sec.)	Muzzle energy (Foot.Lb.)
P I S T O L	St.velocity	40	Lead	984	86
	High vel.	37	Coppered Hollow pt.	1263	131
	Stringer[r]	32	Coppered Hollow pt.	1220	106
C A R B I N E	St.velocity	40	Lead	1217	132
	High vel.	37	Coppered Hollow pt.	1397	160
	Stringer[r]	32	Coppered Hollow pt.	1673	199

- Shooting through a one pound block of wet soap allows closer visualisation of the cavity and occasionally reveals an exterior effect with ejection of matter.   Thus .22 rifle wounding capabilities are comparable with those of more powerful assault rifles with ammunition of small mass and higher velocity.

Three factors contribute to the severity of wounding:

a) the track of the wound with substantial penetration
b) the extensive cavity caused by vibratory phenomena due to the compression wave and the unstable line of flight.
c) ejection of matter.

THE SHOTGUN

Shotgun injuries, ranging from superficial scatter to lethal wounds are proportional to the type of shot and the range.

The Shotgun.   The smooth, long barrelled shotgun is likewise free of restriction in France.   Its calibre or "gauge" refers to the number of hemispherical lead spheres per pound which fits the gun bore.   So .12 gauge is the calibre of one of the twelve bullets weighing a pound.   The usual gauges are .12, .16, .20 and .410. A "choke" is a muzzle constriction reducing the shot spread: at 40 yards a full choke barrel will confine 70% of the pellets in the target; a modified barrel will confine 60% and a cylinder bore about 40%.

Shotgun Shell.   This comprises a cylinder of plastic casing fused into a brass base and containing the primer, including shot charge, wad and powder charge.   The chamber length implies the shell length - $2\frac{1}{2}$ inches, 2.75 inches and 3 inches.

<u>Shotgun projectiles.</u>   The number of pellets per load is defined
by a number, small pellets having a high number.   French shot size
is different to the English shot size (Table 2).

TABLE 2.   Characteristics of .12 gauge shotshells
(Shell length 2 3/4"; shot weight 1 1/4 oz)

English shot size	French shot size	Pellet cal. (inches)	Pellet weight (grains)	Number of pellets / load
BB	0	0.167	6.17	90
1	2	0.147	4.79	114
3	4	0.127	3.08	175
5	6	0.108	1.88	190
8	8	0.088	1.03	530

By substituting projectiles of a larger size (hence giving greater
wounding power) it is possible to adapt shotgun to bigger game.
Reducing projectile weight and increasing muzzle velocity imparts
higher energy to "buckshots" and "slugs".   A 12 bore "rifled
slug", weighing 437 grains, has an energy of 2500 foot-pounds
at 1600 f.p.s.

<u>Shotgun ballistics.</u>   Shot charge progresses from the muzzle in a
cone-like fashion: the cone is dense less than 20 yards.   Within
this range human wounds are serious;   beyond this range the sparse
pattern and reduction in velocity reduces wounding power giving a
simple scattering.   Sherman and Parrish (1963) considering that
shot range is the most important factor contributing to gravity of
injury have classified shotgun wounds into three categories:

Type   I   - beyond 7 yards   :   Penetrating wounds

Type   II - 3 to 7 yards   :   Perforating wounds

Type III   - under 3 yards   :   Massive tissue destruction

Because of their high mass, bucks (whilst responding to the same
ballistic characteristics at short range) conserve their wounding
power until a distance of 55 yards.   Thus a .00 buckshot at 20
yards contains a kinetic energy thirty times greater than a .6 shot
pellet (see Table 3).   This energy would produce a long bone
comminuted fracture at such a range.

TABLE 3.   Characteristics of .12 gauge buckshots
(shell length 2 3/4": shot weight 1 oz)

English shot size	French shot size	Pellet cal. (inches)	Pellet weight (grains)	Number of pellets /load
00 Buck	2	0.33	54	9
0 Buck	4	0.32	40	12
1 Buck	6	0.31	30	16
4 Buck	10	0.24	20	27

J.M.Abbeys, N.Dufeu and A.Margenet

Single projectiles used in shotguns are extremely lethal. A .12
gauge "rifled slug", 437 grains, 1600 f.p.s., maintains a kinetic
energy of 2500 foot pounds at a distance of 20 yards.   At point
blank range it could traverse six deal boards, each one inch thick,
or it could make a twelve litre volume cavity in wet clay.

REFERENCES

Bell M.J. 1971. The management of shotgun wounds. J.Trauma.
11.   522-527.
Demuth W.E.Jr. 1978. Buckshot wounds. J.Trauma. 18. 53-57.
Harto-Garofalides, G. et al. 1968. Traumatismes par fusil de
chasse. Rev.Chir.Orthop. 54. 61-65
Legerwood A.M. 1977. The management of shotgun wounds. Surg.
North Am. 51. 111-120.
Sherman R.T. et al. 1963. Management of shotgun injuries: a
review of 152 cases. J.Trauma 3. 76-86.

Care of the Acutely Ill and Injured
Edited by D. H. Wilson and A. K. Marsden
© 1982, John Wiley & Sons Ltd.

PENETRATING WOUNDS OF THE CHEST

H.M. Stevenson, F.R.C.S.

Royal Victoria Hospital,
Grosvenor Road,
Belfast, BT12 6BA.,
Northern Ireland.

Penetrating chest wounds have challenged the surgeon's skill since
man first learnt to make weapons. In Belfast during a ten year
period of civil disturbances between 1970 and 1980, the preponderance
of gun shot wounds is notable (Table I).

TABLE I. PENETRATING CHEST WOUNDS

Gun Shot Wounds	216
Stab Wounds	10
Wounds Due To Other Missiles	4

Having regard to the greatly improved accuracy of small arms over
this last century, one would have anticipated that there would also
be an increasing incidence of thoracic wounds, since the chest is
the traditional target for the marksman or assassin. In fact, in
most published series of gun shot wounds admitted, the proportion
of chest wounds to the total is remarkably constant at around 10
to 12 per cent (Table II).

TABLE II. GUN SHOT WOUNDS 1970 - 1980

Total number of G.S.W. admitted	1,972	100%
G.S.W. Chest	216	11%

The particular hazards of penetrating thoracic injuries are the
mechanical effects of pneumothorax, haemothorax, and chest wall
disruption upon ventilation, and the possibility of serious
haemorrhage from large systemic or pulmonary vessels. Such
injuries may therefore be immediately fatal, but the facility of
rapid transfer to hospital, has meant that a high proportion of
casualties are in fact admitted, many of whom in other
circumstances would not have survived. In Belfast the average time
between wounding and admission is 30 minutes.

In the Casualty Department, where necessary, a large cannula is
placed in the external jugular vein, which allows a high flow as
well as being useful as a central venous pressure line. After
blood has been taken for cross matching, infusion of crystalloid
solution or dextran may be begun. Unmatched O-Negative blood is

available if necessary.

The routine administration of large amounts of IV fluids in these patients, however, is undesirable and often dangerous. In the case of simple through and through bullet wounds of the chest, the blood loss may be minimal, and the patient is at far greater risk from unrecognised pneumothorax than from a lowered blood volume. Excessive transfusion simply adds pulmonary oedema to his ventilatory problems.

A chest drain is inserted into one or both pleural cavities, where obvious penetration by a bullet has occurred, or where there is any clinical evidence of blood or air in the pleural cavity. An estimate is made of the probable track of the missile or missiles, and careful clinical examination, especially of the abdomen, carried out. Low velocity missiles are often retained, and x-ray films of chest and abdomen should be available.

It is widely accepted that most bullet wounds of the chest can be successfully managed by adequate intercostal drainage and close observation. (Heaton et al., 1966. Oparah and Mandal, 1978). In circumstances however, where numbers of such casualties at any one time have been small, and where full surgical facilities are available, a more aggressive approach for. other than simple cases may well be indicated. Many patients had associated abdominal injury, and in these surgical exploration is mandatory. (Table III).

TABLE III. ASSOCIATED INJURIES

G.S.W. Chest	216	100%
Abdomen	47	21.8%
Liver	26	12.0%
Spleen	7	3.2%
Oesophagus	1	—
Stomach	13	6.0%
Intestine	8	3.7%
Kidney	2	—
Spine	20	9.3%
Limbs	71	32.8%

The indications for open thoracotomy are significant or continued haemorrhage, a dangerous predicted track and associated intra-abdominal injury.

Estimation of the track of a bullet however, is not always reliable.

Case 1 — A young man was admitted with chest wounds, and was found to have an entry wound in his third left intercostal space in front, and an exit wound in his eighth left intercostal space in the posterior axillary line. He responded well to minimal

resuscitation, and only a little blood drained from his left
pleural cavity. There was some guarding however, in the left sub-
costal region. On left thoracotomy, there were two small holes
one above the other in the pericardium, two holes side by side in
the diaphragm and a track through the lingula. Further exploration
showed that the bullet, presumably of very low velocity, had
grooved the left ventricle, traversed the diaphragm, and bounced
back off the spleen which was superficially lacerated.

SURGICAL APPROACH

This is obviously dictated by circumstances. A postero-lateral
thoracotomy gives much better access to the hemithorax than does
an anterior one, and is preferable except under very urgent
circumstances. Where there appears to be serious bleeding into
both pleural cavities, a bilateral trans-sternal anterior approach
has occasionally been used. The low thoraco-abdominal incision
has been useful where abdominal penetration has also occurred, and
this allows good access to the liver or spleen. In general, however,
the abdomen is more satisfactorily explored through a separate
laparotomy, though the chest should first be drained.

One type of injury where the selection of approach may be difficult
is a gun shot wound at the thoracic inlet, where one may be faced
with serious bleeding, both externally and into the chest cavity.
(Graham et al., 1980). Immediate temporary control of haemorrhage
from the sub-clavian artery and vein at the point of injury is
required, but wider access is necessary to allow repair of the
vessels. Median sternotomy with extension up into the neck, with
or without excision of part of the clavicle, is essential. On
the left side extension of the sternotomy into the third left
intercostal space anteriorly gives a wide trap-door type of opening.

TYPE OF MISSILE

The types of gun-fired missiles are commonly divided into low and
high velocity groups. The former are fired from revolvers and
pistols, and a variety of short-barrelled automatic weapons, and
the latter from rifles. The kinetic energy of the missile is
related to its mass, and to the square of its velocity, though
other factors are involved in its wounding potential.

The low velocity bullet is often deflected by soft tissue planes.

Case 2 — A man was admitted with a single bullet wound in his left
anterior axillary fold. His first chest x-ray showed a left
haemothorax, but no bullet, but a second film was taken which showed
it lying over the right acromion process. In view of the projected
track of this missile through the superior mediastinum, the chest
was explored through a median sternotomy. The track was found to
be posterior, and the missile had penetrated the mediastinum

between the oesophagus and the vertebral column, neither of which structures were damaged.

Injury by a high velocity missile is a much more lethal event, and far fewer of these patients have come to surgery. Where a rifle bullet has passed cleanly through the chest, the characteristic effect of a high energy dissipation may not be observed. The low specific gravity, low water content, and tissue elasticity minimize the cavitation effect of high velocity missiles passing through the lung. (De Muth 1968). Where, however, the sternum, ribs or vertebral column is struck, widespread pulmonary effects, such as disruption and rapid development of bilateral pulmonary oedema may occur. Associated spinal cord injuries are common in this type of injury.

PROCEDURE

In the surgical management of pulmonary injuries, the use of a double lumen endotracheal tube for anaesthesia is essential, in order to control excessive air leakage, and minimize aspiration of blood into the other lung. A conservative approach has been adopted, and where at all possible, pulmonary wounds are explored, bleeding and air leaks controlled, and the lung repaired by suture. The diaphragm is inspected with great care, and if perforated it must be opened. Few lobectomies have been performed, and two pneumonectomies.

Few cardiac wounds have come to surgery. Those that have have been preserved from total exsanguination by the temporary effect of tamponade.

Case 3 - A young woman was shot from behind with a large calibre automatic pistol; the bullet traversed her 9th thoracic vertebra, and passed upwards and forwards through both atria. On admission to hospital she was very shocked, and had a right haemothorax, which drained freely after inserting an intercostal tube. On right thoracotomy, a hole was seen in the pericardium, just anterior to the phrenic nerve, and the pericardial cavity was full of blood. The pericardium was opened anteriorly, and a wound in the right atrium was closed. The opening of the pericardium however, increased the blood loss, and a further tear was palpated in the back of the left atrium. While this was controlled with the finger, the lung was displaced forward, and the pericardium opened posterior to the pulmonary vein. It was impossible to apply a clamp, and the use of a Foley catheter proved life saving. A No. 20 Foley Catheter with a 30 ml balloon, clamped and with a syringe full of saline, attached to the balloon, was rapidly inserted in the tear, the balloon was inflated, and gentle traction applied to the catheter. The haemorrhage was completely controlled, and closure was effected by encircling suture pulled tight, as the deflated catheter was removed. This girl survived, though with permanent paraplegia.

The chest wall wounds have mostly been small and have been excised
and closed by delayed primary suture.

POST-OPERATIVE CARE

The post-operative course of most patients was uncomplicated and no
ventilatory assistance was required. Some degree of lung contusion
was present in all, but development of pulmonary insufficiency was
dependent upon the velocity of the missile, the extent of the chest
wall injury, and by the severity of other injuries. These patients
developed this syndrome early, and a decision to institute special
intensive care, including controlled ventilation, was usually taken
at the end of operation. Possible factors responsible for the
development of this syndrome in high velocity injuries to the chest,
were outlined by Wanebo and Van-Dyke in 1972.

RESULTS

The overall mortality during the period was 9.3%, many deaths being
due to associated abdominal injuries. Table IV summarizes the
procedures carried out on the 216 cases.

TABLE IV.   TREATMENT OF G.S.W. TO CHEST.

Thoracotomy	79	36.6%
Thoracotomy and abdominal exploration	27	12.5%
Intercostal drainage	90	41.7%
Intercostal drainage and abdominal exploration	17	7.9%
Superficial chest wounds treated and abdominal exploration	3	1.4%
Died	20	9.3%

STAB WOUNDS

Relatively few patients with stab wounds to the chest have been
seen. Many are trivial, and most that penetrate the pleural cavity
are treated by tube drainage only. Where cardiac or major vessel
injury is suspected, urgent thoracotomy is indicated. (Oparah
and Mandal 1976). There is no place for pericardiocentesis as a
definitive line of treatment in suspected stab injuries of the
heart, though it has been found to be useful on one occasion when a

patient was transferred from a peripheral hospital, and
intermittent aspiration of blood from the pericardium through a
fine cannula controlled tamponade and ensured survival.

Low stab wounds may be associated with injury to abdominal viscera.
A particular hazard is injury to the liver where the knife has
penetrated the diaphragm, and a diagnosis may not be suspected until
a pleuro biliary fistula develops.

OTHER MISSILE WOUNDS

Other missiles come in all shapes and sizes.

Case 4 — A man was a front-seat passenger in a car which crashed
into a fence, and the top cross-post passed through his chest and
out through the rear window. The Fire Authority sawed the post
off at both ends to extract him from the car, but luckily did not
remove it. He also had facial injuries from flying glass. A
standard right thoracotomy was performed to assess the track of the
missile. While the ribs and lower part of the scapula were
shattered, the lung was displaced downwards but was undamaged,
and major vessels were intact. He made a good recovery.

CONCLUSION

In conclusion, gun shot wounds of the chest have become more
common overall in civilian practice. Miller in 1976, reports a
15 fold increase during the last 10 years, as opposed to a 2 fold
increase in stab wounds of the chest treated in a Harlem hospital.
Surgeons will be called upon increasingly to deal with this type
of injury, and except under conditions of organised terrorism, most
wounds are likely to result from relatively low velocity missiles.
While many such patients may be treated conservatively by chest
drainage and observation, the essentially capricious nature of
penetrating thoracic injuries may sometimes justify a more
aggressive approach to their management.

REFERENCES

De Muth, W.E. High velocity wounds of the thorax. Am. J. Surg.,
115 : 616 (1968).
Graham, J.M., Feliciano, D.V., Mattox, K.L., et al. Management
of subclavian vascular injuries. J. Trauma 20 : 537 (1980).
Heaton, L.D., Hughes, C.W., Rosegay, H., et al. Military surgical
practices of the U.S.A. army in Vietnam. Curr. Probl. Surg.,
(1966).
Miller, D.W., Hutchinson, J.E., Malm, J.R. Chest trauma. Its
nature in an urban ghetto. N.Y. State J. Med., 7 : 1103 (1976).
Oparah, S.S., Mandal, A.K. Penetrating stab wounds of the chest.
J. Trauma 16 : 868 (1976).
Oparah, S.S., Mandal, A.K. Penetrating gunshot wounds of the chest
in civilian practice : experience with 250 consecutive cases.
Br. J. Surg., 65 : 45 (1978).

Wanebo, H., Van Dyke, J. The high velocity pulmonary injury :
relation to traumatic wet lung syndrome. J. Thorac. Cardiovasc.
Surg., 64 : 537 (1972).

Care of the Acutely Ill and Injured
Edited by D. H. Wilson and A. K. Marsden
© 1982, John Wiley & Sons Ltd.

GUNSHOT AND STAB WOUNDS OF THE DIAPHRAGM

J.Waninger, G.Spillner and G.Kauffmann

Chirurgische Universitätsklinik
Hugstetterstr.55, D-78 Freiburg

Abstract

Perforation of the diaphragm indicates a combined thoraco-abdominal injury. In the period from 1969 to 1980 25
patients were treated at the Chirurgische Universitätsklinik Freiburg for gunshot and stab wounds of the diaphragm. Chest tube drainage and laparotomy were adequate
treatment in 60 % of the cases. Gunshot wounds had a
higher rate of associated abdominal injury than stab
wounds.

Introduction

During the period from 1969 to 1980 109 patients with
gunshot wounds and 123 patients with stab wounds were
treated at the Chirurgische Universitätsklinik Freiburg.
34 gunshot and 53 stab wounds were confined to the thorax.
The bullet had passed through the thoracic wall in 79 %
and the stabbing instrument in 64 %. 70 % of perforating
wounds below the 6th intercostal space involved the diaphragm. 80 % were on the left side and 20 % on the right
side. The diaphragm itself was perforated in 10 cases by
gunshot wounds and in 15 cases by stab wounds. There was
a preponderance of 19 men over 6 women. 36 % of the patients had more than one wound. 6 gunshot wounds were
caused by criminal assault and 4 were self-inflicted, but
86 % of the stab wounds resulted from an assault and one
was either self-inflicted or caused by an accident.
The trajectory depends on the position of the body and
the direction of the flight at the moment of the impact
of the bullet. This explains why a bullet entering the
thorax even higher than the 5th intercostal space may
penetrate the diaphragm and reach the abdomen.

Diagnosis

There are several diagnostic procedures to rule out addi-
tional abdominal injury, for instance peritoneal lavage
(Thal,1980) and radiographic examination of the wound
(Steichen,1967). These examinations were not performed in

261

our cases. X-ray of the thorax and abdomen in two planes
and a thorough clinical examination are the most important steps in the diagnosis of open thoraco-abdominal
wounds. If the wound is in the thoracic wall and the x-
ray demonstrates the bullet in the abdomen the diaphragm
must be perforated. If several bullets hit the body it is
difficult to reconstruct the trajectory of each bullet.
the first clinical signs of abdominal injury should lead
to the diagnosis of a perforated diaphragm and subsequent
laparotomy. If there is any doubt, exploration of the
thoracic wound under general anaesthesia and extension to
a small thoracotomy which allows inspection of the diaphragm is a safe procedure.

Treatment

Four approaches are possible in the management of diaphragmatic injury. Thoracotomy with exploration of the
abdomen through the diaphragm should not be routine , but
is very helpful in unsuspected diaphragmatic perforations
encountered during thoracotomy. The combined thoraco-
abdominal incision has been reported in individual cases
(Borja,1971). A separate thoracotomy and laparotomy is
the safest procedure but not necessary in all thoracic
injuries. Most of them need a chest-tube only(Borja,1971).
A total of 36 abdominal organs had been lacerated in the
present series. Gunshot wounds had a higher rate of associated abdominal organ injury than stab wounds. Negative
laparotomies were done for stab wounds in 44 % and in
20 % for gunshot wounds. Colonic injuries were responsible for a lethal outcome in 3 cases and a cardiac injury in 2 cases. Repair of the colonic wound with diverting colostomy is a safe procedure to reduce complications following leakage of the suture line.

References

Borja,A.R., and Ransdell,H.T.,1971.Treatment of penetrating gunshot wounds of the chest.Am J Surg,122,81.
Steichen,F.M.,1967.Penetrating wounds of the chest and
the abdomen.Current Problems in Surgery,8,Year Book
Medical Publishers, Inc./ Chicago.
Thal,E.R.,Robert,A.M.,and Beesinger,D.,1980.Peritoneal
lavage. Its unreliability in gunshot wounds of the
lower chest and abdomen. Arch Surg,115,430.

Care of the Acutely Ill and Injured
Edited by D. H. Wilson and A. K. Marsden
© 1982, John Wiley & Sons Ltd.

MISSILE AND STAB WOUNDS OF THE LEFT UPPER ABDOMINAL
QUADRANT ASSOCIATED WITH MULTIPLE ABDOMINAL INJURIES

M.Azzola, R.Azzoni, M.Gavinelli

Surgical Clinic 1, Institute of Emergency Surgery,
University of Milan, Italy.

ABSTRACT

Twenty three cases of penetrating wounds of the left upper abdominal
quadrant are described, with particular consideration of the
mortality and number of injured viscera in the left upper abdominal
quadrant compared with wounds of other abdominal quadrants.

INTRODUCTION

Missile and stab wounds of the abdomen present a multiplicity of
management problems to the surgeon.   Consequently a considerable
number of reports have been published on various aspects of this
problem, but wounds involving the left upper abdominal quadrant
(LUAQ) and their management are poorly documented in the medical
literature.

MATERIALS AND METHODS

From July 1976 to June 1980 the authors observed 23 cases of
penetrating wounds of LUAQ (19 gunshot wounds and 4 stab wounds)
and 35 cases of penetrating wounds of the other abdominal quadrants
(all gunshot wounds) admitted to The Institute of Emergency Surgery
of the University of Milan.

RESULTS

At laparotomy (all patients were submitted to surgery) the authors
observed 75 injured viscera in 23 cases of LUAQ wounds with an
average of 3.6 viscera injured for each patient.

The viscera most often involved were stomach (14 cases), small
bowel (11), liver (9), colon, mesentery and spleen (7), pancreas(6),
and great vessels (4).

Five of the 23 patients injured in LUAQ died, a mortality of 21.7%.
One patient who was previously suffering from chronic renal failure
died on the sixth day.   Four of the deaths occured within the
first 24 hours from irreversible shock.   In wounds of the other
abdominal quadrants (35 cases) 44 injured viscera were observed
with an average of 1.3 for each patient.   In particular 51% had

only one viscus injured and in 3 cases there were no visceral
lesions (8%).

The mortality rate in gunshot wounds of these quadrants was 11.4%
(4 cases).

DISCUSSION

The present study highlights the differences between wounds of
LUAQ and wounds of other quadrants of the abdomen.   In fact in
LUAQ wounds a great number of fiscera were injured every time,
with a high mortality (21.7%) as compared with 11.4% in wounds of
other quadrants.

In wounds of LUAQ the authors observed two or more viscera injured
in 78% of cases as compared with 40% in gunshot wounds of the
other quadrants.   In wounds affecting other quadrants only three
cases without lesions requiring repair were observed - in LUAQ
wounds repairs (frequently multiple) were required in all cases.

The authors underline the seriousness and mortality rate of missile
and stab injuries in LUAQ compared with other abdominal quadrants.
This is primarily due to the numerous organs contained in this
quadrant.

Furthermore the authors stress the importance of an aggressive
approach with laparotomy mandatory in these circumstances.

REFERENCES

Huse J.B. et al. 1979. Gunshot wounds of left upper abdominal
    quadrant associated with multiple abdominal injuries.   The
    American Journal of Surgery. Nov.1979. 135.
Riva R., Castiglioni A., Azzola M., Ronchetti E. 1981. Le Ferite
    d'Arma da Fuoco Addominali.   Incontri Internazionali di Chirur
    gia. Milano. 10-13 Maggio 1981. Personal communication.
Nance F.C. et al. 1973. Surgical judgement in the Management of
    penetrating wounds of the abdomen: experience with 2212 patients
    At the Annual Meeting of the Southern Surgical Association, Hot
    Spring, Virginia. Dec 3-5. 1973.
Riva R., Castiglioni A., Azzola M., Ronchetti E. 1981 Surgical
    Approach to Civilian Colonic Injuries. 5th International Con
    gress of Emergency Surgery. Brighton 7-10 June 1981. Personal
    communication.

Care of the Acutely Ill and Injured
Edited by D. H. Wilson and A. K. Marsden
© 1982, John Wiley & Sons Ltd.

MISSILE INJURIES OF THE LARGE INTESTINE

T.G. Parks

Department of Surgery,
Queen's University, Belfast.

ABSTRACT

One hundred and five patients received treatment for missile
injuries of the large intestine. An average of 3.8 viscera were
injured in each of 18 fatal cases. No patient with an isolated
colorectal injury died.

INTRODUCTION

During the period 1969-1979, 105 patients of whom 95 were male,
were admitted to the Royal Victoria Hospital, Belfast, with missile
injuries of the colon and rectum. The age of the patients ranged
from 13-69 years with a mean of 28.2 years.

INITIAL TREATMENT

Urgent resuscitation was considered to be of paramount importance.
If circumstances permitted, x-rays of the chest and abdomen were
taken to help in localisation of the missile or confirmation of the
presence of intra-peritoneal gas from rupture of a hollow viscus.
However, the absence of abnormal radiology findings cannot be relied
upon to exclude serious intra-abdominal injury.

Unless surgery was contra indicated because of concomitant lethal
injury, e.g. severe brain damage, laparotomy was undertaken as soon
as adequate resuscitation has been achieved. At operation priority
was given to the control of haemorrhage after which a thorough
examination of the abdominal and pelvic cavities to assess the
overall situation was mandatory.

NON-PENETRATING INJURIES

There were 18 cases in which the missile entered or passed through
the abdominal cavity but did not encroach upon the bowel lumen. In
5 of these the sero-muscular layer of the colon was torn and
required only to be over-sewn. In 3 cases a major colic vessel was
damaged resulting in bowel ischaemia which necessitated resection.
Ten patients had either a haematoma or a rent in the mesentery.

PENETRATING INJURIES

In 87 cases the missile or missiles penetrated the large bowel
itself; 82 were due to gunshot and 5 to bomb blast.

Wounds of the right colon were for the most part treated by primary
closure if the injury was limited, or by resection with anastomosis
if the damage was more severe. Resection was essential for injury
resulting from high velocity weapons.

Penetrating injuries of the transverse colon were commonly treated
by exteriorisation; if the injury itself was limited in extent it
was generally converted into a colostomy but if damage was more
severe a segment of colon was excised and both ends were exteriorised.

Various surgical procedures were used in the management of left colon
wounds depending on the circumstances. When trauma was severe
resection without anastomosis was undertaken at the initial
operation. In other cases direct suture was performed or resection
and anastomosis undertaken initially but a proximal colostomy was
usually added. In 6 cases with left sided penetrating wounds a
concominant colostomy was not performed and two of these patients
developed a faecal fistula, one with a fatal outcome.

Intraperitoneal rectal injuries were repaired and where feasible
extraperitoneal rectal wounds were also closed. In all except one
case proximal colostomy was established to allow temporary
decompression.

ASSOCIATED INJURIES

When missiles penetrate the abdominal cavity it is unusual for the
colon alone to be injured. In this series there were only 16 cases
in whom the visceral injury was confined to the large intestine.
None of these patients died.

In 18 patients with fatal injuries there was an average of 3.8
intra-abdominal or intra-thoracic organs injured compared with 2.2
in those who survived. Haemorrhage, sepsis and associated shock
were the most important factors causing death.

DISCUSSION

No single policy of surgical management is applicable to all cases
of missile injury of the large intestine. The policy adopted
depends not only upon the site and severity of the colorectal damage
but also upon the associated injuries and the general state of the
patient. Morbidity and mortality were higher when large bowel
injury was associated with massive haemorrhage, gross peritoneal
contamination, multiple visceral injuries, undue delay in treatment
or when caused by a high velocity weapon.

Care of the Acutely Ill and Injured
Edited by D. H. Wilson and A. K. Marsden
© 1982, John Wiley & Sons Ltd.

GUNSHOT FRACTURES OF EXTREMITIES

Zajic Zivorad, M.D.

Trauma Department of First Surgical Clinic,
Visegradska 26, Belgrade,Yugoslavia.

ABSTRACT

This paper describes the characteristics of firearm wounding in
Peace Time (1975-1980) according to the site and treatment method.
Nineteen patients are reported with injuries caused by pistol,
bomb fragments, military or hunting rifles. Special attention
was paid to fractures in the region of joints. The specific
problems of wounding due to high velocity missiles are presented.
The treatment methods and results are detailed.

INTRODUCTION

Firearm wounds are relatively rare in peacetime. However an
increase occurs as the number of hunting and air rifles rises.
Wounds caused by military rifles are particularly important - data
obtained in modern local wars (Piscevic, 1969) clearly shows that
the destructive power of high velocity missiles is being
intensified. The decrease in bullet weight has increased the
absolute low impact velocity. Low impact velocity missiles cause
small entry and exit wounds while projectiles of high impact
velocity produce greater exit wounds (8 - 10 cm) compared with the
entrance wound (1 cm) - between the two lies the temporary cavity
which may be some 30 times greater than it appears at subsequent
surgical exploration. Formation of the wound canal is termed
"wound ballistics" (Davidovski, 1950 b) a term describing three
zones:

- a central zone of direct traumatic necrosis

- a zone of massive shock with destroyed tissue around the wound
  canal

- a zone of molecular shock in which transient tissue ischaemia
  occurs.

RESULTS

We have experienced the effects of both low and high velocity
missiles in 19 gunshot wounds. We note that low velocity, e.g.
pistol injuries, do not show temporary cavitation and there is
limited tissue damage. High velocity injuries demonstrate a
cavity whose size is proportional to the kinetic energy of the

Zajic Zivorad, M.D.

missile.

In 13 patients there were bone fractures - the remaining six wounds were of soft tissue only.

Pistol wounds prevailed and were found in 6, air rifle injuries in 5, hunting rifle in 4, military rifle in 3 and explosion in 1. In one case with a pistol wound severe bleeding from a fractured tibia occurred (Zajic, 1972 c).

The site and results of the injuries are as shown in the Table.

SITE	No.	RESULTS			
		Cure	Infection	Amputation	Death
Shoulder and Upper Arm	2	2	-	-	-
Elbow and Forearm	3	3	-	-	-
Hand and Fingers	5	3	1	1	-
Hip and Thigh	4	2	1	-	1
Knee and Lower Leg	3	1	-	2	-
Foot and Toes	2	1	1	-	-
TOTAL	19	12 (63%)	3 (16%)	3 (16%)	1 (5%)

Amputations were required in the patients with severe wounds complicated by bascular injury caused by hunting rifles. The explosion victim died from gas gangrene nine days after wounding.

REFERENCES

Piscevic S., Zajic Z., Djuknic M. 1969. Mechanism of Wounding with High Velocity Projectiles. Vojnosanit.Pregl. 26:3,136-.40.
Davidovski I.V., 1950b. Ognestrelnaja rana deloveka. Tom I. Akademija Medicinskih Nauk SSSR, Moskva.
Zajic Z., Micanovic V., Mitic S.: 1972c. Traumatic Osseous Bleeding and methods of Homeostasis. Acta Chir Jugoslavica, 19:2. 443-449.

Care of the Acutely Ill and Injured
Edited by D. H. Wilson and A. K. Marsden
© 1982, John Wiley & Sons Ltd.

INJURY SEVERITY SCORE AND GUNSHOT WOUNDS

D. Beverland

Accident and Emergency Department,
Royal Victoria Hospital, Belfast.

INTRODUCTION

In 1974 Baker et al described the Injury Severity Score (I.S.S.) which, when used for road traffic accidents gave a linear correlation with mortality. The aim of the present study was to test the validity of the I.S.S. for gunshot wounds (G.S.W's).

METHODS

The present study analysed the records of 875 G.S.W's from the Royal Victoria Hospital, Belfast, over a two year period. This included post-mortem records of those patients dead on arrival. Their injuries were graded, as in Baker's study, using the Abbreviated Injury Scale (A.I.S.), each injury receiving a separate grade from 1 to 5 according to severity. The I.S.S. was then calculated by adding the sum of the squares of the highest A.I.S. grade in each of the three most severely injured areas.

RESULTS

The overall mortality in Baker's study was 11% as compared to 22% in the present study. The mortality by A.I.S. grade of most severe injury was comparable for both studies; in Baker's study when the most severe injury was A.I.S. Grade 5 the mortality was 64%, similar to the 58% found in the present study. However, when Baker analysed this group and looked at the mortality according to the grade of the second most severe injury, a steadily increasing mortality rate was found, from 22% when the second injury was A.I.S. Grade 1 to 100% when the second injury was A.I.S. Grade 5. However, in the present study when the second injury was A.I.S. Grade 1 the mortality was much greater, 57% with no significant increase in mortality until the second injury was Grade 5 when the mortality was 76%.

When the I.S.S. was calculated for the present study there was no linear correlation with mortality.

CONCLUSION

At present the Injury Severity Score without suitable modification to the Abbreviated Injury Scale is not valid for gunshot wounds.

D. Beverland

DISCUSSION

The essential differences between the two studies are that in the
present study a single A.I.S. Grade 5 injury carries a much higher
mortality and that further injuries unless also of a A.I.S. Grade 5
severity do not alter the mortality. The Figure shows the marked
variation in mortality by body area within the present study where
each patient received the same A.I.S. Grade (5).

In the Table we can see further marked variation in mortality within
the two body areas shown depending on the presence or absence of
vascular injury. Possibly the essential difference between gunshot
wounds and road traffic accidents is the penetrating nature of the
gunshot injury leading to direct major vascular injury and more
rapid haemorrhage and death.

FIGURE

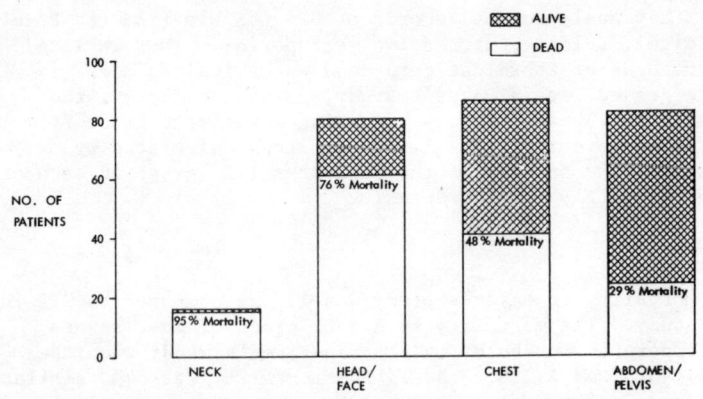

TABLE

	Overall Mortality	Mortality for Major Vessel Heart/Liver	Mortality for all other Internal Injuries
Chest	48%	95%	27%
Abdomen	29%	63%	10%

REFERENCE

Baker, S.P., O'Neill, B., Haddon, W. Jnr. and Long, W.B., 1974.
Journal of Trauma, 14, 3, 187-196.

Care of the Acutely Ill and Injured
Edited by D. H. Wilson and A. K. Marsden
© 1982, John Wiley & Sons Ltd.

STAB INJURIES IN GLASGOW

I. J. Swann

Accident and Emergency Department,
Royal Infirmary, GLASGOW

ABSTRACT

The features of stab injured patients presenting to an Accident and
Emergency Department in 1978 were studied prospectively. The
incidence of penetrating injuries to the trunk and the volume of
blood transfused were compared with those of a previous study of
stab injuries carried out in the sixties.

INTRODUCTION

The prevalence of stabbing in the east end of Glasgow was previously
studied retrospectively by Batey and MacBain. They showed that the
incidence of victims admitted to Glasgow Royal Infirmary was
increasing between 1962 and 1965.

METHOD

I carried out a prospective study of patients with stab injuries who
presented to our Accident and Emergency Department during the year
1978.

RESULTS

The study comprised 142 patients, representing 0.3% of all cases of
trauma presenting to the Accident and Emergency Department. The
commonest group were young men in their twenties, and injuries were
most often sustained on a Saturday night. Three quarters of the
patients claimed to be innocent victims of assault, but only half
of the cases were reported to the Police. Three quarters had been
drinking and 15 of the 97 admitted patients signed their own
discharge against doctors advice. Police information reveals that
over 61% of all patients had a criminal record and that over 16%
had a record for serious assault.

A wide variety of weapons had been used and there was no simple
relationship between the length of the skin wounds and the severity
of injury. Over two thirds of the wounds were anterior, and most
were left sided which may be due to the commoner use of the right
hand by the assailant.

59 patients had chest wounds; 15 of these were not admitted, and 5 patients were neither admitted nor X-rayed. Most of the 18 patients with thoracic complications were managed by insertion of a chest drain or observation, thoracotomy only being necessary on one occasion.

The abdomen was the site of injury in 50 patients. 42 were admitted and almost half of these (20) had laparotomies, one quarter of which were negative.

There were 3 deaths — 2 of which had cardiac tamponade and 1 had transected the superior mesenteric vessels and pancreas.

Almost one third of the patients had limb wounds and one tenth had wounds of the head or neck.

A total of 90 units of blood was given, almost 5 units of blood per patient transfused, compared with the study by Batey and MacBain when 37 units of blood per year were transfused, an average of 4 units per patient.

There were almost double the number of lesions of the thoracic and abdominal cavities in 1978 compared with the average yearly figures of the sixties (table 1).

TABLE 1   Penetrating Trunk Wounds

	1962-65 (Average/year)	1978
Chest Lesions	11	18
Abdominal Lesions	12	22

DISCUSSION

The study shows that the phenomenon of stabbing in 1978 was at least as prevalent at the Glasgow Royal Infirmary as it was in the sixties. It casts doubt about the credibility of many of the patients who claim to be innocent victims of assault. It raises questions of management, including the admissions policy and the use of diagnostic methods, e.g. wound exploration and peritoneal lavage.

REFERENCE

Batey, N.R. and MacBain, G.C. Injury by Stabbing.
    Scot. Med. J., 1967, 12, 251. Reproduced by permission
    of the Scottish Medical Journal.

Care of the Acutely Ill and Injured
Edited by D. H. Wilson and A. K. Marsden
© 1982, John Wiley & Sons Ltd.

THE SEVERITY OF INJURY IN ABDOMINAL
AND CHEST STABBINGS

L.A. Donaldson* I.G. Findlay A. Smith

Departments of Surgery:
Welsh National School of Medicine*, Heath Park, Cardiff
and Glasgow Royal Infirmary, Castle Street, Glasgow.

ABSTRACT

In this study there was no relationship between the admission findings and the subsequent severity of injury. In particular, 5% of the
patients with a perforated viscus had a normal blood pressure, pulse
rate and bowel sounds on admission. These factors contribute to the
problems associated with the management of stab victims.

INTRODUCTION

This study compared the admission findings with a final assessment of
the severity of the injury. The incidence of alcohol ingestion and
time of admission was recorded.

METHOD

Over a two year period 89 stab victims were admitted to Glasgow Royal
Infirmary. They were assessed on admission for the presence or
absence of 'clinical shock' (BP<100 Pulse>100) and the presence or
absence of bowel sounds. This resulted in the patients being designated into one of four groups. The severity of injury was assessed
as follows; SEVERE (major haemorrhage or visceral perforation),
MODERATE (minor liver laceration, bruised bowel, haemo/pneumo thorax)
MILD (never shocked, no laparotomy or a negative laparotomy).
Assessment of 'tenderness' was ignored due to the high incidence of
alcohol ingestion.

RESULTS

The mean age of the patients was 28.4 years with a male : female
ratio of 7 : 1. Seventy nine percent were admitted after 2300 hours
and 73% were admitted on either a Friday, Saturday or Sunday. Eighty
percent of the patients had consumed alcohol, 38% were clinically
drunk. Twenty two percent of the patients had more than one entry
wound and 33% had sustained injury of more than one organ or viscus.

L.A. Donaldson I.G. Findlay A. Smith

TABLE

	Admission Findings	Final Severity of Injury		
Group I	(Clinical shock and absent bowel sounds)	7 severe		
Group II	(Clinical shock and bowel sounds present)	8 severe	2 moderate	
Group III	(Not shocked and absent bowel sounds)	3 severe	4 moderate	1 mild
Group IV	(Not shocked and bowel sounds present)	12 severe	12 moderate	34 mild
	Total	30 severe	24 moderate	35 mild

Sixty four of the 89 patients in this study were in group IV on admission. However, 30 of these 64 patients (47%) were subsequently shown to have suffered severe or moderate injury. This included one quarter of all those patients with injury producing haemorrhage and half of those patients subsequently shown to have a visceral perforation.

DISCUSSION

There was a high incidence of significant injury in stab victims admitted with normal BP, pulse and audible bowel sounds (Donaldson et al 1981). Since this included many patients with a perforated viscus we consider a laparotomy is the optimum diagnostic procedure, providing experienced anaesthetic support is available.

REFERENCES

Donaldson, L.A., Findlay, I.G., and Smith, A., 1981. A retrospective review of 89 stab wounds to the abdomen and chest. Brit. J. Surg. (In press).
Reproduced by permission of the British Journal of Surgery and John Wright & Sons Ltd.

Care of the Acutely Ill and Injured
Edited by D. H. Wilson and A. K. Marsden
© 1982, John Wiley & Sons Ltd.

STAB-MISSILE INJURIES IN A DOWNTOWN HOSPITAL
IN MUNICH : ANALYSIS AND LATE RESULTS

J.Kleinschmidt, W.L.Brückner, and W.Heltzel

Surgical Policlinic of the University of Munich,
GERMANY

ABSTRACT

73 patients suffering from stab (52) or missile (21)
wounds during the past decade have been reviewed and
controlled. Males outnumbered fenales; the age-group
20 to 30 years was predominant. 70 percent had recovered
completely, whereas 16 percent revealed minor or major
disablement. 14 percent could not be traced down.

INTRODUCTION

Criminal activities result in more violence. Facing this
fact, a review of the injury-pattern as well as late results after emergency and/or elective surgery seemed
useful.

METHODS

73 medical recordings during the past decade have been
evaluated. At control, a physical check-up as well as
blood chemistry controls were performed; X-rays and
specialist check-ups were added when necessary.

RESULTS

Stab assaults (52) were more frequent than missile injuries. Fifty percent were age 20 to 30 years. Half of
the patients showed chest and/or abdominal injuries.
Small bowel and gut perforations were frequent. Fifty
percent had to be hospitalized. Two thirds could be
dismissed within 2 weeks. 50 percent received antibiotics

up to 7 days. Hemotherapy was necessary in less than 20 percent. Complications occurred in 34 percent (shock, pneumothorax, peritonitis). At control 1 to 10 years later, 70 percent had completely recovered. Recurrent hepatitis, respiratory deficiency, and hemiplegia were among the poor results.

DISCUSSION

Stab-missile-injuries require an experienced surgical emergency team in order to handle injuries of all topographic regions adequately. Rescue from vital threat ranks first; definite (reconstructive) surgery may be performed after stabbing, but must be postponed after shooting, because of contaminated tissue.

REFERENCES

Fischer, H., 1979. Schußverletzungen im Frieden und
        ihre Behandlung. Fortschritte der Medizin 2,
        49 - 52

Schwerd, W., 1975. in: Kurzgefaßtes Lehrbuch der Rechts-
        medizin für Mediziner und Juristen (Deutscher
        Ärzteverlag GmbH; Köln), 28-32, 58-64

Rehn, J., and Müller-Färber, J., 1979. Offene Brustkorb-
        und offene Bauchverletzungen, in: Hefte zur
        Unfallheilkunde; 42. Jahrestagung (ed.
        J. Probst). Springer-Verlag Berlin

SECTION SIX

INJURIES TO THE EXTREMITIES

Care of the Acutely Ill and Injured
Edited by D. H. Wilson and A. K. Marsden
© 1982, John Wiley & Sons Ltd.

TRAUMA TO MAJOR LIMB VESSELS

P.R.F. Bell

Department of Surgery,
Clinical Sciences Building, Royal Infirmary, Leicester, UK

Major limb vessels can be damaged in a variety of ways. Penetrating injuries caused by knife or bullet wounds provide over 80% of cases presenting in most series. (Bole et al, 1976). This type of injury is frequently associated with a high incidence of limb salvage, usually in the region of 90-95%. (Robbs and Baker, 1978) In contrast major limb vessel damage associated with blunt injury carries a much greater chance of limb loss varying between 25% and 77%. (Doty et al, 1967), Waddell and Lenczner, 1974) These figures apply to the lower limb where exploratory procedures for vascular damage are usually required if the leg is to be saved. In contrast, blunt trauma to the upper limb does not usually cause severe peripheral ischaemia. Operative intervention is, however, usually required where bleeding is a problem, with supra condylar fractures of the humerus and where arterio-venous fistulae have formed. This paper deals with factors that may help to avoid loss of the lower limb in patients with blunt trauma and vascular injury.

Fractures of the shaft of the femur and upper tibia are most common-ly associated with vascular trauma (Robbs and Baker, 1978). Vessels can be damaged in a number of different ways, presumably as a direct result of injury from the broken bone. Damage can result in a partial or complete tear, and compression can cause contusion and thrombosis. Alternatively, especially in patients with atheroma, the arterial intima can be fractured and lead to dissection with occlusion of the vessel. The reasons for a significant incidence of limb loss are many, but the more important are outlined below.

Delay in Diagnosis. Because of pain from fractures and other injuries, the usual symptoms and signs normally associated with vascular damage are not always noticed. Pallor and reduced tempera-ture are often attributed to shock. Pulses may be absent, but dis-regarded because of the patient's general condition and the possi-bility of vascular trauma forgotten. The situation may only become clear much later when the general clinical condition improves but the leg does not. The only way to avoid delay is to have a high index of suspicion. If there is any possibility of vascular injury, then the patient should be assumed to have such an injury until proved other-wise. Spasm is not an acceptable diagnosis. Valuable time should not be wasted sending the patient to the Xray Department for an

arteriogram. This can be done either in the emergency room or the
operating theatre by direct injection into the femoral artery. If
the arteriogram shows no arterial obstruction, then the other
injuries can be dealt with confidently. Alternatively, if there is
obstruction or any doubt, the vessel must be explored.

In many institutions, the fracture is next dealt with by internal
fixation and the artery repaired later. Because of the risk of
increasing muscle damage from ischaemia, the vessels should be
repaired first and the bones afterwards.

The type of repair used will depend upon the injury sustained by the
artery. If a small area of artery is contused and crushed, it can
often be excised and an end to end anastomosis performed. If this
is done, it is imperative that tension is avoided. In order to do
this, it may be necessary to divide one or two branches, but if
there is any tension at all, the gap should be bridged with a vein
graft, which should be taken from the arm or the opposite leg. If
the injury is due to intimal fracture, the vessel should be opened
longitudinally, the damaged intima removed, and the distal layer
stitched down with interrupted sutures. The incision in the vessel
should then be closed with a patch of vein which should extend
across the distal limit of the intima.   (Figure 1).

Associated Venous Injury. If the main vein accompanying the artery
is divided or damaged, then the prognosis for the limb is poorer.
(Robbs and Baker, 1978). An attempt should always be made to repair
the vein. Artificial materials are of little use for this purpose
as the repaired vessel usually thromboses. Instead, a vein graft
should be used to bridge the defect: the long saphenous, cephalic
or external jugular veins are suitable for this purpose. If the
long saphenous vein is used, the graft should be taken from the
opposite leg as the superficial veins in the damaged limb may be
essential for venous drainage. If large veins like the femoral are
damaged, then they can often be salvaged by using the veins mentioned to patch part of the lumen. If a complete portion needs to be
replaced, the graft can be tailored to a larger size by slitting it
open longitudinally and dividing it in two equal halves, which are
then stitched end to end and formed into a tube(O'Reilly et al,1980).
(Figure 2)
Muscle Oedema - Fasciotomy. After ischaemia, the muscles, particularly of the calf, become oedematous within fairly rigid fascial
compartments, causing further ischaemia due to compression. A
solution to the problem is to perform a fasciotomy, remembering that
all compartments must be opened for almost the whole length of the
lower leg. A common mistake is to open only one of the four compartments, which will lead to necrosis of muscle in the other three.
All four compartments: anterior, superficial posterior, deep
posterior and lateral, can either be dealt with by two separate
lateral and medial incisions, or all compartments can be reached by
removing the middle segment of the fibula through a lateral incision.
(Ernst and Kaufer, 1971)   (Figure 3).

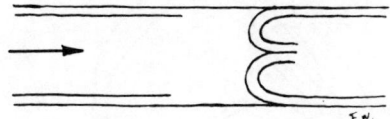

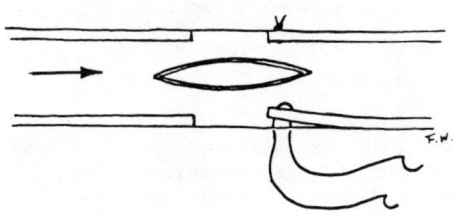

Fig. 1 The dissected atheroma
        should be removed, the
        distal intima stitched
        down and the incision in
        the artery closed with a
        vein patch

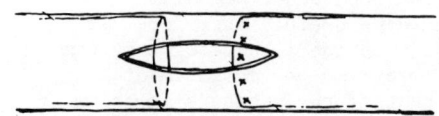

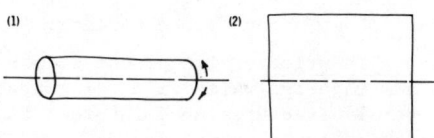

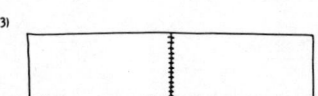

Fig. 2 Method used to convert a
        length of long saphenous
        vein into a short length
        of wide bore vein

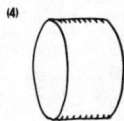

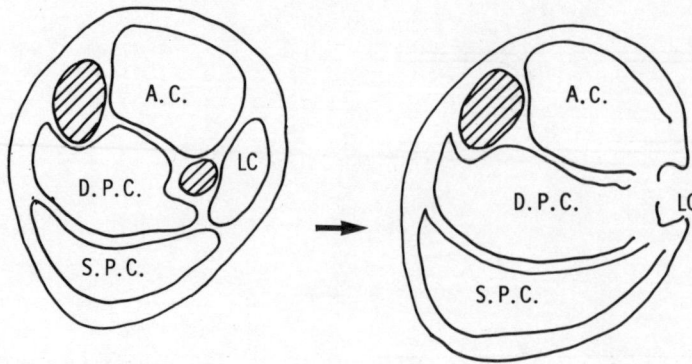

FIG. 3   Removal of a segment of fibula allows access to all four
                compartments. Anterior (A.C.)   Deep Posterior (D.P.C.)
                Superficial Posterior (S.P.C.) and Lateral (LC)

Surgeons do not always perform a fasciotomy when they should because
of the large incisions involved and the occasional need for
secondary suture or grafting. It would be useful, therefore, if
some method existed to help the surgeon decide if a fasciotomy was
necessary. Matsen et al (1980) have measured the compartmental
pressures in such cases and suggest that if the pressure is 45 mm of
Hg or more then the limb should be decompressed. This observation
remains to be substantiated as pressure measurements are notoriously
unreliable. If the calf muscles have been ischaemic for more than
4-6 hours, the patient should probably have a four compartment
fasciotomy as described earlier.

Other Injuries.   The prognosis for the limb will also depend on
other injuries which will, of course, need appropriate therapy. In
general, fractures need internal fixation, nerves secondary suture
if there is extensive damage, and dead muscle needs to be excised if
a successful outcome is to occur. Recognising dead muscle is
another problem, and if there is any doubt, excision is the rule.

          SUMMARY

In summary, penetrating injuries are associated with a good prognosis
for the limb because vessel damage is readily appreciated and treated.
With blunt trauma, limb loss is much greater because vessel trauma
is often missed for too long. Results can only be improved if the
surgeon has a high index of suspicion and avoids delay. This can be
done by doing arteriograms in the emergency room, repairing the
vessels before the fracture, repairing associated venous injury,
fasciotomy, excision of dead tissue and internal fixation of bone.

REFERENCES

Bole, P.V., Purdy, R.T., Munda,R.T., Moallem, S.H.A., Devanesan, J.
    and Clauss, R.H., 1976. Civilian arterial injuries. Annals of
    Surgery, 183, 12-23.

Ernst, C.B., and Kaufer, H., 1971. Fibulectomy - Fasciotomy:- an
    important adjunct in the management of lower extremity arterial
    trauma. The Journal of Trauma, 11, 365-377.

Doty, D.B., Treiman, R.L., Rothschild, P.D., and Gaspar, M.R., 1967.
    Prevential of gangrene due to fractures, Surgery Gynecology &
    Obstetrics, 125, 284-288.

Matsen, F.A., Winquist, R.A., and Krugmire, R.B., 1980. Diagnosis
    and management of compartmental syndromes. Journal of Bone and
    Joint Surgery, 62A, 286-291.

O'Reilly, M.J.G., Hood, J.M., Livingston, R.H., and Irwin, J.W.S.,
    1980. Penetrating injuries of the popliteal vein: a report on
    34 cases. British Journal of Surgery, 67, 337-341.

Robbs, J.V., and Baker, L.W., 1978. Major arterial trauma: review
    of experience with 267 injuries. British Journal of Surgery, 65,
    532-538.

Waddell, J.P., and Lenczner, E.M., 1974. Arterial injury associated
    with skeletal trauma. Injury, 6, 28-32

Care of the Acutely Ill and Injured
Edited by D. H. Wilson and A. K. Marsden
© 1982, John Wiley & Sons Ltd.

A SIX YEAR REVIEW OF ARTERIAL INJURIES

W.E.G.Thomas, R.J.Lusby, V.Yamin and R.N.Baird

Department of Surgery
Bristol Royal Infirmary, Bristol, UK

INTRODUCTION

Although arterial injuries form a small percentage of the work load of a vascular unit, they assume a vital importance as they tend to affect a young population in whom rapid surgical intervention can salvage a limb that might otherwise be condemned to amputation. A review of all such injuries has been undertaken in the Bristol hospitals.

METHODS

All patients presenting to the Bristol Royal Infirmary and Frenchay Hospital with peripheral arterial injuries between 1974 and 1980 were studied. Injuries to the heart and thoracic aorta were excluded, as were negative operative explorations and isolated venous injuries.

RESULTS

Sixty-three arterial injuries were treated in 58 patients. Their ages ranged from 6-73 years (median 22 years) with the majority (over 70%) occurring in teenagers and young adults. The causes were road traffic accidents - 28, stabbing - 16, (both domestic and assault) glass - 8 and iatrogenic injuries - 6. Of these latter cases 4 followed cardiac catheterisation, I hip replacement and I laparoscopy. Concomitant fractures or dislocations occurred in 27 and nerve injuries in 19.

Penetrating injuries were explored without delay. Some closed injuries were diagnosed late, especially if distal pulses were transiently restored as occurred after reduction of a fracture/dislocation (twice) or with a stab wound (once). In these cases the decision to explore the vessel rested on a high index of suspicion and arteriography. The other indications for operation were uncontrolled bleeding, acute and chronic limb ischaemia, and arterio-venous fistula.

Reconstructive operations were done in 51 (81%) and major amputations were necessary for combined arterial and brachial plexus injury (2), crush injury (2) and irreversible ischaemia (I). Two reconstructions were initially less than ideal and were detected and corrected by intraoperative monitoring using arteriography and a pulse volume recorder. Postoperatively 48 of 51

285

reconstructions remained patent. However combined artery and nerve injuries commonly resulted in a poor functional result.

DISCUSSION

In order to produce good clinical results following arterial injuries, early diagnosis and good operative techniques are vital. Early diagnosis depends on a high index of clinical suspicion and we would emphasise the need and importance of arteriography. All penetrating wounds should be explored without delay, and in stab injuries both anterior and posterior walls of the vessel should be inspected for possible entry and exit holes. Operative techniques involve preliminary bony fixation and repair of any concomitant venous injury. Excision of the damaged portion of the artery may be necessary and we would recommend the use of vein grafts in injuries of the limb vessels as all anastomoses must be performed without tension. The functional result can be assessed by intraoperative monitoring using pulse volume recordings of the wave form and on-table angiography. These are simple and quick methods of assessing the arterial blood flow in the grafts, and can be used for out-of-hours emergencies. They allow immediate correction of any reconstruction that is less than ideal and the pulse volume recorder can be used for monitoring in the recovery room as well. The final functional outcome often depends on concomitant nerve injuries. With combined artery and nerve injuries for which arterial reconstructions were performed, 8 out of 11 patients had prolonged poor sensory and motor function, although limb perfusion was satisfactory. In two brachial plexus injuries, the nerves were irrecoverably damaged and in consequence the associated arterial injury was not repaired and an amputation done.

In conclusion, the successful management of arterial injuries depends on painstaking diagnosis, with a high index of clinical suspicion and early arteriography. The cornerstones of operative repair are removal of the damaged segment and the avoidance of undue tension at the anastomoses, with prior bony fixation and concomitant repair of damaged veins. Intraoperative monitoring by arteriography and pulse volume recordings are valuable adjuncts to surgical repair. Successful arterial repair is rewarded by long term patency, the final outcome depending on the severity of any associated nerve injury.

Care of the Acutely Ill and Injured
Edited by D. H. Wilson and A. K. Marsden
© 1982, John Wiley & Sons Ltd.

USE OF THE CORACO—CLAVICULAR HOOK
IN ACROMIO—CLAVICULAR DISLOCATION

W. N. F. Boughey, F.R.C.S.

Pilgrim Hospital, Boston, Lincolnshire.

Acromio—clavicular dislocations have been treated by many methods
none of which are satisfactory and the Coraco—Clavicular Hook
was designed to deal with this. It is an entirely new concept
and consists of a curved area which fits under the coracoid
with a male and female size for the male and female coracoid
processes. This continues into a screw thread with a washer
and nut.

A hole is made through the clavicle and the screw thread allowed
through this freely, then the washer is countersunk, the bolt
applied and the whole of the bolt screwed down so that the
clavicle apposes the coracoid and thus reduces the acromio-
clavicular dislocation.

This, in fact, mimics the action of the conoid and trapezoid
portions of the coraco—clavicular ligament. The excess screw
thread is removed with a cutter.

The incision is from the tip of the corocoid directly backwards
over the clavicle and almost down to the spine of the scapula.
This incision is medial to the usual shoulder incisions such as
for Putti—Platt operation etc. The incision is made so that
this corresponds to the strap area in the female. This is
sometimes difficult to attain but every effort should be made,
particularly in the female, to place the incision in such a
position. The incision is deepened down to the sub—cutaneous
tissues and the muscles. These are the muscles overlying the
coracoid process and the muscles and aponeurosis over the
clavicle. This is by a blunt dissection along the line of the
muscle fibres overlying the coracoid. The coracoid is exposed
from base to tip. Next an incision is made down and through
the aponeurosis to the clavicular bone and the area of the
clavicular bone is stripped by periosteal elevator both medially
and laterally as far as the acromio—clavicular joint. The
acromio—clavicular joint will be found usually to have a loose
meniscus and the superior acromio—clavicular ligaments are not
very strong and found to be disrupted. At the same time it
will be found that the conoid and trapezoid portions of the
coraco—clavicular ligament will, in the case of an acromio-
clavicular dislocation, be completely torn and this can be

287

demonstrated at operation. The whole of the area of the
clavicle, i.e. the superior, inferior and other two surfaces
should be completely mobilised. Having mobilised both the
corocoid and the clavicular area and the acromio-clavicular
joint and exposed this area there is still some tissue between
these two areas including a leash of vessels. The leash of
vessels has to be cauterised and the area cleared between the
base of the coracoid and the clavicle. This is a very small
area.

Having done this it can be demonstrated that the clavicle can
be easily pulled up by use of a bone hook. As all attachments
and ligaments are torn the lateral end of the clavicle can be
easily pulled upwards. This is in order eventually to be able
to place the tip of the screw thread through the lower surface.
An incision is made into the lateral side of the coracoid and
a MacDonald's inserted. This enables the hook to be placed as
near the bone as possible. Having mobilised this area the hook
area is slipped under the bone by use of the fingers. This has
to be snugly placed under the bone so that the curve of the
hook completely encompasses the lower part of the coracoid
process. Having done this the line of the screw thread should
then be orientated towards the clavicle at a suitable point.

Once this is lined up a hole may be made in the clavicle. This
hole has to be larger, of course, than the screw thread to
allow the screw thread to pass through freely. The hole is
started with an awl and then the hole drilled in line with the
screw thread through the clavicular bone. This line should not
be too near the edge of the bone otherwise problems will occur.
The hole is usually made with the largest Muller drill bit
(suitable for the large cancellous screws). A periosteal
elevator is always used when drilling to protect the under
surface of the clavicular bone and the vessels beneath it. Once
the hole is made the bone hook is used to pull up the clavicle.
The clavicular hook is steadied in the area of the coracoid
process with the forceps and the screw thread gently slid
through the clavicular bone till it comes through the superficial surface. The screw thread is then put through the bone
and a countersink instrument either attached to a drill or hand
used is then used to make some depression in the surface of the
clavicular bone. This is to enable the washer and nut to be
countersunk somewhat so that it does not project too much. It
is important that this amount of bone should not be too much
otherwise the clavicular bone will be weakened. So long as a
small depth is attained then this is satisfactory for the
purpose. Once the countersink instrument has been used then the
washer is placed on, then the nut and the nut and washer screwed
down with the instrument. If none is available then the edge
of a pair of pliers or even some other form of gripping tool
would be satisfactory to turn the nut suitably. If a countersink instrument is not available then the cannulated drill used
in pinning femurs can be used. The nut is then turned and the

clavicular bone is seen to gradually appose the coracoid
process and this goes on until the lateral edge of the
clavicular bone is level with the acromium, in other words the
acromio-clavicular joint dislocation is suitably and rigidly
reduced. The excess screw thread is then cut off with a
Berberker wire cutter.

Having done this the muscle and aponeurosis and muscle over the
clavicular bone and over the nut and washer area is sewed with
interrupted Ethiflex sutures. It is best to use unabsorbable
sutures in this situation. Occasionally it is worth firstly
removing the torn meniscus if it has not already disappeared in
the dissection from the acromio-clavicular joint and secondly
if there is some tissue left round the joint it is worth putting
one or two Ethiflex sutures in what was the area of the superior
acromio-clavicular ligament. A Zimmer drain is then placed in
the sub-cutaneous tissues and the fat sutures inserted.
Interrupted Mersilk sutures are used for the skin and a dressing
applied. A sling is applied immediately at the end of the
operation. The drain is removed at forty-eight hours. It is
not sutured in usually and is just slid out through the dressing.
The arm is kept in a sling, the patient can go home when matters
have settled usually in four or five days and be seen a week
later, i.e. at twelve days for removal of some or all of the
sutures. The sling is kept on another week, a total of three
weeks. Active movements are then started by the patient himself
or herself and there is no need for physiotherapy except in
resistant cases. Usually movements are attained very rapidly
and at the time of eight weeks there is full movement, full
power and the patient is usually able to go back to work.

This technique can be used in early or later cases. In early
cases the patient is seen and put on the next operating list
which may be two, three, four or five days later. These cases
can be done at any time particularly in females who have a
deformity and wish to exchange deformity for a scar that can be
hidden. It makes no difference in late cases whether the
situation is two months, four months or even six months old.

In the past eight years this technique has been used for forty
cases of acromio-clavicular dislocation particularly in patients
who are involved in extremely heavy work such as in the farming
community etc. This can be considered a permanent implant. All
shoulders are satisfactory at eight weeks with full movements
and all patients have been back to work from six to eight weeks
and to full, heavy work at the end of eight weeks. In only two
cases has the hook had to be removed because of sepsis, one
early and one late.

The scar falls backwards in the strap region in the female and,
therefore, is cosmetically satisfactory. There have been no
problems with the scar cutting through the coracoid, breaking
of the hook, avulsion of the bolt or breaking of the washer etc.

In fact, none of what might have been expected problems have
occurred. It can, therefore, be considered to be a very
satisfactory method of dealing with the problem of the acromio-
clavicular dislocation.

Hooks and the two instruments can be obtained from Howmedica
(U.K.) Ltd. A film of the technique may be loaned if the author
can show it.

Care of the Acutely Ill and Injured
Edited by D. H. Wilson and A. K. Marsden
© 1982, John Wiley & Sons Ltd.

KAESSMANN COMPRESSION NAIL IN FRACTURES

J.Stapert, C.R.v.d.Hoogenband, J.M.Greep, H.A.J.Lemmens

Department of Traumatology, St.Annadal Hospital,
University of Limburg, Maastricht, The Netherlands.

Intramedullary fixation of fractures has been practiced for a long
time. Since Nicolaysen 1897 described this treatment, many systems
of intramedullary stabilisation have been developed.
The work of Küntscher resulted in a world-wide use of his technique.
Küntscher devoted a surgical lifetime perfecting his method based on
the principle of achieving stability by the impingement of an elastic
nail in the medullary canal.
The Swiss A.O. group advocated a method of osteosynthesis based on
the principle of interfragmentary compression.
In 1966 Kaessmann developed an intramedullary nail by means of which
interfragmentary compression could be given and thus combined the
Küntscher concept with the A.O. principles.
In intramedullary fixation of fractures, the method of osteosynthesis
is to a large extent defined by the relation of the fracture site to
the isthmus of the medullary canal. We used three methods of intramedullary fixation.

1. KUNTSCHER NAIL.
This nail can only be applied to a segment of the femoral shaft where
after reaming of the medullary canal, enough cortical bone remains in
order to achieve stability by the elastic impingement of a Küntscher
nail. This segment contains the potential isthmus. After reaming this
potential isthmus or artificial isthmus should be long and wide
enough to ensure internal locking of a Küntscher nail strong enough
to take all the strain it will be subjected to.
Fractures in this potential isthmus are preferably treated with a
Küntscher nail. About two thirds of all femoral fractures are within
the limit of this potential isthmus. About one third however is not
located within this segment and together with the very oblique and
comminuted fractures insuitable for the Küntscher technique.

2. KAESSMANN NAIL.
The second method we used is the Kaessmann nail. With this nail axial
directed interfragmentary compression can be obtained.
Stability is obtained by interfragmentary compression and securing
axial deformity by the nail.

In this method bone and nail together bear the external stresses they
are subjected to. In consequence the nail can be smaller and reaming
of the medullary cavity is no longer essential to obtain stability.

3. KAESSMANN NAIL IN COMBINATION WITH CERCLAGE WIRES.

If it should prove necessary to stabilize comminuted fractures or
very long oblique fractures, we use our third method of stabilization
by adding encircling wire loops to the Kaessmannnail.
First of all it is impossible to obtain perfect stability by the use
of encircling wire loops alone for osteosynthesis. Moreover, in this
type of fracture the fragments will tend to splay outwards and considerable shortening is to be expected if axial directed interfragmentary pressure is applied.
Perfect stability can however be achieved if such splaying is controlled by a number of cerclage wires.

RESULTS.

143 Femoral fractures in 139 patients, 37 female and 96 male, have
been stabilized by intramedullary fixation in a ten years' period in
our 780 bed hospital. 11 Patients died, 4 because of the trauma, 7
because of an unrelated disease.
9.1% Of the fractures were open, 17.5% comminuted. 60% Of the patients
were under 30 years old, 10% over 70 year.
97 were re-examined, one patient ten year after the trauma.

COMPLICATIONS.

In the 79 "Küntscher patients" two (2.1%) had an infection. No pseud-
arthrosis was seen. In the 33 "Kaessmann patients", four (11.7%)
suffered from an infection. Two patients had a non-union, one pseud-
arthrosis was infected. In the 31 "Kaessmann cerclage patients" two
(6.4%) got infected, three patients (9.6%) had a non-union and one
patient (3.2%) had an infected non-union.
Looking to the healing of these fractures, we see that in the
"Küntscher patients" non-weight bearing walking could be started 2.5
weeks after operation. Full weight bearing was allowed after 7 weeks.
Radiological union was achieved in 14.7 weeks.
Patients resumed their work after 6.8 month.
In the Kaessmann cerclage group the consolidation period was almost
the same.

FUNCTIONAL RESULTS.

The functional results were called good if full return to work and/or
sport was achieved. If normal daily activities were possible, sometimes with complaints of pain or slight restricted function, the
functional results were called moderate. Patients with bad functional
results had severe complaints or influence on the daily activities.
There was no bad result in the Küntscher group, in both Kaessmann
groups one patient had a bad outcome of his treatment. Looking at
these figures one thing is clear: if you have to perform an internal
fixation on a transverse or short oblique femoral fracture within the

potential isthmus, use a Küntscher nail.
But fractures unsuitable for treatment with a Küntscher nail are
difficult and in many hospitals an indication for plating.
The results of the fractures treated with a Kaessmann nail should be
compared with the results of plate osteosynthesis for femoral
fractures.
In our material we compared the results of intramedullary stabilized
comminuted and long oblique fractures with the results of plate
osteosynthesis of other authors.

		Infection	Pseudarthrosis
Koudi	100 (51 A.O. + 33 K. nail)	6 %	6 %
1977			
Tscherne	comminuted femur		
1977	160 (127 A.O. + 33 K. nail)	8.6%	13.1%
Roberts	35 A.O. plate	2.8%	11.4%
1977			
Taillard	80 A.O. plate	4 %	5 %
1976			
Kootstra	43 A.O. plate	7 %	13.5%
Maastricht	34 intramedullary	2.9%	8.8%

In our opinion the Kaessmann cerclage system offers to the surgeon
familiar with intramedullary fixation, a safe alternative to plating.
Undoubtedly the eldery patient with a low energy injury resulting in
a long oblique fracture, can benefit from this method.

CONCLUSION.
For femoral fractures where osteosynthesis with a Küntscher nail is
impossible, Kaessmann compression and cerclage wiring is a safe and
simple method of treatment.

Care of the Acutely Ill and Injured
Edited by D. H. Wilson and A. K. Marsden
© 1982, John Wiley & Sons Ltd.

THE PLANNING AND ORGANISATION FOR THE MANAGEMENT OF HAND
INJURIES.

N. J. Barton

The University Hospital, Queen's Medical Centre,
Nottingham. NG7 2UH

THE PROBLEMS

The problems to be solved in organising a service for the treatment
of hand injuries can perhaps be shown most clearly by comparing them
with those presented by abdominal injuries.

Injuries to the abdomen are uncommon. They may seem fairly minor,
but must always be treated seriously because the damage may be more
extensive than appears at first sight. However there is no doubt
as to who should deal with them: this is the province of the
abdominal surgeon, and he should be called to see all such injuries.

In contrast, injuries to the hand are very common, comprising about
25% of all injuries. Moreover it is not immediately obvious which
type of specialist is best equipped to deal with them, since many
hand injuries require in-patient treatment and specialised surgical
skills and facilities which are beyond the scope of the Accident
and Emergency Department, and they may have both orthopaedic and
plastic components. Having decided on the appropriate specialist,
one faces the central and most difficult problem of all in planning
a hand injury service, which is that hand injuries are so common
that it is quite impractical to call the specialist to see them all.

Casualty Officers. In practice they will be treated in an Accident
and Emergency Department by a junior doctor with no more than six
months experience of such matters, usually less, sometimes none at
all. Some hand injuries are minor and can safely be treated by
these junior doctors. Others are obviously major and must be
admitted, or referred immediately to some more experienced surgeon.
Many seem minor, like some abdominal injuries, but in fact need
skilled treatment: for example, Lipscomb has said of phalangeal
fractures: "Too often they are treated as minor injuries and major
disability results".

Second Line Of Defence. It is therefore necessary to have a more
senior doctor, i.e. someone in a permanent post to provide continuity
and experience and to be responsible for organising the service.

THE PLAN

It is not necessary or even desirable that every hospital should
organise its hand service in the same way. The needs and facilities
of a small hospital are different to those of a large one, though
a very isolated hospital should be able to offer more treatment
than is necessary in a hospital which is close to another centre
with a specialised department of hand surgery.

Who should be the specialist responsible for treating hand injuries?
It is not necessary to specify that he should come from a particular
speciality: what he must have is -

1. A genuine and keen interest in hand injuries, and a willingness
    to undertake primary treatment, because in all hand injuries,
    and especially the more serious ones, the result depends to a
    great extent on getting it right first time.

2. Knowledge about hand injuries and training in their treatment.
    In practice, this means that he must have an adequate background
    in the relevant parts of orthopaedic and plastic surgery.
    Since plastic centres are few, but all District General
    Hospitals have an orthopaedic department, an orthopaedic surgeon
    is the most likely person to fill this role in the average
    hospital. It is now recommended that a District General
    Hospital should have at least three orthopaedic consultants,
    one of whom has a special interest in hand injuries.

3. Time, not only to operate on badly injured hands, but to do
    regular hand clinics as a screen behind the junior Casualty
    Officers. Ideally all patients with hand injuries should be
    screened by the senior doctor, but it may be more realistic to
    specify certain categories of patients who must be referred to
    the next specialist clinic. It is important to avoid delay:
    two weeks after the injury, it may be too late to change the
    treatment.

Specialist Hand Surgeons. In America, hand surgery is well
established as a surgical speciality. In Europe, few hospitals
have surgeons whose work is confined to hand surgery, though in
most large centres it is recognised that better results are obtained
by surgeons who devote a large proportion of their time to this
type of work.

A Hand Surgery Team. The British Society for Surgery of the Hand
considers it "unlikely, in the foreseeable future, that hand surgery
will become a separate speciality in this country. Hand surgery is
undertaken, to a large extent, by the orthopaedic and plastic
surgical specialities and in both these disciplines there are
surgeons with a particular interest in surgery of the hand to whom
cases are channelled". However, it is necessary that these
specialists work together, not only with each other, but with
Accident and Emergency specialists, to provide a team for the
treatment of hand injuries. This is the system we use at the

Nottingham University Hospital and it works well (Fig. 1).

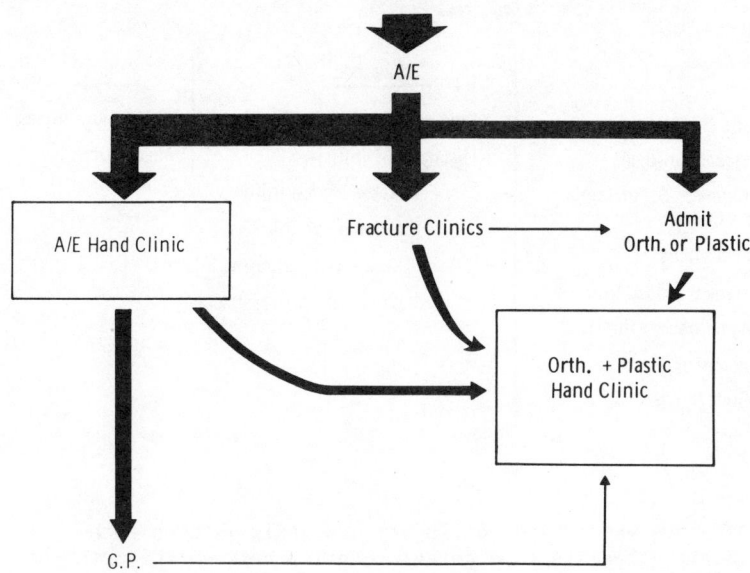

Fig. 1. Flow chart for hand injuries in Nottingham.

The A.&E. consultant does a hand clinic in his department every afternoon at 3.00 p.m., to which patients are referred by the Casualty Officers. In addition, an orthopaedic consultant does a Fracture Clinic every morning to which all fractures from the previous day are referred. Once a week there is a combined hand clinic at which one particular orthopaedic consultant and one particular plastic consultant, each of whom has a special interest in hand surgery, work simultaneously in adjoining rooms, consulting together as necessary. These two are on call alternately for the care of major hand injuries requiring admission to hospital.

If this is to work there must be an agreement as to who will normally treat what, and this agreement must be honoured. There must also be goodwill and a free interchange of patients and ideas between the different specialists, who must meet and talk to each other regularly. Sometimes they will work together on one patient.

The other essential member of the team is the hand therapist: not just any physiotherapist, but one with a special interest and experience in the hand. The surgery needs a specialist and the therapy needs a specialist too, because the hand is not the same as the leg or back and the techniques of treatment are not the same either.

TABLE 1. The distribution of different types of hand
injuries between different specialists in
Nottingham.

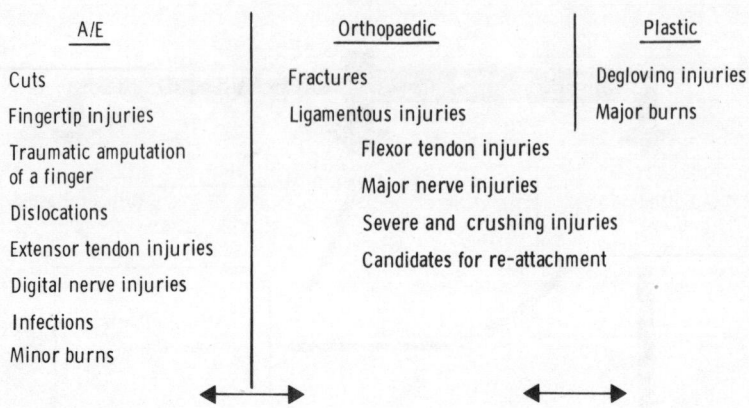

A/E	Orthopaedic	Plastic
Cuts	Fractures	Degloving injuries
Fingertip injuries	Ligamentous injuries	Major burns
Traumatic amputation of a finger	Flexor tendon injuries	
Dislocations	Major nerve injuries	
Extensor tendon injuries	Severe and crushing injuries	
Digital nerve injuries	Candidates for re-attachment	
Infections		
Minor burns		

Table 1 shows which types of injury are dealt with by each
department: there is considerable overlap between the orthopaedic
and plastic departments. Fractures in the hand are best treated by
specialists in the treatment of fractures and should be referred to
the next Fracture Clinic to see an orthopaedic surgeon. The only
exceptions are fingertip fractures where the bony injury should be
ignored and the condition treated as a soft tissue injury in the
A.&E. Department.

TRAINING

How are we to train the doctors who will be treating hand injuries?

Casualty Officers. This is the critical area, because if the
Casualty Officer fails to realise the significance of an injury,
the best opportunity to treat it has been missed. However, if he
correctly diagnoses the injury but then tries to treat the injury
himself when it is beyond his level of competence, he will do
permanent and irreparable harm because once an area of scarring and
adhesions has been introduced into the hand it can never be removed.

However, it is very difficult to train Casualty Officers because
they change every six months, they have to deal with a wide range
of accidents and emergencies and they are under great pressure, not
only in the busy Casualty Department, but because they are often
studying for higher exams.

As far as hand injuries are concerned, the minimum training must
include:

a) **An initial indoctrination** given to all new Casualty Officers on

arrival, either in the form of a talk from the head of the
department, or a document, or preferably both. The principles
to be got across are that hand injuries are potentially very
disabling and are therefore important ("small does not mean
minor"); that lacerations over a tendon or nerve must be assumed
to have cut that tendon or nerve until proved otherwise, not by
poking around in the wound but by a careful and informed
clinical examination of the parts distal to the wound; that
common operations are not necessarily easy operations; and that
operations on the hand require care, fine instruments, a
tourniquet etc.

Most important of all, they must be given clear and written
instructions as to which type of injury may be treated in the
A.&E. Department, and which must be referred to the hand
specialist or specialists (see Table 1). Stress must be laid
on the necessity to get the treatment right first time, i.e.
to call the specialist then, not days or weeks later. Similarly,
they must be instructed to refer patients whom they have treated
for minor hand injuries to a senior colleague within the next
few days, so that the diagnosis and treatment can be checked.

b) Lectures or seminars on the systematic examination of the hand
    (including lacerations of the wrist) and recording of findings,
    and on how to treat those conditions (see Table 1) which are
    suitable for management within the A.&E. Department. It is
    possible to obtain recorded tape-slide presentations on these
    topics. It is also desirable that the common operative
    procedures, such as terminalisation after a traumatic amputation,
    should be demonstrated and taught to the Casualty Officer before
    he does them on his own.

c) As an optional extra, Casualty Officers should be encouraged to
    attend suitable courses. The British Society for Surgery of the
    Hand holds regional courses in Basic Hand Surgery for S.H.O.s
    and registrars: each year there is one course in the South-
    West, one in the Midlands and one in the North-East of England,
    usually lasting two days. Details may be obtained from the
    Secretary of the British Society for Surgery of the Hand, whose
    offices are at the Royal College of Surgeons in Lincoln's Inn
    Fields.

Accident and Emergency Specialists. The training programme for
this speciality, as laid down by the Joint Committee on Higher
Medical and Surgical Training, specifies that training and
experience should include "The initial assessment of hand infections
and injuries and their initial management only". It is thus
recognised that the surgical treatment of injuries to flexor tendons,
the median and ulnar nerves, or the crushed hand, requires
specialised skills and experience which cannot be provided in the
A.&E. Department.

Orthopaedic and Plastic Surgeons. The Specialist Advisory
Committees for these specialities require training in hand surgery

as part of the training of every orthopaedic or plastic surgeon.

Hand Surgeons. The Sub-Committee on Training of the British
Society for Surgery of the Hand recommends that "Senior Registrars
anxious to pursue their interest in hand surgery as part of their
career as a consultant in either orthopaedic or plastic surgery,
should be encouraged to obtain a rotation or exchange with a Senior
Registrar in a plastic/orthopaedic unit. This would complement the
trainee's basic experience and enable him to rectify any defects in
his overall training. Six months or one year are the suggested
times for such an exchange. It would be necessary to designate
certain Units for such further training viz., those where there is
a sufficient volume of hand surgery available as well as the
necessary facilities. There may well be difficulties because of
the preponderance of orthopaedic to plastic trainees. At the
present time, it is sometimes necessary for trainees to seek a
period of further training overseas".

However, although a period of training overseas is often very
beneficial, it should also be possible to obtain specialist training
in hand surgery in Great Britain, not only for our own Senior
Registrars but for surgeons from other countries which still look
to Britain for their training in medicine and surgery. The
Department of Health and Social Security should create about ten
special posts, equivalent to Senior Registrar, to provide advanced
training in hand surgery. These posts would be held for six or
twelve months, which would constitute additional training but would
not affect the manpower situation, as the holders would then proceed
to existing consultant posts in orthopaedic or plastic surgery, or
would return to their own country overseas.

REFERENCES

British Society for Surgery of the Hand (Sub-Committee on Training
in Hand Surgery). Memorandum on Training in Hand Surgery. May
1981.
Joint Committees on Higher Medical and Higher Surgical Training.
Accident and Emergency Medicine: Full Training Programme.
Lipscomb, P. R., 1963. Management of fractures of the hand. The
American Surgeon, 29 : 277

Care of the Acutely Ill and Injured
Edited by D. H. Wilson and A. K. Marsden
© 1982, John Wiley & Sons Ltd.

ACUTE HAND PROBLEMS - BONE AND JOINT INJURY

P.J.Mulligan, F.R.C.S.(G), F.R.C.S.(Eng.).

The Royal Orthopaedic Hospital,
Birmingham and Birmingham General Hospital.

      The acute hand injury interferes dramatically
with the life of the patient. Immediate care should
be of the highest quality available. I will describe
difficulties that I have encountered when dealing with
patients.

ASSESSMENT

The assessment must deal with three main factors.

    A. The injury sustained.

    B. The functional loss.

    C. The functional requirement of the patient.

All of these aspects must be accurately documented and
the appropriate treatment thereafter undertaken by
someone who can envisage the result in the weeks and
months ahead.

PITFALLS

The inexperienced member of a medical team will
frequently undertake the treatment of such injuries
without recognising the dangers until it is too late.
Examples would be:-

    a). Preoccupation with fractures, neglecting
    the soft tissues.

    b). Mis-diagnosing the 'closed crush injury'.

    c). Failing to recognise joint instability
    and allowing early movement.

INTERIM CARE - SPLINTAGE AND REHABILITATION

After the initial interview, proper care should be
given to the elevation, prevention of swelling and
splintage in position of protection. The physiotherapist

P.J.Mulligan, F.R.C.S.(G), F.R.C.S.(Eng.).

involved must be fully acquainted in the amount of active and passive movement that can be allowed and active deformities which should be prevented.

PRINCIPLES OF TREATMENT OF SOME SEVERE INJURIES.

The Major Crushed Hand

By early transfixtion of digits in severely crushed injury, with multiple compound fractures, stabilisation and early movement can be achieved. Examples will show how many fingers are saved by this technique and how it can be applied to single finger injuries and those requiring skin grafting.

Phalangeal Fractures.

Fractures in the medulla of the phalanges should only be reduced if there is rotation or angulation. Internal fixation should always be applied where there is gross involvement of the joint.

Metacarpal Fractures.

Assessment of these is frequently poor and shortening, rotation or malalignment are good indications for internal fixation.

Joint Instability.

Instability in the proximal phalangeal joints after injury is probably the commonest cause of progressive deformity, pain and stiffness and it is often poorly managed. Early mobilisation should not be undertaken until the stability of the joint is fully assessed. It should be immobilised in extension for inspection by a qualified hand surgeon. Metacarpal phalangeal joint ligament injuries should be repaired.

Mulligan, P.J. and Scott, M.M., 1980
    Les Fractures des Phalanges a Fragments Multiples
    Communitives (Hand Surgery - Roaul Tubiana).
Scott, M.M. and Mulligan, P.J., 1980.
    Stabilising Severe Phalangeal Fractures.
    The Hand, 12:1, 44-50, 1980

Care of the Acutely Ill and Injured
Edited by D. H. Wilson and A. K. Marsden
© 1982, John Wiley & Sons Ltd.

THE TREATMENT OF NERVE AND FLEXOR TENDON INJURIES

F.D.Burke, F.R.C.S.

Consultant Hand Surgeon,
Derbyshire Royal Infirmary, Derby.

The hand is an unforgiving area of the body and is particularly so
in cases where there has been nerve or tendon injury.   When
discussing the treatment of such injuries it is, I feel, necessary
to spend a short period of time on the question of diagnosis,
because the treatment depends entirely on whether a diagnosis is
made on the patient's first visit to the Accident and Emergency
Department, or at a later date.

When the patient is first seen in the Accident and Emergency
Department he is examined and a history taken.   The Doctor should
then be in a position to identify all the damaged structures and to
plan his treatment programme.   It is a programme which can be
altered as events unfold, but I think it is important that a plan
should be made by the Doctor before an exploration of the hand takes
place.   We sometimes tend to forget that the patient also expects
something of this initial interview and should be informed of the
likely damage that he has sustained and how it will affect him over
the next few weeks or months.

Assessment involves the predicted injury to the various systems in
the hand, skin, bones, joints, tendons, nerves and blood vessels.
There are also other important factors that have already been
mentioned, notably the patient's age, occupation and dominant hand.
The cut/crush ratio is an important fact to establish, the length
of time since injury, and the degree of contamination of the wound
are clearly also significant.   The position of the hand at the
time of injury is particularly important from the point of view of
the flexor tendons and will be mentioned a little later.

Should the repair of nerves and tendons be performed at the time of
injury?   I believe where facilities are available for the primary
repair, this is the treatment of choice.   This applies both to
nerves and tendons.   The majority of severe hand injuries attending
Accident and Emergency Departments in this country arrive within an
hour or two of the injury itself and the degree of contamination is
not great.   I believe that all but the most grossly contaminated
injuries can be treated by primary repair.

A secondary repair is required for that small number of patients who present late with a grossly contaminated wound, or in whom the diagnosis has been overlooked at their first assessment.   Why are such cases overlooked in the Accident and Emergency Department? - frequently because the examination is inadequate.   The patient is emotionally shocked and can be a poor witness.

In dealing with sensory loss, I believe it is important to stroke the finger tip that is being examined and to ask the patient whether it feels the same as another uninjured finger.   In this way one is comparing two different fingers and asking the patient if the sensation is the same.   This seems to me a satisfactory way of assessing sensation and one is less likely to be misled.   The phrase to avoid in examining for sensory loss is "Can you feel this?" stroking the tip of the involved finger.   If the patient feels any sensation over the tip of the finger, or indeed is conscious of any movement of the finger, however slight, he is likely to say "Yes", even in the presence of a nerve injury.

When examining a hand one naturally looks at the position of the fingers and whether the normal cascade of increasing flexion from radial to ulnar border of the hand is present or not.   Motor testing of the abductor digiti minimi - supplied by the ulnar nerve, is best done by not only testing abduction of the small finger but by placing an examining finger on the muscle itself to ensure it is contracting.   Movement of the long finger from side to side is a good quick test of the ulnar intrinsic, supplied by the deep motor branch.   More recently the capacity to cross one's fingers has been described as a useful test in this regard.   Checking the motor branch of the median nerve, abductor pollicis brevis, again the thumb is laid on the muscle itself, checking that that particular muscle is contracting and responsible for the movement. Similarly, I would test the profundus and superficialis function across all the fingers.   This examination may cause the patient a certain amount of discomfort, but I still think it is required. I do not think it is acceptable to explore a hand and see what is divided, I think one should have a very clear idea before exploration occurs, what structures are likely to be damaged.

From the Accident and Emergency point of view, I think the most important thing is to have a high index of suspicion in these cases and a sufficient knowledge of anatomy to appreciate the structures which lie under any particular laceration.   The amount of gross anatomy taught in our medical schools in this country has been markedly reduced over the last few years and I think it important that the anatomy of the upper limb and hand particularly should be stressed, as it is injury to this area that the Casualty Officer is going to have to frequently deal with.

Coming now on to nerve repairs, should it be epineurial or fascicular?   Up to recent years, surgeons have been fairly content to repair the epineurium alone.   It is a relatively easy thing to do, the epineurium forming a fairly thick sheath around the nerve, which takes a stitch fairly satisfactorily.   Theoretically,

objections to this are that the fascicles may not be correctly
aligned inside and if too much tension is placed on the repair,
the fascicle ends may buckle and reduce the number of axons crossing
to the distal portion of the nerve.

To overcome this, the fascicular nerve repair was then put forward,
where the epineurium is cut back over a short segment and the
fascicles themselves are sutured, using finer suture material.
I favour the epi-perineurial suture, where a suture is placed
through a peripheral fascicle, then through the epineurium, the
stitch is then carried back through the epineurium of the distal
portion of the nerve and then through the appropriate fascicle.
This technique seems to give one the best of both worlds, where the
fascicles are aligned and yet the stitch is in firm fibrous tissue.
One can place two or perhaps three fine fascicular sutures at the
centre of the nerve to align the more central fascicles.

I believe the repairs should not be performed under any significant
tension, that the eight-O or ten-O mono-filament nylon should be
used as a suture and that nerves the size of the median or ulnar
should be repaired with the operating microscope.   Digital nerves
I would simply repair with the aid of magnifying loupes of 2½ times
magnification.

Where the treatment of nerve injury is delayed, either due to a
failure of diagnosis or gross contamination, a secondary repair
would be required.   Diagnosis of these lesions is not usually a
problem.   There may be an obvious motor deficit and there is usually
a fairly obvious sensory loss.   There may be marked tenderness over
the scar, indicating an underlying neuroma.   O'Riain's test is
useful in cases where there is an element of doubt.   When the hand
is immersed in warm water for 25-30 minutes, the characteristic
wrinkling of the skin occurs, but not in an area which has been
denervated.

An excruciatingly painful papilloma appearing in the scar may
indicate a cutaneous neuroma.   In such cases the proximal end of
the divided digital nerve is left on the skin surface at the time of
injury.

When one explores a late nerve injury, one often finds a large
neuroma and I find that I almost invariably need to cable graft the
defect.   To repair the nerve under tension is felt by most people
to grossly prejudice the result.   By the time one has trimmed back
to good material on both sides, there is usually a 3cm gap which
requires a cable graft.   I normally use the sural nerve from the leg
or perhaps one of the cutaneous nerves of the forearm.   The
procedure is done with an operating microscope, ten-O or eight-O
nylon sutures being used to hold the cables in place.   Partial nerve
injuries similarly require exploration under the operating microscope,
with the preservation of the continuity of the intact fascicles and
the repair or grafting of the damaged ones.

Turning now to flexor tendon injuries, our problems here relate
particularly to the flexor tendon in the finger.   The problems
arise largely because of the flexor tendon sheath which intimately
invests the flexor tendons and permits them to work so effectively
in flexing the finger joints.   The hand and wrist have been
divided into five zones.   Zone 1, where the profundus tendon alone
lies in the sheath, creates some difficulties, but the most
difficult area of all is Zone 2, where both profundus and superficialis are running within the flexor tendon sheath.   It is this
area particularly that has caused difficulties in the past and is
consequently regarded as no-man's land.

The problem is to bring the tendon ends together with sufficient
tension to hold them in contact but not to permit any significant
bunching of the tendons to occur, because it will then be unable to
move up and down the flexor tendon sheath.   Adhesions between one
of the flexor tendons and the sheath, or indeed between the flexor
tendons themselves, as their excursion differs, will result in
reduced range of motion in the fingers.

Treatment again consists of making the correct diagnosis at the time
of original assessment.   There is usually an alteration in the
cascade of the hand.   Each of the flexor tendons should then be
tested to assess function.   I think it is useful to splint the
wrist in about 30^0 of flexion with a plaster backslab prior to
surgery.   This may reduce the chances of the proximal end of the
tendon migrating into the palm.

The position of the hand at the time of laceration is particularly
important.   If the fingers have been cut in flexion, then there
will be effectively a short tendon distally and the laceration will
need to be explored distally rather than proximally.   If the
fingers have been cut in extension, as with the hand going through a
glass window or door, then there will be no need to expose the
finger more distally, simply flexing the finger will deliver an
adequate amount of distal tendon at the laceration site.   These are
important points, because one aims to keep the area of tendon
exposed and the amount of sheath resected to a minimum during such
procedures.

At exploration it is reasonable to flex the wrist and try and milk
the tendons from proximally.   If this is not successful, then a
fine tendon retriever is invaluable.   Failure to retrieve the
tendon means a further exploration more proximally to identify the
tendon and to pass it back down the sheath.   As to the stitch
itself, I favour a modified Kessler suture, which seems to me to
achieve reasonable grip without bunching the tendons.   I use a
four-0 Ethibond suture for the Kessler stitch itself and if the join
is a little untidy, I would consider a running six-0 nylon suture,
but rarely in fact feel the need to put this in.   I try to excise
as little as possible of the flexor tendon sheath but do not try
and stitch it at the end of the operation.

As to post-operative management, there are several ways to do this, and the majority of people probably rest the hand in a plaster with the wrist and fingers somewhat flexed for $3\frac{1}{2}$ to 4 weeks, then mobilise the hand passively for perhaps a week and then more actively with physiotherapy.   Alternative methods of passive physiotherapy from the time of surgery can be performed, but patient selection is important if good results are to be obtained.

The other method more recently in vogue is the method described by Kleinert, where the affected finger is exercised against an elastic band.   The theory behind this technique is that as the finger extends against the elastic band, there is reflex relaxation of the flexor muscles, so permitting the tendon repair to move up the flexor tendon sheath with a minimum of force on the repair. When full extension of the finger is achieved, the patient simply relaxes the finger and allows the elastic band to draw the finger back down.   The ambition of this technique is that the repair moves up and down the flexor tendon sheath with a minimal loading on the tendon but with a reduced risk of significant adhesions developing.

If this technique is used, I think on completing the tendon repair the tourniquet should be let down, haemostasis obtained and then the wound closed well with frequent fine interrupted nylon sutures. I find two or three elastic bands, in series, are required to permit sufficient excursion of the finger tip.   The patient is placed in a plaster hood with the wrist slightly flexed at $30\text{-}40^{\circ}$ and similar flexion of the metacarpophalangeal joint.   However, full extension of the proximal interphalangeal joint and the distal interphalangeal joint should be possible.   Exercising against the elastic band starts at 24 to 48 hours post-operatively and cannot be achieved if there is a bulky dressing on the finger.

Attachment of the elastic band to the finger tip is a problem. I tried gluing brassiere hooks to the nail and sticking false finger nails to the nail with the elastic band attached to the false finger nail.   Neither of these methods has been very satisfactory in my hands and I am still, when using this technique, putting a stitch through the tip of the finger nail.   This is not particularly satisfactory because in full extension the nylon of the stitch tends to rub against the tip of the pulp, causing discomfort. I have not found a very satisfactory way of getting round this problem.

At $3\frac{1}{2}$ weeks the splint is discarded and the patient continues to use the elastic band for a further week without plaster support, effectively mobilising the wrist.   At $4\frac{1}{2}$ weeks the check rein is discarded and physiotherapy is commenced.

In conclusion, I have attempted to outline the options available in the management of nerve and tendon injuries, stressing the importance of early diagnosis and accurate assessment.   They are crucial because I believe the optimum management of both nerve and tendon injuries is primary repair.

Care of the Acutely Ill and Injured
Edited by D. H. Wilson and A. K. Marsden
© 1982, John Wiley & Sons Ltd.

THE USE OF BONE SCANNING FOR THE DIAGNOSIS
OF FRACTURE OF THE SCAPHOID.

N. Pyrgos and P.A. Griffiths.

Departments of Accident & Emergency and Medical Physics,
Lincoln Hospitals, Lincoln, UK

ABSTRACT

This paper describes a study of 44 patients who presented with
suspected fractures of their scaphoids. Bone scanning was found to
be more sensitive in the assessment and more useful in the
management than X-ray techniques.

INTRODUCTION

Although bone scanning is a well established technique, there have
been relatively few reports of its use to demonstrate peripheral
bone trauma and its role in the subsequent management of patients.
Its use in the diagnosis and management of fracture of the scaphoid
was selected because of the difficulties experienced with this
particular condition.

METHODS

Patients. 44 patients (24 female and 20 male) between the ages of
15 and 73 who attended within 14 days of injuries to their wrists
were studied. On examination they all had clinical signs of
fracture of the scaphoid with sufficient symptoms to justify
treatment with plaster of paris. Their initial X-ray however,
showed no bony injury.

Investigative Procedures. Soon after their initial X-rays
radionuclide images of both hands and wrists were taken by gamma
camera, 2 hours after the injection of 5 mCi of Technetium — 99m
labelled Methylene Diphosphonate. Anterior views were obtained
containing 100,000 counts.

Two to 5 weeks after their initial X-ray, all patients were
assessed clinically and radiologically. Normal scaphoid views were
taken and in addition many had macro-radiographic films.

RESULTS

The results are summarised in the table

PATIENTS	X - RAY		SCAN	DIAGNOSIS
	Initial	Follow-up		
16	Negative	Negative	Negative	No fracture
5	OA	OA	OA	OA - ?fracture
3	Negative	Positive	Positive	Fracture wrist
3	Negative	Negative	Positive	Fracture wrist
9	Negative	Positive	Positive	Fracture Scaphoid
8	Negative	Negative (later X-rays positive)	Positive	Fracture Scaphoid

DISCUSSION

Out of 44 cases only 17 were proven to have fractured their scaphoids. Allthese were demonstrated on the bone scan, but only 9 were shown on their follow-up X-rays. The remaining 8 cases were all confirmed on X-rays taken several months later. There were a further 6 cases who had a fracture of other bones in their wrists and again all were demonstrated on scan but only 3 on their follow-up X-rays.

Sixteen bone scans showed no abnormality and in all these the final diagnosis was no fracture. Five patients were also diagnosed as having no fracture, but X-rays showed osteoarthritic (OA) changes. Their scans also showed abnormalities consistent with OA changes, although these were more extensive than those shown on X-rays.

The bone scan was valuable, therefore, not only in demonstrating the existence of a fracture but also in excluding one.

The major shortcomings of the scan lay in the non-specific nature of the results. The relatively poor resolution in distinguishing different anatomical sites and the greater complexity of the technique compared with X-rays.

Care of the Acutely Ill and Injured
Edited by D. H. Wilson and A. K. Marsden
© 1982, John Wiley & Sons Ltd.

COMPLICATIONS OF EMERGENCY HAND SURGERY
IN LAGOS NIGERIA

H. Olusanya Adeyemi-Doro

Hand Rehabilitation Clinic
Lagos University Teaching Hospital, Nigeria.

ABSTRACT

Surgical management of hand injuries in Nigeria is not
infrequently followed by complications of acts of
omission or comission at the initial treatment. An
intensive educational campaign would reduce the incidence
of such misguided initial treatment.

INTRODUCTION

Injuries and acute pyogenic infections are the common
surgical hand conditions treated as emergencies in Lagos.
The results of such management are frequently attended
by complications because of improper emergency care by
the primary medical personnel. Since the initial
management determines the extent of subsequent reconstruction and functional recovery of the hand, such personnel
constitute a most important group, particularly in Nigeria
where there are only three hand surgeons to a population
of eighty million people (Table 1).

TABLE 1.

	Doctor	:	Population	Surgeon	:	Population
1970	1	:	30,000	1	:	860,000
1980	1	:	13,000	1	:	220,000
				Hand surgeon	:	Population
				1	:	26,000,000

CASE ILLUSTRATIONS

The most severe singular loss of hand function occurs
when one of its three major nerves is injured (figs.1 & 2).
10 cases (57%) of 17 lacerated peripheral nerves of the
hand and forearm (excluding digital nerves) were not
recognized at the initial treatment.
Fig.1 shows the claw dominant hand of a fifteen year old
girl caused by an unrecognized ulna nerve transection in
the healed wrist laceration.

311

H. Olusanya Adeyemi-Doro

Fig.2 demonstrates failure of proper pulp to pulp
opposition in the left hand of a 23 year old man due to
missed median nerve injury in the forearm laceration.

Fig.3 shows the boutonniere deformity of the middle finger of a
35 year old woman caused by the undiagnosed rupture of the central
slip of the extensor mechanism.

Fig.4, Primary suturing of human bite lacerations
resulted in spreading infection of the hand and
amputation of the gangrenous fifth finger.

DISCUSSION

The primary medical personnel that provide the initial
care for the injured hand in Nigeria is shown in table 2.

TABLE 2.   Nigeria Primary Medical Personnel

1. Native surgeons
2. Community health officers
3. Nurses and mid-wives
4. Nursing superintendents
5. Nigeria youth service corps(NYSC)
6. Casualty officers
7. Private practitioners

The exhibition of a low index of suspicion for injured
vital structures in the hand is not restricted to the
lower cadre of personnel but includes doctors and
surgeons without special interests in hand problems. The
importance of native surgeons in Nigeria as described by
Elebute (1971) has not diminished. Hence methods for
incorporating them in the Nigeria medical structure for
specific functions as advocated by the World Health
Organization (WHO) should be explored. An intensive
educational campaign to disseminate pertinent knowledge
to the primary medical personnel and the Nigeria
population should significantly reduce the "...........
..misguided initial treatment which may doom the patient
to life-long disability" (Grant, 1980).

REFERENCES

Elebute, E.A., 1971. The problem of under-doctored areas
    J. Royal College Surgeons Ed. 16: 177-184 July.
Grant, G.H., 1980. The hand and the psyche. Journal of
    Hand Surgery 5: 5, 417-419, Sept.

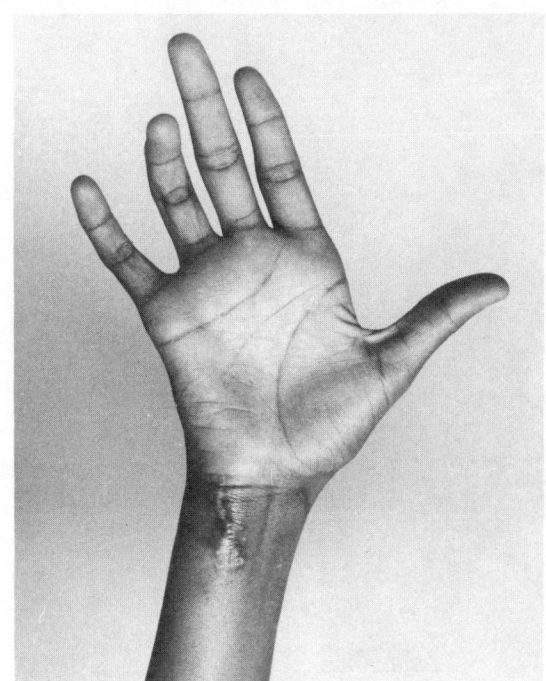

Figure 1

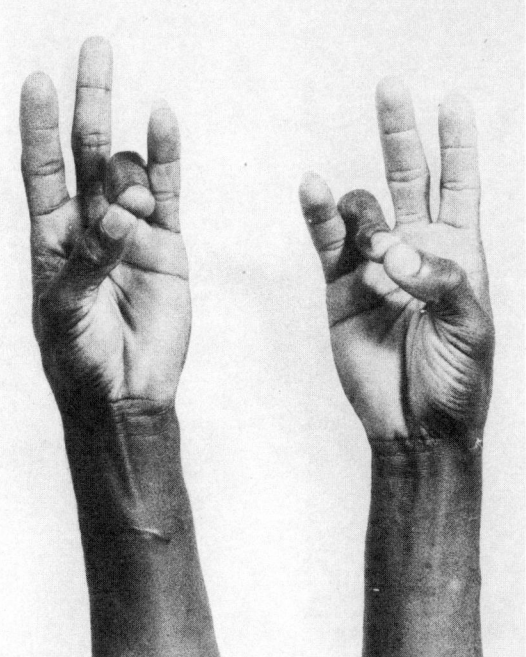

Figure 2

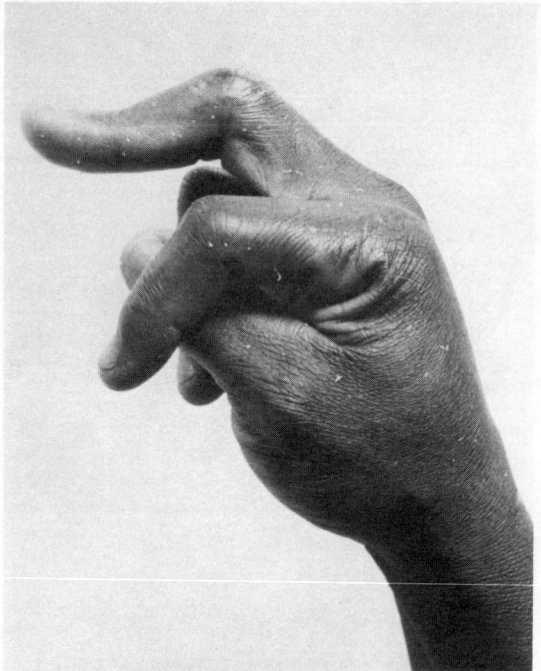

Figure 3

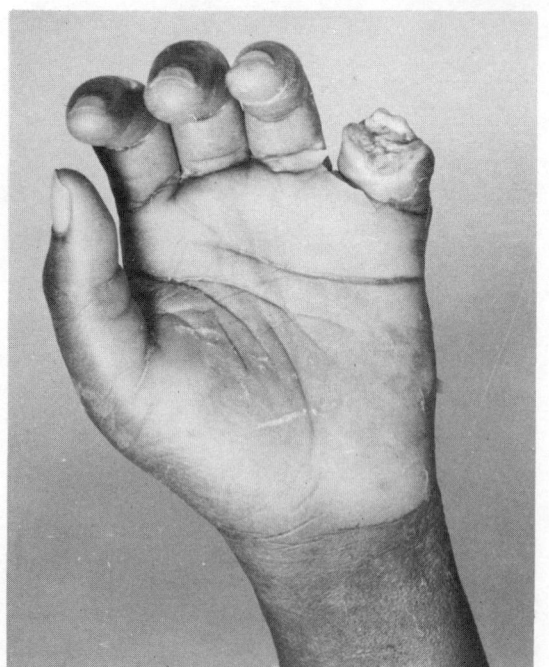

Figure 4

Care of the Acutely Ill and Injured
Edited by D. H. Wilson and A. K. Marsden
© 1982, John Wiley & Sons Ltd.

A FRESH LOOK AT 'COAL SCUTTLE SHIN'

A. K. Marsden

Pinderfields General Hospital, Wakefield,
Yorkshire, UK.

ABSTRACT

A multicentre study has examined 218 Pre-Tibial Lacerations.
180 such injuries were treated uniformly with adhesive skin
closures and achieved a median healing time of 25 days.   There
do not appear to be any identifiable factors in the aetiology or
nature of these wounds which contribute significantly to the small
number of failures of the treatment method.

INTRODUCTION

The pre-tibial laceration is a common injury of elderly women and
can be produced by the most trivial trauma such as a glancing blow
against furniture or a stationary household object - the nickname
"Coal Scuttle Shin" implies a simple domestic incident with
presumably simple resolution.   Left untreated the injuries are
unsightly and, although healing by granulation will eventually
occur, there is an intervening morbidity with sloughing of the
skin, gravitational oedema,infection and pain.

The accident is almost exclusively one of post menopausal women
although flap lacerations can occur at any age in either sex.
The proximally based flap predominates.   Anatomical and pathological factors contribute to the nature and quality of these injuries.
The thin skin of the shin overlies bone and there is a peculiar
blood supply.   Retraction of wound edges occurs readily.   With
ageing the skin becomes stiffer, less elastic and more likely to
disruption - the effects reproduced by therapy with corticosteroids.

A number of studies have been undertaken to determine how best to
deal with these lesions.   Early trials (Tandon and Sutherland
1973) advised wound excision and split skin grafting with the
patient admitted to hospital;   recent treatments (Crawford and
Gipson 1977) have aimed to encourage mobilization and independence.

Direct closure of the wound by suture is not acceptable as tension
is produced and dehiscence readily follows.   The idea of adhesive
wound closures came from the ancient Egyptians who employed linen
strips with flour and water paste.   Modern wound closure strips
are comprised of plastic or porous synthetic tapes lined with

315

acrylic adhesives.   Sneddon in 1972 advised the use of adhesive strips for corticosteroid-induced wounds.

In 1979 in a pilot study of 50 pre-tibial lacerations treated in The General Infirmary at Leeds the author reported a mean healing time of 23 days achieved by utilising adhesive strips alone.

THE PRESENT STUDY

The simple technique of wound closure with adhesive strips was followed prospectively at nine Accident and Emergency centres in order to sample a large heterogenous population.

Protocol   The technique can be undertaken by any trained member of staff.   Aseptic wound toilet with saline removes blood clots underlying the flap so that closure can be effected without tension - a gap of one strip is always maintained between adjacent closures. If the wound edges cannot be completely approximated a small area is left for granulation.

Review   The injuries were followed on a specially constructed trial form including a metric grid indicating the nature and size of the wound.   Wounds were inspected weekly until final healing obtained - this being defined as occurring in a closed stable wound requiring neither support nor supervision.

RESULTS

218 trial forms were returned showing a mean age of 64 and a female-male ratio of 6 : 1.   180 injuries fulfilled the entry criteria for collaborative study.   Predisposing factors are listed in the table.

TABLE   Aetiological factors in 180 Pre-Tibial Lacerations

	%
Cardiac oedema	13.8
Corticosteroid therapy	14.7
Diabetes mellitus	2.0
Peripheral vascular disease	11.9
Distally based flap	23.9
Wound area in excess of 10 sq.cm.	15.0

Fourteen patients were deemed failures of treatment in that they did not achieve primary healing or had failed to achieve this by 99 days.   Notwithstanding this the median healing time was 25 days with an average of four return visits per patient.

A gross scrutiny of the failure group is not able to reveal any obvious causative factors - there is no apparent relationship between, for example, corticosteroids or a distally based flap and a failure of the treatment method.   The results of a multiple regression analysis which may clarify the position are still awaited.

CONCLUSIONS

The study has proven that a simple technique of wound closure for pre-tibial lacerations can be applied in different centres with uniformly good results.   It has not been possible to predict which patients will not do well by the method but their numbers are small and perhaps negligible when related to the overall success of the technique.

ACKNOWLEDGEMENTS

Thanks are due to the medical and nursing staff of Birmingham Accident Hospital; The General Infirmary at Leeds; Glasgow Royal Infirmary; The General Hospital, Birmingham; Hope Hospital, Salford; Hull Royal Infirmary; Kent and Canterbury Hospitals; Pinderfields General Hospital, Wakefield; Selly Oak Hospital, Birmingham who have participated in the trial.

REFERENCES

Crawford B.S. and Gipson M. 1977 The Conservative Management of Pre-Tibial Lacerations in Elderly Patients.   Brit.J.Plastic Surgery 30 174-176.

Sneddon J. 1972   Skin Trauma and Corticosteroids.   Brit.Med.J. 3 113

Tandon S.W. and Sutherland A.B. 1973   Pre-Tibial Lacerations. Brit.J.Plastic Surgery 26 172-175

Care of the Acutely Ill and Injured
Edited by D. H. Wilson and A. K. Marsden
© 1982, John Wiley & Sons Ltd.

PRE-TIBIAL FLAP LACERATION

A K Maitra, FRCS (Eng. and Edin.)

Consultant-in-Charge, Accident and Emergency
Department, Royal Victoria Infirmary,
Newcastle upon Tyne, UK

ABSTRACT

Sixty-one pretibial lacerations in 60 patients were prospectively
studied. All were treated conservatively using sutures and adhesive
tapes ('steristrips') with or without 'viscopaste' (bleached cotton
bandage enmeshed with zinc oxide paste). It is concluded that the
combination of 'steristrips' and 'viscopaste' bandage is an effective, practical method of treatment well-accepted by these elderly
female patients.

INTRODUCTION

The management of pretibial lacerations had been well summarised
elsewhere (B.M.J 1978). The aim of the present study is to present
clinical details of patients treated at the Accident and Emergency
department of this hospital with a view to establishing (a) percentage of skin flap necrosis, (b) features of patients with delayed
wound healing and (c) simple, effective and acceptable methods of
treatment.

PATIENTS AND METHOD

Sixty patients with 61 lacerations have been included in the study.
The clinical details are summarised below:

Age – average 69 (42 – 89), 80% in their sixties and seventies.
Sex – exclusively female.
Nature of trauma – minor knocks and falls, 60% indoors.
Twenty-one per cent had some form of pre-existing medical condition
(lower limb oedema, etc) or were on drug therapy (e.g. steroids).

Nature of skin flaps – 76% were proximal and 24% distal. Eighty
per cent were longitudinal (↓↑) of which 89% were either 'U' or 'V'
shaped. Twenty per cent were transverse flaps (⇌). Lower ⅓rd
(60%) and left leg (56%) were more affected than the middle (37%)
and upper ⅓rd (3%) and right leg (44%). The size of wounds varied
from 2.0 x 2.0 to 17 x 8 cm.

Treatment – (a) primary (i) steristrips 74% (ii) suture 19%

(iii) dressings only 3%. Supporting bandage: (i) Crepe and tubular elastic bandage only 73% (ii) with 'viscopaste' bandage 27%.
(b) secondary: dressings with Milton/paraffin solution, Betadine ointment, porcine dermal graft.
Complications – (a) skin flap necrosis 23% (b) discharging wound 63% 35% with +ve bacterial (mainly staph. Aureus and Albus) culture.

Results – the average healing time was 46 (10 – 168) days; number of hospital visits 6 (2 – 28): 'viscopaste' treated group did better than those without – 42 (21 – 86) to 48 (10 – 168) days.

Analysis of 15 patients with delayed healing, 95 (58 – 168) days, showed that about 50% were on drugs or had underlying disease, 75% of the wounds were on lower 3rd of leg, and relatively larger in size (3.5 x 3.5 to 17 x 8 cm.) Eighty per cent had been treated without 'viscopaste' and 28% sutured. All suffered from wound discharge, 75% underwent skin flaps necrosis, 35% showed +ve bacterial culture.

DISCUSSION

Woodyard (1968), Tandon and Sutherland (1973) advocated primary excision of skin flaps and splint–skin grafting which reduced healing time but required in-patient treatment. This radical approach was opposed by Crawford and Gipson (1977) who recorded survival of the skin flaps and reasonable healing time by adopting a conservative regime ('steristrips' and 'viscopaste'). The present study supports this view. The 'problem' wounds with delayed healing time are also likely to benefit as long as further trauma to the wound is avoided (no local anaesthetic or sutures). The underlying rich vascular tibial periosteum probably determines the survival of the flap once the tissue oedema is effectively controlled by 'viscopaste' bandage. All patients readily accepted this regime and rejected skin-grafting when offered.

REFERENCES

Crawford, B.S. and Gipson, M., 1977. The conservative management of pretibial lacerations in elderly patients. British Journal of Plastic Surgery, 30, 174 – 176.
Leading article, 1978. Flap lacerations. British Medical Journal 1, 4 – 5.
Tandon, S.N. and Sutherland, A.B., 1973. Pretibial lacerations. British Journal of Plastic Surgery, 26, 172 – 175.
Woodyard, J.E., 1968. A commonly neglected soft-tissue injury of the lower limb. Practitioner, 200, 533 – 536.

Care of the Acutely Ill and Injured
Edited by D. H. Wilson and A. K. Marsden
© 1982, John Wiley & Sons Ltd.

THE USE OF FREE SKIN FLAPS

M. D. Brough, F.R.C.S.

St. Andrew's Hospital,
Billericay,
Essex.

Skin loss in the limbs resulting from trauma is often best treated
with the application of split-skin grafts.   In the long term,
though, they may contract; they may remain unstable particularly
if subjected to further trauma; they may show a different degree
of pigmentation from surrounding skin and their quality is inferior
to normal skin.   Further, there are occasions when there is an
inadequate vascular bed for them to survive at all.   In general,
when bare nerve, tendon, bone or joint is exposed, a skin flap is
necessary for skin cover and a flap may be needed to improve
function or cosmesis.

In the hand there are many small local skin flaps available but
when a large skin flap is required for any part of the upper limb,
it is usually obtained from the trunk.   In the lower limb, the
cross-leg flap has for long been the standard technique for
introducing a large area of flap skin to a skin defect.   When this
flap is inappropriate as, for example, when there has been trauma
to the opposite limb or the donor defect is not acceptable as in a
young girl, a tube pedicle from the trunk is used.   These two
techniques have been well proven over several decades, but they both
involve multiple surgical stages and a prolonged period of
hospitalisation (Stranc, Labandter, Roy, 1975).   During the last
decade they have been superseded as a result of, firstly, the
recognition of axial pattern flaps and, secondly, the technical
development of the operating microscope.

For long it was taught that the length of a skin flap should not be
greater than its breadth.   This was because its blood supply was
random. In 1944 Shaw described the hypogastric flap with a high
length/breadth ratio (Shaw, 1944).   In 1965 Bakamjian described
the deltopectoral flap with a 2/1 ratio (Bakamjian 1965).   The
reason for the reliability of these flaps was not fully appreciated
until 1970 when McGregor and Jackson explored the potential of the
extended deltopectoral flap (McGregor and Jackson, 1970), and then
subsequently described the groin flap (McGregor and Jackson, 1972).
Their detailed investigation of the latter in conjunction with
Smith and Foley, revealed that this flap constantly had a specific
artery and vein in its base which passed along its axis (Smith et
al, 1972).   They designated the term "axial pattern" to this flap.

321

Since that time, several other cutaneous axial pattern flaps have
been described.

The length of an axial pattern flap is dependent on the vascular
territory supplied by the axial vessels while the pedicle can be
very narrow providing it contains the axial artery and vein.
Indeed, it need only consist of the artery and vein (or veins)
themselves. With the development of microvascular surgery so these
flaps can be transferred distally as free flaps and revascularised
in their distant site by anastomosing their artery and vein to
suitable local vessels in one operation. The realisation that
axial pattern flaps not only exist in skin but also in muscle, bone
and other structures has led to an explosion of reconstructive
techniques over the past few years.

The first flap to be used extensively as a free flap was the
superficial groin flap. The superficial circumflex iliac artery
is its axial artery and this arises from the femoral artery some
2 cm. below the inguinal ligament. It usually arises as a single
vessel but may arise from a common trunk with the superficial
epigastric artery. The vessel passes below and parallel to the
inguinal ligament (Smith et al, 1972), but may pass more obliquely
upwards towards the anterior superior iliac spine (Harii et al, 1975)
The artery pierces the deep fascia at a variable point, but well
before reaching the anterior superior iliac spine. The veins are
more superficial than the artery and drain into the saphenous bulb.

The skin overlying the anterior iliac crest is usually thin making
it an ideal flap for transferring to the distal part of either upper
or lower limb. The pedicle though may be bulky as the artery and
vein may be separated by a significant amount of fat at their origin.
If this is so, the pedicle may have to be trimmed at a second stage.
One particular advantage of the flap is that the donor defect can
nearly always be closed primarily.

The deep groin flap (Taylor, Townsend and Corlett, 1979) is based
on the deep circumflex iliac vessels. The artery is given off the
external iliac artery just above the inguinal ligament and passes
up towards the anterior superior iliac spine before passing around
the internal circumference of the crest. It is usually accompanied
by a single vein. The area of skin supplied and drained by these
vessels overlaps that of the superficial vessels but is more
posterior, reaching back to the erector spinae. In raising the flap
a cuff of muscle along the iliac crest needs to be raised with the
flap to be sure the vessels are incorporated. The donor defect
posteriorly may not close primarily and may have to be grafted.

The dorsalis pedis flap can occasionally be used as a pedicled flap
for skin defects around the ankle. It has a greater value as a
free flap (McCraw and Furlow, 1975), particularly for defects on the
dorsum of the hand. The flap is based on the dorsalis pedis artery
to which it has a very tenuous attachment. The venous arch on the
dorsum of the foot should be included in this flap as this drains

into the long saphenous vein which acts as the flap vein.   These
two vessels can be dissected out for a significant distance which
can provide this flap with a long, mobile pedicle.   Inclusion of
the superficial peroneal nerve can provide sensation to the flap
if this is linked appropriately.   The main disadvantage of the flap
is that the donor site must be grafted and at its best the cosmetic
defect is significant.

The tensor fascia lata flap is a myocutaneous flap as its vessels
are those which supply and drain the tensor fascia lata muscle,
(Hill, Nahai and Vasconez, 1978).   The artery is given directly off
the cruciate anastomosis and it has an accompanying vein.   The flap
is useful as the muscular component is small and the cutaneous
element is large.   The flap can include skin on the lateral aspect
of the thigh down to the lower third.   It must include the fascia
lata which supports the vessels and may include the lateral
cutaneous nerve of the thigh to provide a sensory flap (Cason, 1980).
The flap is more useful in males where there is less subcutaneous
fat but because of this the donor defect more commonly has to be
grafted.

There are several other cutaneous flaps which have been described
recently.   The place of these in trauma is currently being
evaluated indicating the rapidly developing field of reconstruction
which is now taking place.

REFERENCES

Bakamjian, V.Y., 1965.   A two staged method for pharyngo-oesophogeal
    reconstruction with a primary pectoral flap.   Plastic and
    Reconstructive Surgery 36, 2, 173-184.
Cason, A., 1980.   Personal Communication.
Harii, K., Ohmori, K., Torii, S., Murakama, F., Kasai, Y.,
    Sekiguchi, J., and Ohmori, S., 1975.   Free groin skin flaps.
    British Journal of Plastic Surgery, 28, 225-237.
Hill, H.L., Nahai, F., and Vasconez, L.O., 1978.   The tensor fascia
    lata myocutaneous free flap.   Plastic and Reconstructive
    Surgery 61, 4, 517-522.
McCraw, J.B., and Furlow, L.T., 1975.   The dorsalis pedis
    arterialised flap.   Plastic and Reconstructive Surgery, 55, 2,
    177-185.
McGregor, I.A., and Jackson, I.T., 1970.   The extended role of the
    deltopectoral flap.   British Journal of Plastic Surgery, 23,
    173-185.
McGregor, I.A., and Jackson, I.T., 1972.   The groin flap.   British
    Journal of Plastic Surgery, 25, 3-16.
Shaw, D.T., 1944.   Open abdominal flaps for repair of surface
    defects of the upper extremity.   Surgical Clinics of North
    America, April,   293-308.
Smith, P.J., Foley, B., McGregor, I.A., and Jackson, I.T., 1972.
    The anatomical basis of the groin flap.   Plastic and
    Reconstructive Surgery, 49, 1, 41-47.
Stranc, M.F., Labandter, H., Roy, A., 1975.   A review of 196 tubed
    pedicles.   British Journal of Plastic Surgery, 28,1, 54-59.

Taylor, G.I., Townsend, P., Corlett, R., 1979.   Superiority of the
deep circumflex iliac vessels as the supply for free groin
flaps.   Plastic and Reconstructive Surgery, 64, 6, 745-759.

Care of the Acutely Ill and Injured
Edited by D. H. Wilson and A. K. Marsden
© 1982, John Wiley & Sons Ltd.

MICROSURGERY : TRAINING, RESEARCH AND DEVELOPMENT

C.J. Green

Division of Comparative Medicine,
M.R.C. Clinical Research Centre,
Northwick Park, Harrow, Middx.

ABSTRACT

All surgeons should have microsurgery included in their training
programme.   A new polyglactin absorbable microsuture is described
and simpler techniques for end-to-end and end-to-side anastomoses
reported.   Attention is drawn to the possibilities opened up by
the use of vascularised nerve auto- and allografts, and by further
development of the pseudosynovial sheath for nerve regeneration.
The need for further research into avulsion injury, monitoring of
free flap perfusion, prevention of ischaemic injury, the use of
novel vasodilator and anti-thrombotic drugs, and for lymphatic
reconstruction is emphasised.

TRAINING

The operating microscope has for many years been an essential tool
in ENT and ophthalmic surgery, and in the past fifteen years has
been increasingly accepted as an aid to reconstructive surgery of
small blood vessels, nerves and the urogenital tract.   Nevertheless,
its use is still limited to a few specialties, and widespread
acceptance is probably inhibited as much by the belief that microsurgical techniques are difficult to master as by the initial cost
of instruments and the prolonged periods spent in theatre at each
individual operation.   It is high time that the mystique
surrounding microsurgery be discarded and all surgeons whatever
their proposed specialty should be given at the least an introductory course in basic technique as early as practicable in their
career.   A few days of intensive practice under a microscope is
almost invariably sufficient to dispel the aura of difficulty,
adding a new and exciting dimension to experience and an enhanced
appreciation of gentle atraumatic technique in handling tissues.

Having suggested that microsurgical techniques are not particularly
difficult, it must be added that they cannot simply be picked up
by observation and it is essential that the basics should be
taught properly in selected animal models.   This in turn requires
properly organised laboratory and animal holding facilities.   It
is probably unrealistic for each hospital or centre to have its

own training unit but there should be suitable laboratories at
regional level where basics can be taught by experienced personnel
and where surgeons can afterwards return for say one day per week
to practice and enhance their skills.   In an ideal world, the
best training would probably be gained by one year attachment to
a clinical unit with its own laboratory and with time divided
roughly equally between the two as provided in Melbourne by Dr.
B. O'Brien.   Alternatively, a flexible training programme could
be developed in the U.K. to cater for more surgeons wanting
exposure to microsurgery.   Short 3 to 5-day introductory courses
or workshops are useful in sifting those really interested from
the less motivated.   Subsequent development tends then to be self-
selecting and the enthusiasts return for further training or want
to do 6 or 12-month periods of training combined with experimental
and clinical work.   The emphasis must be on flexibility because
of difficulties in taking time away from clinical work whilst
attempting to make a career in surgery.   To avoid wasting time,
highly trained technical staff are essential to provide continuity
and skills in handling, anaesthesia and surgery of the animals.
Microscopes and instruments should be similar to those available
in the clinic but should be kept in the laboratory exclusively for
animal work.

In those countries which allow the use of animals for the
acquisition of surgical skills, a range of technical exercises have
been evolved in laboratory rats and rabbits.   In the U.K., such
work is illegal so it is necessary for the aspirant to obtain a
license to do experimental work.   Rabbits have vessels (carotids,
jugulars, femorals, epigastrics and renal) which approximate those
most commonly encountered in clinical microsurgical practice both
in size and quality.   The female uro-genital tract is ideal for
studies involving reconstruction of, for example, the fallopian
tubes and translocation of the ovaries on a vascular pedical.   The
equivalent vessels in rats are smaller ranging from 1mm down to
0.3mm diameter. We favour this species since the training exercise
is itself difficult and it is then relatively easy to anastomose
a vessel of 1.5mm diameter in man afterwards - the clinical
situation of course presents other difficulties in positioning and
working at depth in a cavity which can be avoided in the laboratory
so we feel that the basic skills should be obtained on the smallest
vessels practicable.   Small pigs up to 15kg body weight are also
useful experimental animals for microvascular surgery.

There are numerous experimental models which can be used for
example for: evaluation of skill; development of new microsurgical
techniques and suturing materials; assessment of immunosuppressive,
vasolidator or anti-thrombotic agents; or for studying mechanisms
of injury or rejection of allografted tissues.   Those most useful
involve microsurgical anastomoses of the femoral or carotid vessels,
and vessels attached to renal and cardiac grafts, groin flaps,
rabbit ears, ovaries and fallopian tubes.   The essential of a good
microvascular model is that immediate and long-term patency can be

assessed by perfusion and subsequent viability and physiological function of a tissue or organ.   Perhaps the groin flap in rats is the most useful of all since its viability can be easily assessed visually.

RECENT RESEARCH AND DEVELOPMENT

Materials.   Further miniaturisation of technique can only follow improvement in optical facilities and refinement of sutures.   The early microvascular work was done using ophthalmic instruments and sutures but advances in polymer chemistry have since allowed the development of very fine gauge (10-20 μ diameter) monofilament polyamide and polypropylene sutures with atraumatic needles especially designed for delicate tissues.   The newest advance in the field of fine sutures is the synthetic absorbable co-polymer of glycolytic and lactic acids (polyglactin 910 or Vicryl[R]).   This has been tested in animals comparing monofilament 0.2 metric (10/0) polyglactin with the same sized monofilament nylon sutures on the following criteria: tissue reaction around the suture, tensile strength of the anastomosis, endothelial regeneration, regeneration of the anastomosed section, formation of thromboses and eventual haemodynamic efficiency.   These showed that under similar conditions the polyglactin suture possessed adequate tensile strength to withstand the intravascular pressure in a vessel of 1.5mm outside diameter and that tissue reaction had disappeared after 42 days, whereas inflammation of the media and hyperplasia of the intima persisted even after 70 days with the nylon.   There was no difference in thrombogenesis, and complete endothelial regeneration had taken place within 3 weeks.   The sutures, which are broken down hydrolytically, had disappeared completely by 60 days. The only disadvantage apparently was that the polyglactin suture was less visible under the operating microscope (Ippisch et al., 1981; Dahlke, Dociu and Thurau, 1981).

Another advance to be developed recently by Ethicon Ltd., is a new 12/14 μ diameter nylon suture swaged to a 3mm needle.   This is still being evaluated in a number of laboratories but is likely to be useful in lymphatic and microneural reconstruction.   Also likely to be useful in neurosurgery is a new 100 μ diameter needle with a cutting tip developed by the same company.

Techniques.   Conventional end-to-end techniques (Jacobson & Suarez, 1960; Buncke & Schulz, 1966) have proved reliable in experimental and clinical situations.   However, they are not always convenient and there is a need for simpler techniques to be developed.   The cuff-ligature anastomosis technique is useful for experimental work but has not proved popular since it was first described (Malt & Harris, 1965) even though it is easy and quick to perform.   A new and easier way to anastomose microvessels has been described recently (Lauritzen, 1978) in which the proximal portion of an artery is telescoped within the lumen of the distal part and held by 2 sutures at 180° apart.   In experimental rats this proved successful and had the great advantage that it was done quickly and with minimal intimal dissection.   It remains to be seen whether this can be repeated in other experimental animals and in the clinic.

There are many clinical applications such as extracranial to intracranial micro-revascularisation where good end-to-side anastomoses
are required. End-to-side techniques are also useful if there is a
major discrepancy in vessel diameters making end-to-end apposition
difficult. The best method is still not established but it was
recently shown (Nam, Roberts and Acland, 1978) that angling of the
donor vessel was not important as had been previously thought and
that a slit arteriotomy was as effective as a disc taken out of the
recipient wall. By placing the first suture in the back row it may
be easier to ensure patency than in the standard practice of starting with stay sutures at either end of the anastomosis (Greenhalgh,
Rossi and Hoare, 1981). Again with the intention of simplifying
the procedure, we recently described a new method for arterial
end-to-side anastomosis termed the 'wrap-around' technique and
found it to be efficient in vessels down to 0.5mm outside diameter.
This involved no intimal handling and only 3 sutures were needed
(Sanders, Green and Tan, 1981).

Nerve reconstruction where gaps have to be bridged as for example
after brachial plexus injuries is to date limited to autografted
material and hence to the availability of donor sites such as the
sural nerve. The demonstration that vascularised nerve is more
likely to survive and provide a pathway for neo-axonal regeneration
than simple grafts (Taylor & Ham, 1976) has given fresh impetus to
clinical attempts to correct severe deficits usually associated
with avulsion injuries. If the experiments of Lundborg & Hansson
(1980) in which it was shown that axonal regeneration would take
place down preformed pseudo-synovial sheaths can be repeated in
other species, an exciting field of experimental endeavour will be
opened up and other methods of grafting may be rendered obsolete.

Clinical Problems. Many clinical problems have not yet been solved
but perhaps the most important of these involve: the nature of
avulsion injury and prediction of the outcome after reconstruction;
how soon an axial pattern free flap is able to survive without its
axial vessels; how best can good flow in the microvasculature of a
free flap or replanted digit be monitored; how long will an amputated and ischaemic extremity remain viable at ambient temperature
and how best should it be preserved both for transport and during
the long surgical procedures to follow; is there any value in
treating the recipient with anticoagulant or anti-platelet agents
to prevent microcoagulopathy and thrombosis in the vasculature; is
the outcome more successful if vaso-dilator drugs are used to
improve initial perfusion of the graft; and is lymphaticovenous
reconstruction a realistic way of relieving chronic lymphoedema.

Avulsion lesions affect the nerves and vasculature as well as other
structures. Recently, Jamieson and Eames (1980) showed that even
after an avulsion injury, there is significant regeneration of
motor axons across an anastomotic repair, but that there was no
regeneration of sensory axons into the cord after repair of avulsed
dorsal rootlets. They suggested that until further advances are
made by producing sensory regeneration within the spinal cord

along the lines suggested by Wilson & Jagadeesh (1976), attempts at
reimplantation of avulsed spinal roots should be abandoned.
Avulsion injuries involving vessels necessitate the interposition
of micro-venous grafts and these have been used to replant an
avulsed scalp (Miller, Anstee and Snell, 1976) and an experimental
study to investigate combined crushing and degloving injuries has
also been reported (Kurata, O'Brien and Black, 1978).

Many free skin myocutaneous flaps are based on axial vessels and
there is a need to know how soon after transfer a collateral circulation sufficient to support the tissue is established. It may
be necessary to thin the flap for cosmetic or functional reasons
or to do secondary surgery on structures below the flap. This
involves either a peripheral or central incision on the flap but
in clinical practice it is often poorly tolerated and necrosis may
ensue. Failure may be due to inadvertant damage to axial vessels
or to lack of capillary ingrowth perhaps because hypoxic stimulation is lacking. Black et al., (1978) raised rectus abdominus
flaps based on the superficial epigastric artery in pigs and showed
that axial vessels could be ligated at 8 days with complete flap
viability but this is at variance with much clinical experience.

Monitoring the circulation in free flaps is important since success
depends on achieving primary perfusion and maintenance of flow
across the microvascular anastomosis. Thrombosis at the vascular
junction should be relieved within 12 hours - it is important
therefore to monitor circulation within the flap by non-invasive
means. In a recent study (Harrison, Girling and Mott, 1981), a
comparison was made between various monitoring techniques including
the percutaneous PO_2 monitor (Achauer, Black and Litke, 1980) and
it was concluded that a highly sensitive photo-plethysmograph provided the most accurate system.

The rat groin flap model has been used to study the long-term
effects of new vasolidator drugs (Finseth & Adelberg, 1978, 1979;
Zide, Buncke & Finseth, 1980). A comparison of the effect of
isoxuprine, guanethidine, hydralazine and phenoxybenzamine in preventing the standard pattern of necrosis in extended flaps showed
that isoxuprine was the most effective if it was given for at
least 13 days prior to flap elevation and at least 7 days post-
operatively. The same group (Finseth & Cutting, 1978) showed that
the delay phenomenon in flap surgery could be due to adrenergic
denervation or to ischaemia independent of each other.

FUTURE RESEARCH AND DEVELOPMENT

It is only possible in such a brief survey to make a few suggestions where future studies might prove rewarding.

Clearly, much remains to be done in improving neural reconstruction
particularly after avulsion injuries of the brachial plexus.
Further exploitation of vascularised nerve autografts as well as
the preformed pseudo-synovial sheaths mentioned above may improve
the presently disappointing clinical results in dealing with these

lesions. Perhaps, since a graft would only be necessary to provide a pathway for neo-axonal growth, cadaver material could be used as allografts accompanied by a short period of immunosuppression. This would avoid creating donor site deficits and the problem of a limited supply for grafting - at least it should be done in experimental animals.

Avulsion injury to microvessels also needs further experimental study. If possible, the clinician would welcome some simple technique for assessing how much vessel should be resected before interposing vein grafts. Perhaps this could be done by seeing whether spasm is reversible after bathing the apparently intact vessel in lignocaine solution - if it proves irreversible then it is likely that the intima of the vessel is irreversibly damaged.

The whole question of monitoring needs further study, but this is particularly true of free skin and myocutaneous flaps where secondary surgery is required for thinning or other reasons. Before making a decision to incise an apparently successful flap, it is important to know whether collateral circulation is truly established or whether the flap has retained axial flow characteristics. Perhaps the circulation could be mapped by improved photo-plethysmograph monitoring.

Finally, it is time that the information gained from preservation of organs, particularly the kidneys, should be applied to amputated digits and free flaps. At present, it is normal practice to place the tissue to be replanted in a bag of sterile isotonic saline solution surrounded by ice so that the temperature is lowered to about $2^{o}C$ in time. However, it is then difficult to prevent rewarming to ambient temperature during lengthy operations so the tissue may be subjected to warm and cold ischaemia which is likely to damage endothelial cells in the microcirculation. This in turn is likely to result in the no-flow phenomenon commonly experienced in transplantation of poorly preserved kidneys. Perhaps experiments should be designed to find ways of preventing warm and cold ischaemic damage. Carefully done, there is no obvious reason why initial vascular flush with a properly designed fluid such as hypertonic citrate solution or other balanced salt solutions rendered hyperosmolar to prevent endothelial cellular swelling should not improve viability in the same way as was achieved with kidneys many years ago.

REFERENCES

Achauer, B.M., Black, K.S., and Litke, D.K. (1980). Transcutaneous PO_2 in flaps : a new method of survival prediction. Plastic and Reconstructive Surgery, 65, 738-742.
Black, M.J.M., Chait, L., O'Brien, B.McC., Sykes, P.J., and Sharzer, L.A. 1978. How soon may the axial vessels of a surviving free flap be safely ligated : a study in pigs. British Journal of Plastic Surgery, 31, 295-299.

Buncke, J.J., and Schultz, W.P. 1966.   Total ear reimplantation
    in the rabbit utilizing microminiature vascular anastomoses.
    British Journal of Plastic Surgery 19, 15-22.
Dahlke, H., Dociu, N., and Thurau, K. 1981.   Synthetic absor-
    bable and non-absorbable sutures in microvascular surgery
    (a study of experiments in animals).   Hand Surgery 6,
    1-22.
Finseth, F., and Adelberg, M.G. 1978.   Prevention of skin flap
    necrosis by a course of treatment with vasolidator drugs.
    Plastic and Reconstructive Surgery 61, 738-743.
Finseth, F., and Adelberg, M.G. 1979.   Experimental work with
    isoxuprine for prevention of skin flap necrosis and for
    treatment of the failing flap. Plastic and Reconstructive
    Surgery 63, 94-100.
Finseth, F., and Cutting, C. 1978.   An experimental neurovascular
    skin island flap for the study of the delay phenomenon.
    Plastic and Reconstructive Surgery 61, 412-420.
Greenhalgh, R.M., Rossi, L.F.A., and Hoare, M.R. 1981.   The
    precise technique of end-to-side microvascular anastomoses
    with a suitable experimental model. Annals of the Royal
    College of Surgeons of England 63, 28-30.
Harrison, D.H., Girling, M., and Mott, G. 1981.   Experience in
    monitoring the circulation in free flap transfers. Plastic
    and Reconstructive Surgery (in press).
Ippisch, A., Duspiva, W., Wriedt-Lubbe, I., and Blumel, G. 1981.
    Microsurgical sutures of nerves and vessels with absorbable
    suture material.   Ethicon Research and Development
    Bulletin, May, 1981.
Jacobson, J.H., and Suarez, E.L. 1960.   Microsurgery in
    anastomosis of small vessels. Surgical Forum II, 243-245.
Jamieson, A.M., and Eames, R.A. 1980.   Reimplantation of
    avulsed brachial plexus roots : an experimental study in
    dogs. International Journal of Microsurgery 2, 75-80.
Kurata, T., O'Brien, B.Mc.C., and Black, M.J.M. 1978.   Micro-
    vascular surgery in degloving injuries : an experimental
    study. British Journal of Plastic Surgery 31, 117-120.
Lauritzen, C. 1978.   A new and easier way to anastomose micro-
    vessels : an experimental study in rats. Scandinavian
    Journal of Plastic and Reconstructive Surgery 12, 291-294.
Lundborg, G., and Hansson, H.A., 1980.   Nerve regeneration
    through preformed pseudosynovial tubes. The Journal of
    Hand Surgery 5, 35-38.
Malt, R.A., and Harris, W.H., 1965.   Monograph I. Reimplantation
    of Limbs,   Ethicon, Inc. Sommerville New York 1965, p12-13.
Miller, G.D.H., Anstee, E.J., and Snell, J.A. 1976.   Successful
    replantation of an avulsed scalp by microvascular anastomoses.
    Plastic and Reconstructive Surgery 58, 133-136.
Nam, D.A., Roberts, T.L., and Acland, R.D. 1978.   An experimental
    study of end-to-side anastomosis. Surgery, Gynecology &
    Obstetrics 147, 339-342.

Sanders, R., Green, C.J., and Tan, W.T.L. 1981. The wrap-
    around end-to-side anastomosis for micro-vessels. British
    Journal of Plastic Surgery 34, 148-180.
Taylor, G.I., and Ham, F.J. 1976. The free vascularised nerve
    graft. Plastic and Reconstructive Surgery 57, 413-425.
Wilson, D.H., and Jagadeesh, P., 1976. Experimental regeneration
    in peripheral nerves and the spinal cord in laboratory
    animals exposed to a pulsed electromagnetic field.
    Paraplegia 14, 12-20.
Zide, B., Buncke, H.J., and Finseth, F. 1980. A study of the
    treatment necessary for the vasolidator drug isoxuprine to
    prevent necrosis in a skin flap. British Journal of
    Plastic Surgery 33, 383-387.

Care of the Acutely Ill and Injured
Edited by D. H. Wilson and A. K. Marsden
© 1982, John Wiley & Sons Ltd.

RATIONALE OF A NEW TREATMENT FOR HYDROFLUORIC ACID. BURNS

H.Bartels, W.Erhardt[+], G.Blumel[+]

Department of Surgery and[+]Department of Experimental
Surgery Medical Centre, Klinikum r.d. Isar
8000 München 80, Ismaninger Str. 22. Germany.

ABSTRACT

Through experimental studies we have developed a new treatment for
hydrofluoric acid chemical burns. Intra-arterial injection of
20% calcium into the main artery supplying an injured area is
superior to the common treatment of local calcium infiltration.
This treatment has proven acceptable in clinical practice in burns
of the hand and fingers.

INTRODUCTION

Hydrofluoric acid burns are becoming increasingly common with the
widespread use of the chemical in industry. The burns show a
progressive tissue necrosis often resulting in permanent tissue
loss because hydrofluoric acid (HF) is extremely corrosive and the
fluoride ion has a specific toxic effect on inhibition of enolase
activity resulting in depressing of cell metabolism and reduction
of oxygen uptake.

Carney demonstrated that the concentration of fluoride ions sank
below the toxic level by the addition of calcium salts to his model.
This effect is due to the reaction of toxic fluoride ions into non-
toxic, insoluble calcium fluoride - an effect which we have been
able to confirm by isotope studies: standardised H.F. burns and
thermal burns to rabbit ears were treated with identical doses of
labelled Ca^{47}. A 48 hour radioactivity count revealed more
radioactivity on the HF burned ear than on the control - indicating
the presence of non soluble CaF_2. The recommendations for the
clinical treatment of H.F. burns have varied over the years - the
present accepted regime consists of local infiltration of calcium
into the injured area - a painful and traumatic procedure.

METHOD

We examined the therapeutic effects of calcium injection into the
main artery of a H.F. burned area. Standardised amounts of H.F.
were applied to rabbit ears and both treatments performed using
differing concentration of calcium salts and differing time
intervals between exposure and therapy. Our results were interpreted by planimetrical, histological and microangiographical
studies. (After whole body perfusion of the rabbits with

macropaque we radiographed the dissected ears).

RESULTS

Local calcium infiltration results in a reduction of the H.F.
specific necrosis when compared with untreated ears but intra
arterial injection of calcium proved superior.   The effect of
20% calcium is more pronounced than that of 10%.   The earlier the
injection takes place the better the result - an injection of 20%
calcium within 2 hours of burning results in total restoration of
the burned area.   Between 2 and 8 hours after exposure injection
is more effective in preventing tissue destruction than infiltration
- beyond 8 hours there is no significant difference between the
two methods.

There is no transient or permanent damage to the vascular system
after injection of up to 25% calcium salts.   Peri-arterial
injection results in perivascular inflammation but there is no
clotting within the central artery.   We monitored the systemic
effects of calcium injection into the descending aorta of dogs.
Although noting the "instant digitalis effect" we found no signs
of cardiotoxicity even after digitalisation.

Since 1974 81 H.F. burns were seen at the Medical Centre r. d. Isar
in Munich.   Twelve patients with injuries to hand and fingers were
treated with intra arterial injections.   The injection of 10 ml
20% calcium takes about five minutes.   The new technique appeared
to be as successful clinically as it was in the animal models.
Thermographic studies showed that the burning sensation experienced
during intra arterial calcium injection is not related to any rise
of surface temperature.

CONCLUSION

We recommend that, in major hydrofluoric acid burns to hand and
fingers, where local calcium infiltration is impossible to apply,
the practice is followed of early injection of 20% calcium salt
into the main artery of the affected area.

REFERENCES

Bartels, H.: 1980. Treatment of Chemical Injuries by Hydrofluoric
    Acid - An Experimental Study. Toxicology letters.S.I. No.1. 154.
Bartels H.: 1981. How to Handle Injuries by Hydrofluoric Acid
    Burns - Experimental and Clinical Studies. European Surgical
    Research Vol.13. No.1. 101.
Carney S.A.: 1974. Rationale of the treatment of Hydrofluoric Acid
    Burns. Brit.J.Industrial Medicine. 31. 317-321.
Iverson R.E.: 1971. Hydrofluoric Acid Burns. Plastic and Recon
    -structive Surgery. 48. 107-112.

Care of the Acutely Ill and Injured
Edited by D. H. Wilson and A. K. Marsden
© 1982, John Wiley & Sons Ltd.

SYNTHETIC WOUND DRESSINGS - AN APPRAISAL OF
PATIENTS WITH CHRONIC LEG ULCERS

J.Kleinschmidt, W.L.Bruckner, W.Heltzel

Surgical Policlinic of the University of Munich,
Germany.

ABSTRACT

Repeated failures in the local treatment of chronic leg ulcers
resulting from venous insufficiency may lead to therapeutic
nihilism. Temporary wound dressing by means of XENOGRAFTS
(EPIGARD, SYS-PUR-DERM, COLDES) is an effective approach to the
healing of the defect, as detritus and bacteria are rapidly removed
and granulation tissue is induced (Weller, 1981).

INTRODUCTION

The two layers of the polyurethane-synthetic will show physical
interaction with the wound base after direct contact with the ulcer
(Kleinschmidt and Bruckner, 1980; Bruckner and Kleinschmidt 1981).

METHODS

Patients with chronic leg ulcers have been locally treated with
EPIGARD or SYS-PUR-DERM during the past three years. The
synthetic dressing is shaped into the wound when necessary. With
superficial wounds the patches are applied without shaping. No
further medication is involved. The daily change of the dressings
was documented by photographs at 3-4 day intervals.

CASE HISTORY

The course of a 45 year old, 14 kg female is described. After 20
years of circular ulcer defects above both ankles she had been
referred for amputation. Eight weeks after daily xenograft renewal
staged autologous skin transplantation could be performed on good
quality graft beds. After 12 weeks of hospitalisation this patient
required no further dressings nor orthopaedic aids.

CONCLUSION

Xenografts may be expensive but they are useful in the successful
treatment of long-lasting or recurrent leg ulcers.

REFERENCES

Weise, K., Weller, S.: 1981 Behandlungsergebnisse einer
    Vergleischsstudie von Hautersatzmaterialien aus Polyurethan.

Aktuelle Traumatologie 1. 1-6.
Kleinschmidt J., Bruckner W.L.: 1980. Interimsdeckung von
    infizierten Weichteildefekten. Berlin: Symposium "Moglichkeiten
    der temporaren Wunddeckung" (S.Weller). March 1980.
Bruckner, W.L., Kleinschmidt J.: 1981. Hautersatz zur langfristigen
    Deckung von Defektwunden. Symposium on Temporary Wound Dressing,
    Sindelfingen, GFR. April,1981. (S.Weller).

SECTION SEVEN

HEAD INJURIES

Care of the Acutely Ill and Injured
Edited by D. H. Wilson and A. K. Marsden
© 1982, John Wiley & Sons Ltd.

SEVERE DIFFUSE BRAIN DAMAGE : PRIMARY AND SECONDARY
FACTORS INFLUENCING ULTIMATE OUTCOME

D.J. Price

Department of Neurosurgery, Pinderfields Hospital,
Wakefield, England.

INTRODUCTION

Diffuse brain damage may result from neuronal tearing, ischaemia
or hypoxia.   It has been presumed in the past that trauma to the
brain causing death and disability occurs at the time of impact
and is therefore untreatable.   Neuropathologists have repeatedly
emphasised however, that in a high proportion of deaths, neuronal
tearing is minimal and the overriding pathological picture is that
of ischaemia and hypoxia which in theory at least are preventable.

PRIMARY IMPACT INJURY

In a road traffic accident a single deacceleration brain injury is
unusual.   At a crash at 70 m.p.h. the head may, without the body
restraint of a seat belt, accelerate to over 400 m.p.h.   At the
subsequent sudden deacceleration impact less than a second later,
the first phase injury occurs.

First and Second Impact Injuries

Neuronal injury results from transient distortion due to any
combination of surface impact disruption (causing contusions),
neuronal stretching, twisting, shearing or temporary trans-
compartmental herniation.   Second phase impact injury occurs
some 200 milliseconds later as a result of a ricochet with a
higher proportion of rotational components.   The range of
mechanisms within the first second of impact accounts for the wide
variation in initial findings on clinical examination, CT scan and
at autopsy.

Degree of Primary Brain Injury

This depends on the velocity on the first and subsequent phase
impact injuries, the proportion of rotational components and the
distribution of the kinetic energy absorption.   If this kinetic
energy is absorbed entirely by the skull, extensive fractures may
occur with no primary brain damage and conversely many patients
with severe head injuries have no skull fracture but have
devastating injury to the brain.

SECONDARY BRAIN INJURY

In a series of 151 fatal head injuries 138 had histological
evidence of ischaemic brain damage and there was often a known
preceding period of hypoxia (Graham et. al., 1978).   They inferred
that a significant proportion of these patients had minimal
primary injury and death was due to preventable secondary events
occurring in the hospital emergency room or ward.

Hypoxia

In a report from the United States 37% of patients admitted to a
neurosurgical department in coma had a pO2 below 60 mmHg.   A poor
outcome occured in 35% of those without hypoxia as compared with
59% with.   (Miller et. al., 1981).   This confirms earlier work
suggesting that a hypoxic incident is associated with a four times
reduction in chance of returning to work some two years after
injury.   (Price and Murray, 1972).   It would be naive to imply
simple cause and effect in all the patients but the association
cannot be ignored.

Ischaemia

Cerebral perfusion is related to the pressure difference between
the capillary bed and surrounding interstitial tissue.   The
cerebral perfusion pressure is traditionally expressed as the
difference between mean arterial pressure and mean intrcranial
pressure   (fig. 1).

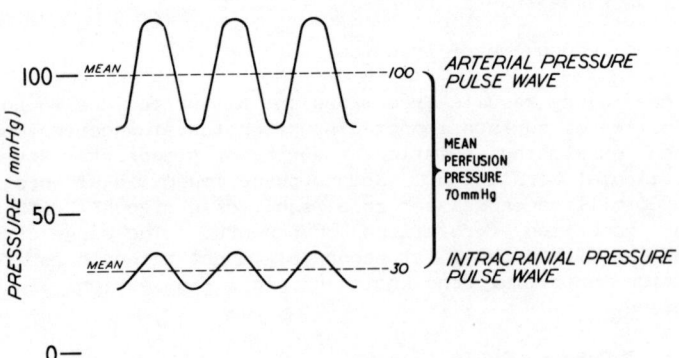

Fig. 1.   The mean cerebral perfusion pressure is the
difference between mean arterial pressure and mean
intracranial pressure.

Such a simple concept however ignores the presence of significant
pressure gradients along the arterial tree or within the brain
substance and in freshly injured brains, both are present.   Initial

management is aimed to maintain adequate perfusion of well oxygen-
ated blood to prevent secondary ischaemia.

Arterial Pressure Gradients

Systemic arterial hypotension invariably influences the pressures
measured along the arterial tree.   If in addition, the pressure
gradient from cerebral artery to capillary becomes abnormally
steep, ischaemia of the part of the brain supplied by that artery
becomes even more likely.   The two sites of partial obstructions
causing steeper pressure gradients are at the cerebral arteries
and the arterioles.   The arterial constriction in calibre following severe head injury can be demonstrated by angiography
(Macpherson and Graham, 1978) and the pial arteriolar damage by
electron microscopy after experimental injury (Wei et. al., 1980).
The discrete necrosis of the endothelial cells occurs shortly
after injury and may in part be caused by the transient arterial
hypertensive episodes and to a greater extent be due to the
generation of free oxygen radicals.   We have yet to prove
whether the early infusion of mannitol might enhance the flow
through the microcirculation to good clinical effect by its action
as a free radical scavenger or by its known effect on blood
viscosity (Burke et. al., 1981).

Interstitial Pressure Gradients

The normal brain is isobaric but following injury, pressure
gradients rapidly develop in the vicinity of contusions.   If any
area of contused brain is represented by a very simplified diagram
(Fig. 2) the pressure measured on the surface by a subdural senson
may be 30 mmHg. but in the centre of the contusion it could be
50 mmHg.

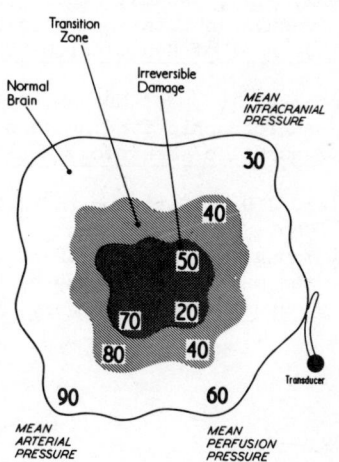

Fig. 2.   A very simplified
diagram of an area of brain
around a recent contusional
haemorrhage.

With a normal arterial pressure gradient from the surface vessels
inward, the perfusion pressure falls well below the 50 mmHg.
'safety' limit.   The only hope of reversing the developing
ischaemia in the intermediate zone is by reducing the pressure
as measured by the surface sensor in order to procure a similar
offset of the deeper interstitial pressures.   Such pressure
control is only a practical possibility if continuous measurement
is instituted in comatosed patients preferably within an hour of
injury.   The final outcome following head injury seems directly
related to the ability to control intracranial hypertension.
Professor Douglas Miller reported a poor outcome in 95% of patients
with intracranial pressure rising above 20 mmHg. despite all
attempts to control it as compared with 27% in those with pressure
below 20 mmHg.   (Miller et. al., 1981).   Although it would be
incorrect to claim that poor outcome is always entirely the result
of uncontrolled pressure, pathological evidence of ischaemia
contributing to this in most patients favours this presumption
for the majority.

CONCLUSION

We may not be able to rescue the thousands of neurons injured at
impact but with immediate transfer to an emergency department
capable of full cerebral rescusitation, we may prevent the
unnecessary devastation of millions of neurones by secondary
injury.

REFERENCES

Burke, A.M.,   Quest, D.O.,   Chien, S., and Cerri, C., 1981.   The
    efects of mannitol on blood viscosity.
    Journal of Neurosurgery, 55,   550 - 553.

Graham, D.J.,   Adams, J.H.,   Doyle, D., 1978.   Ischaemic brain
    damage in fatal non-missile head injuries.
    Journal of Neurological Sciences, 39,   213 - 234.

Macpherson, P., and Graham, D.I.,   1978.   Correlation between
    angiographic findings and the ischaemia of head injury.
    Journal of Neurology Neurosurgery and Psychiatry, 41, 122 - 127.

Miller, J.D., Butterworth, J.F.,   Gudeman, S.K.,   Faulkener, J.E.,
    Choi, S.C.,   Selhorst, J.B.,   Harbison, J.W.,   Lutz, H.,
    Young, H.F., and Becker, D.P., 1981.   Further experience in
    the management of severe head injury.
    Journal of Neurosurgery, 54,   289 - 299.

Price, D.J., and Murray, A., 1972.   The influence of hypoxia
    and hypotension on recovery from head injury.
    Injury, 3,   218 - 224.

Wei, E.P., Deitrich, W.D., Povlishock, J.T., Navari, R.M.,
    and Kantos, H.A., 1980.   Functional, morphological, and
    metabolic abnormalities of the cerebral microcirculation
    after concussive brain injury in cats.
    Circulation Research, 46,   37 - 47.

Wei, E.P., Kontos, H.A., Dietrich, W.D., Povlishock, T.J., and
    Ellis, E.F., 1981.   Inhibition by free radical scavengers
    and by cyclooxygenase inhibitors of pial arteriolar
    abnormalities from concussive brain injury in cats.
    Circulation Research, 48, 95 - 103.

Care of the Acutely Ill and Injured
Edited by D. H. Wilson and A. K. Marsden
© 1982, John Wiley & Sons Ltd.

MINOR HEAD INJURIES -
WHOM TO X RAY AND WHOM TO ADMIT

P. A. M. Weston

Accident and Emergency Department,
University Hospital, Nottingham.

INTRODUCTION

In this country 100,000 patients out of a total of 1,000,000
out-patient head injury attendances to hospital are admitted to
hospital each year (Field 1976).   This is in order to diagnose
and treat early those patients who may develop an intracranial
infection or an intracranial haematoma.

It is necessary therefore that we look carefully at this vexed
problem, because with increasing demand and lessening resources
we shall be forced to make some kind of compromise if we are to
maintain the standard of care for all the patients in the
communities we serve.   Unfortunately statistics may only help us
in assessing the overall pattern of patient care, but we as
doctors are committed to the care of the individual, so that
individual case histories (anecdotes if you like)must have a
place when we are discussing the indications for X Ray and admission.

There are three general points that I would like to make.   Firstly
no system that we devise is going to be infallible - even if all
patients who have been briefly unconscious were admitted, and even
if all patients with a history of a blow to the head were X Rayed,
some patients would inevitably escape the net.   This may be
because neither signs nor symptoms were apparent on attendance at
hospital, or because of faulty history from patient, relatives or
their attendants or because of human failings which will be
mentioned later.   Secondly the problems in children are in some
ways rather different from those in adults and this is not always
brought out in the published discussions.   These differences will
be noted during the course of the discussion.   Finally the use of
the CAT scanner (or better still the NMR scanner when that becomes
available) will not be discussed here because, although the use of
a scanner greatly facilitates the management of patients following
head injury, scanners are not generally available in this counttry
and in any case are most unlikely to replace skull X Rays in the
foreseeable future.

WHOM TO ADMIT - TO PRIMARY HOSPITAL AND TO NEUROSURGICAL UNIT

(a) <u>To primary hospital</u>   If all patients who have been briefly

unconscious following a head injury were to be admitted, skilled
nursing time would be diluted in carrying out observations on
patently healthy folk.   It is likely that observations carried out
under these conditions will be perfunctory and that the early
critical signs of deterioration may be missed.   In addition there
will be less time available for those more seriously injured
patients who may need meticulous observation and continuous nursing
care.   From the patient's point of view moreover, unnecessary
admission may be distasteful - particularly if they are nursed in
the same ward or bay alongside very sick and sometimes very anti-
social patients.   In recent years (Scottish Head Injury Management
Study, Jennett 1977 and McMillan et al, 1979) it has been shown that
unless there is some complicating factor the likelihood of a patient
developing an intracranial haematoma when he has no skull fracture
and has been only briefly unconscious is negligible.   There would
seem to be good common-sense as well as economic reasons therefore
for not admitting every head injury who was only briefly unconscious.
On the basis of this information therefore, and in the face of a
desperate shortage of acute hospital beds in Nottingham, the policy
for admission following a head injury was changed on 1st January,
1978.   Until this time we had admitted all patients who had been
even briefly unconscious but from this time patients were only
admitted if they presented one of the criteria illustrated
(Fig. 1):

      Admission criteria following head injury
      (Nottingham)

---

   1.   Prolonged amnesia or unconsciousness at site.

   2.   Depressed level of response on arrival.

   3.   Neurological abnormality on arrival.

   4.   Clinical or X Ray evidence of fracture.

   5.   Fits, vomiting or severe headache.

   6.   (When in doubt, admit).

Fig. 1.

The protocol indicated however that any patient thought fit for
discharge must have a responsible adult in attendance at home and
must be able to follow the instructions on the head injury card
(Fig. 2) with which he or she had been issued.   The fact that
this card has been given to the patient must be recorded on the
clinical case sheet.

Nottinghamshire Area Health Authority (Teaching)
SOUTH NOTTINGHAM DISTRICT
ACCIDENT AND EMERGENCY DEPARTMENT

GENERAL HOSPITAL
PARK ROW
NOTTINGHAM
Telephone: NOTTINGHAM 46161 Ext. 507/8/9

CHILDREN'S DEPARTMENT
UNIVERSITY HOSPITAL
QUEEN'S MEDICAL CENTRE
Telephone: NOTTINGHAM 700111

CARE AT HOME OF PATIENTS WHO HAVE SUSTAINED HEAD INJURIES

He/she should rest quietly at home for..............................day(s)

Bring him/her back to hospital IMMEDIATELY under the following circumstances:

If he/she:

    (a) Has a convulsion or fit

    (b) Complains of severe headache

    (c) Vomits repeatedly

    (d) Becomes increasingly drowsy and difficult to rouse. (Children should be woken every two hours during the first twelve hours after the injury to make sure that they are still rousable).

If you are worried about the patient's condition at any time.

4/79   SN/77

Since this policy was adopted in adults, the total admission rate has been halved (Table 1) while the number of serious injuries has remained constant.

TABLE I.

	1977	1978	1979
All new attendances (aged 13 or above)	67,110	72,020	69,200
Head injury attendances (aged 15 or above)	6,980	6,240	5,810
Admissions following head injury (adult)	941	536	460
Death due to head injury (adult)	40	49	45

In spite of careful scrutiny of the autopsies in Nottingham and admissions to other accident beds during the subsequent two years I have not come across any patients who have suffered as a result of this change in policy. However, there was one young man who arrived in the early hours of the morning saying that he had been hit on the head but had not been unconscious. His mates corroborated this story. He was carefully examined and the only abnormality was a small recent bruise behind the right ear; there was no neurological abnormality and no blunting of consciousness,

although he had obviously had a few drinks. He was allowed home
and rang for a taxi. He was neither X Rayed nor admitted. His
mother found him dead in his bed the following morning and autopsy
showed a large extradural haematoma underlying a fine fissured
fracture. This boy had given a totally misleading history because
it was found later that he had been "ridden down" during gang
warfare by one of his opponents on a motorcycle and that he had
been unconscious for 15 minutes. The patient would have been
admitted had this history been available. This case illustrates
the difficulties of laying down reliable guidelines. It is quite
possible moreover that the very fine fissured fracture would not
have been seen even if an X Ray had been taken. One author
(Galbraith 1976) examined 87 patients with intracranial haematomas
who had no fracture. Four of these patients had neither a fracture
nor any initial symptoms or signs of injury to the brain (i.e. had
not been unconscious etc). Ironically the only one of these four
who died was the patient who was initially admitted to hospital.
You see how complex the problem becomes. However, I repeat that
so far I am not aware that any patient has suffered as a result of
the change in admission policy that we have adopted in Nottingham.

(b) To neurosurgical unit. If then we accept that in this
imperfect world selective admission policy of this sort is
justifiable we must decide which of these patients carried a
sufficiently high risk of developing complications to warrant
transfer immediately or within a short while to specialist
facilities in a neurosurgical unit. This in turn depends not only
on medical factors but on the beds and facilities which may be
available in neurosurgical centres, on the proximity of the centre
to the primary hospital and on the interest which may be shown in
these patients by the neurosurgeons. In this country about 95%
of all head-injured patients are looked after outside neurosurgical
units but Jennett (1979 and 1981) has shown that many patients die
as a result of delay in diagnosis and operation (associated
sometimes with delayed transfer to neurosurgical units) as well as
from the effects of extra-cranial factors (hypoxia, hypovolaemia
etc). He suggests therefore (Jennett 1979) that with careful
selection and a few more beds in neurosurgical units the vast
majority of intracranial haematomas and open head injuries could
be dealt with in neurosurgical units. Jennett, however, does not
specify which groups of patients he thinks should or should not be
transferred. In an attempt to define these groups a retrospective
study of patients admitted with head injuries to the Nottingham
University Hospital was carried out. Using the indications for
admission to the neurosurgical unit shown in Fig.3 we estimated
that instead of the present transfer rate of 15 patients per annum
approximately 150 high-risk patients would need to be transferred
to the neurosurgical unit - and that these patients could occupy
approximately 3-4 additional beds.

We would suggest that there are two contra-indications to transfer.
These are patients who deteriorate very rapidly within two hours
of admission and patients who have serious injuries to other parts
of the body which require urgent resuscitation and treatment.

FIGURE 3. Head injuries: indications for transfer to
           neurosurgical unit

---

1. Delayed deterioration (hours or days)

2. Failure of improvement in neurological status

3. Fracture of the vault or base of skull (whether open or
    closed)

4. Complications: including CSF leaks, evidence of infection,
    pulsating exophthalmos,etc

The implication of this is that the surgeons in the primary
hospital who are responsible for the immediate care of these
patients must also be willing and able to do emergency burr-
holes and to manage acute cerebral oedema.   The training
implications will not be discussed further here.

WHOM TO X RAY

It is generally accepted in this country that one of the indications
for admission to hospital following a head injury is the presence
of a fracture of the skull - whether this is diagnosed on clinical
or radiological grounds; whether it is open or closed; whether
it involves the vault or the base of the skull, or both.   This is
because it has been shown (Jennett 1979) that 90% of extradural
haematomas in adults are associated with a fracture of the vault of
the skull.   There have been a number of very persuasive papers
written in which the authors have shown that statistically at least
it is possible to define groups of clinical symptoms and signs which
are likely to be associated with a skull fracture. (Figure 5).

FIGURE 5. X-rays and head injuries (all ages):

           Clinical factors associated with a "high yield"
           of positive X-rays (1:10 or less)

---

1. Unconscious or amnesic $>$ 5 minutes at site.

2. Neurological abnormality
    (Stupor, semi-conscious,   on arrival in hospital.
    comatose)

3. Clinical evidence of fracture of skull - base vault.

4. Vomiting.

5. Accident at work or G.S.W.

Conversely there are groups of signs or symptoms which are very
unlikely to be associated with a skull fracture (Figure 6)
(Bell and Loop 1971).   These authors point out that in the

United States some 15 million dollars a year might be saved if
unnecessary X Rays of the skull were omitted.   In support of
this argument a random sample of children's skull X Rays in
Nottingham showed that 95% of films were normal.   Furthermore
some of our young patients had had several skull series and it is
said that repeated skull X Rays may cause damage to the lens in a
child's eye - subsequent cataracts may develop in early middle age.

FIGURE 6.   X-rays and head injuries (all ages):

Clinical factors associated with a "low yield"
of positive X-rays ($>$1:10)

1.   Confusion or drowsiness

2.   Intoxication

3.   Haematoma or swelling

4.   Laceration

5.   Headache

6.   Fits

Other authors (Boulis et al 1978) have added all scalp wounds to
the list of "high yield" factors.   These authors point out that
not only may the quality of skull X Rays taken in the middle of
the night in a restless patient be poor but the interpretation by
harassed junior doctors at such times may be inaccurate.

However only a few of these studies are prospective (Phillips
1979) and the numbers of patients involved are insufficient to
give adequate information about the admittedly rare occurrence of
intracranial haematoma.   None of these authors has sought to find
out what happens to patients who do not have an X Ray and who are
discharged home (Royal College of Radiologists' report 1980).
But one study (Lassen 1979) reports on a series in which 5 patients
who required surgery for an intracranial haematoma (including one
extradural haematoma) would not have been X Rayed had the stringent
criteria advocated by Bell and Loop been adopted.   So the case
for a drastic reduction in the number of skull X Rays does not
seem to be proved.   Furthermore the problem is much less clear
in children, in whom extradural haematomas are much less common
relative to subdural haematomas, than in adults; and in whom a
fracture is associated with an intracranial haematoma in only 40%
of cases - and even then the fracture is often not on the same
side as the haematoma.

The following 2 case histories illustrate the special problems in
children.   Both of these children had had an injury to the head -
in neither case was there a history of unconsciousness at any
stage but both had had an X Ray of the skull which did not show a
fracture.   The first patient vomited in the taxi on the way home.
His level of consciousness began to deteriorate but because it was
the rush hour the father was unable to get him back quickly to the
hospital and he was dead on arrival.   Autopsy showed an extra-

dural haematoma underlying a fine fissured fracture which even in
retrospect was not visible on the X Ray.   The other child was
recommended for discharge but the father insisted that the child
should be admitted because the impact seemed to him to have been
quite severe.   Two hours following admission an extradural
haematoma was removed and the child recovered completely.   In
neither case were clear indications present for X Ray or for
admission.

Certainly therefore it is incumbent on us to try to ensure that
when X Rays are taken the quality is good - even if this means
delaying X Rays for a few hours with the patient under observation.
It is also our responsibility to educate our junior staff in the
value of X Rays, for it is certainly not true, as some authors have
suggested (Evans 1977), that X Rays are of little value.   In
Nottingham a tape-slide presentation illustrating what information
can be obtained from such X Rays is available in the teaching room
within the A and E Department.   In addition a half-hour weekly
meeting between radiographers, a radiologist and the medical staff
in the A and E Department provides education in this and other
aspects of radiology in the department.

How then can we give guidance to our junior staff as to which
patients should be X Rayed since even the most enthusiastic
exponents of taking more skull X Rays do not advocate that all
should be X Rayed (and indeed in Glasgow only some 50% of all head
injury attenders are X Rayed and in Nottingham only about one third).
I would suggest that the following criteria (which must not be
interpreted too rigidly) might merit your consideration and
discussion, bearing in mind that most of the criteria are
dependent in some degree on an accurate history (and as we have
seen this is not always available) and that human or technical
failings may invalidate any such series of criteria (Figure 7).

FIGURE 7.   Suggested criteria for skull X-ray following
head injury

1. When the impact is known to have been severe

2. Most scalp wounds

3. Penetrating wounds in which a foreign body is suspected

4. The presence of any of the criteria for admission (already
enumerated)

SUMMARY AND CONCLUSIONS

The suggestions that I have made are a compromise which would
result in fewer admissions and fewer X Rays.   I have also
suggested that more patients should and could be admitted to
neurosurgical wards - and more beds and additional staff should
be made available for this purpose.

It is important that we should instruct our junior staff in the
reading of skull X Rays and their value.   The early observation of
patients should be carried out meticulously.   It is equally
important that action (including urgent operation or transfer to a
neurosurgical unit) should be taken at the earliest signs of
deterioration.   It is too late to wait until the patient is
comatose or until the pupils are unequal or fixed and dilated.
Finally I would suggest that further large-scale multi-centre
prospective studies should be carried out of all head-injured
patients - whether or not they have had a skull X Ray - in order
to test the validity of the criteria that are selected in each
centre.   The presence or absence of these criteria (one of which
must be the severity and mechanism of injury) should be measured
against the incidence of complications and their effect on outcome.

REFERENCES

1. R.S.Bell, J.W.Loop: New England Med J. 1971. 284. 236-239.
2. F.Boulis, R.Dick, N.R.Barnes, B.J.Rad. 1978. 51. 851-854.
3. K.T.Evans, B.J.Rad 1977. 50. 299.
4. Field - Epidemiology of head injuries in England and Wales,
    1976. HMSO.
5. S.Galbraith, R.McMillan, B.Jennett, Lancet. Jan 31.1981. 272.
6. S.Galbraith, J.Smith, Lancet. March 6 1976. 501-503.
7. B.Jennett et al. BMJ 20 Oct.1979. 955-988.
8. B.Jennett et al. Scot HI Management Study - Lancet March 1979
    75-81; Oct.1977. 696-698.
9. B.Jennett, R.McMillan. BMJ 1981. 10 Jan. 101-104.
10. B.Jennett, R.McMilland: "Medicine" 35. Nov.77. and Health
    Bulletin March 1979. 75-81.
11. K.T.Lassen, D.F.Koziol. JACEP Oct.79. 8. 393.
12. A.D.Mendelow, M.Z.Karni, K.S.Paul, G.A.G.Fuller, F.J.Gillingham.
    BMJ 12 May 1979, 1240-1242.
13. L.A.Phillips, JACEP 8. 106-109. March 9 1979.
14. R.Coll Rad Report. Hosp Practice, Lancet Dec 6. 1980. 1234-1236.

Figure 1 and Table 1 reproduced by permission of the British Journal
of Surgery and John Wright & Sons.

Care of the Acutely Ill and Injured
Edited by D. H. Wilson and A. K. Marsden
© 1982, John Wiley & Sons Ltd.

A PRACTICAL COMA SCALE FOR MONITORING HEAD INJURIES

D.J. Price and A.K. Marsden

Pinderfields Hospital, Wakefield, England.

INTRODUCTION

The introduction of computerised tomography scanning has made
less impact on the management of the majority of head injured
patients than was first anticipated.   The patients at greatest
risk of developing an intracranial haematoma are often restless
and uncooperative and both the intolerance of movement and
restrictions on immediate availability of a scanner impose
serious limitations on its use as a monitoring device for most
patients seen in an emergency department.   Despite this
technological advance, we are therefore still faced with the need
to recognise patients who might develope a haematoma by using
clinical information.

The selection of patients for CT scanning necessitates the
repeated monitoring of the level of risk of a complication
occurring.   This correct principle has been traditionally
accepted as an essential feature of head injury management for
many years but unfortunately little attention has been given to
quantify this level by clearly associating any clinical trend with
a change in definable risk.

The current well-meaning but haphazard approach has led to
indiscriminate use of expensive diagnostic resources to patients
with very small risk of a complication and unnecessary delays in
referral to a neurosurgeon in others with much higher risk.
In two British series, unnecessary delays were thought to be the
most important contributing factors in 33% and 39% of head injury
deaths.   (Jeffreys and Jones, 1981. Jennett and Carlin, 1978)
Mendelow (Mendelow et. al., 1979) confirmed that in a group of
patients with extradural haematoma, the final outcome was directly
related to the length of time from the first report of a falling
conscious level to evacuation of the haematoma.   A similar
conclusion was reached in the United States (Seelig et. al., 1981)
where   mortality resulting from acute subdural haematomas was
found to be three times higher if evacuation was delayed beyond
four hours after injury.   There is little doubt that the most
useful clinical indicant of a developing complication whether due
to a haematoma or raised intracranial pressure per se is a fall in
conscious level.

COMA SCALES

In the last decade two coma scales have been internationally
accepted.   The simplest is a binary scale discriminating by
definition between patients 'in coma' and 'not in coma'.   This
provides a simple clearly defined criterion for management
decisions.   In practice, many would agree that all patients in
coma should, after systemic resuscitation, be urgently transferred
to a neurosurgical department.   The second scale known as the
Glasgow Coma Scale (Teasdale and Jennett, 1974) is designed
primarily for use in comparative studies for evaluation of
different treatment regimes.   When used for this purpose the
three component scores should not be summated as they are non-
parametric and this has rightly been discouraged by displaying the
three coma scale scores on separate graphs but on the same sheet
as two independent motor function graphs.   This scale is
fortunately now widely used for both predictive and comparative
studies, but the five separate graphs are cumbersome for
inexperienced nurses to visualise at a glance and this method of
data collection is more appropriate as a research tool than a
trend detector in the acute situation.

The frequent monitoring of head injured patients during their
transit through emergency departments and observation wards demands
much higher sensitivity for early detection of deterioration,
particularly if there is no neurosurgical service within that
hospital.   The application of a research tool for routine clinical
use is attractive to doctors but before considering its use for
 monitoring by nurses its effectiveness as a trend detector must
first be objectively evaluated.   This aspect of its function has
not been previously challenged.   As the outcome of patients with
intracranial haematoma is so dependent on the early recognition
of deterioration, we thought it essential to define the dangers
and limitations of any scale used.

Requirements of a Scale

The optimum size of definable increments on any scale is usually
dependent on the combined influence of three factors:-

1.   Inter-observer variability
2.   The minimum sensitivity required
3.   Effort

To take an example, asking a nurse to measure heart rate by
counting each pulse beat during a whole minute may well provide a
reliable figure accurate to the nearest one or two beats per minute.
To ask her to count during ten seconds and then multiply by six
reduces both effort and sensitivity but increases inter-observer
variability.   A compromise is required to satisfy all three
factors and nurses instinctively select an optimum.

SELECTION OF COMA SCALE

The selection of a practical coma scale primarily for monitoring
in a busy emergency department requires evaluation of all three
factors.   If used only for trend recognition, the non-parametric
subscores may be summated and displayed as a single graph for the
most junior nurse to understand.

1.   Inter-Observer Variability

Earlier work based on a study of 6,000 observations recorded on
a 0 - 50 scale had shown a coefficient of observer reliability of
95% allowing an error of plus or minus 5%   (Price, 1976).   This
suggests that a fall of three or more points on this scale
indicates a greater than 95% chance of it being relevant.

2.   Minimum Sensitivity Requirement

Seven different numerical scales were examined in detail.   They
varied from the simplest five level scale to the more complex
multi-score systems.   We had previously adopted the 50 point
scale for routine use in the neurosurgical ward presuming it to be
the most sensitive.   It includes 12 aspects of consciousness and
had the advantage of being 'translatable' to all the other known
scales in current use in Britain.   It was accepted by the
nursing staff who welcomed a structured system and had been in use
since 1973.   We randomly selected 100 patients with deterioration
in conscious level of four or five points.   Computer analysis of
the subscores provided translations to seven other coma scales and
for every deteriorating patient, we recorded as to whether the four
or five point fall on the 50 point scale would be detected as a
one or more point fall on each of the seven other coma scales.
If the percentage of patients detected is plotted against the
scale spans, the relationship proves logarithmic below a span of
40 but minimum sensitivity gain was achieved above this.   It was
not surprising that the 12 point Glasgow Coma Scale only recognised
40% of the patients to be deteriorating (Cranswick et. al., 1979).
(Fig. 1)

3.   Effort

We found a wide variation in the time a nurse took in observing
and recording each aspect of consciousness.   This time depended
on both training and previous knowledge of the patient.   The time
taken varied from 8 to 16 seconds for each subscore and the total
time to assess and record the conscious level compared with that
of routine physiological parameters.   For patients with only a
head injury, it would seem reasonable to delegate at least as much
nursing effort on monitoring brain function as cardiovascular
function.

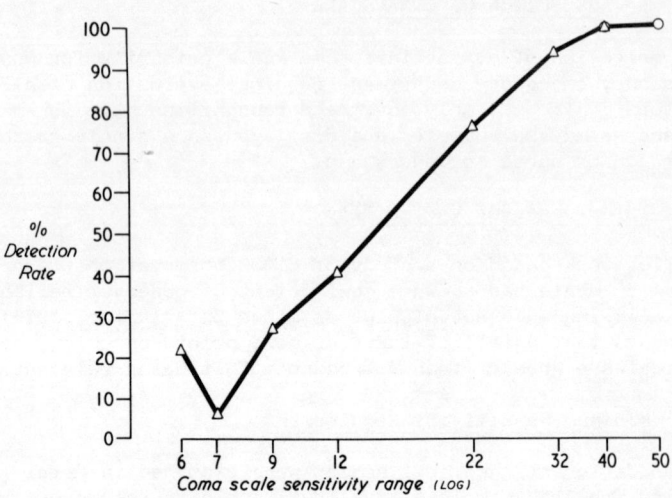

Fig. 1.   The relationship between the coma scale
sensitivity range and the percentage of patients detected
to be deteriorating (detection is defined as a one or more
point fall on each scale reflecting a four or five point
fall on the 0 - 50 scale).

THE SELECTED SCALE IN USE

Following this preliminary work we concluded that a score span of
just over 30 produced a compromise to satisfy the three basic
factors considered.   We therefore designed a coma scale using
seven subscores with a single graph display.   This has now been
used for head injury observations in an accident and emergency
department for a year and has been readily accepted by both
nursing and medical staff.   (Fig. 2).

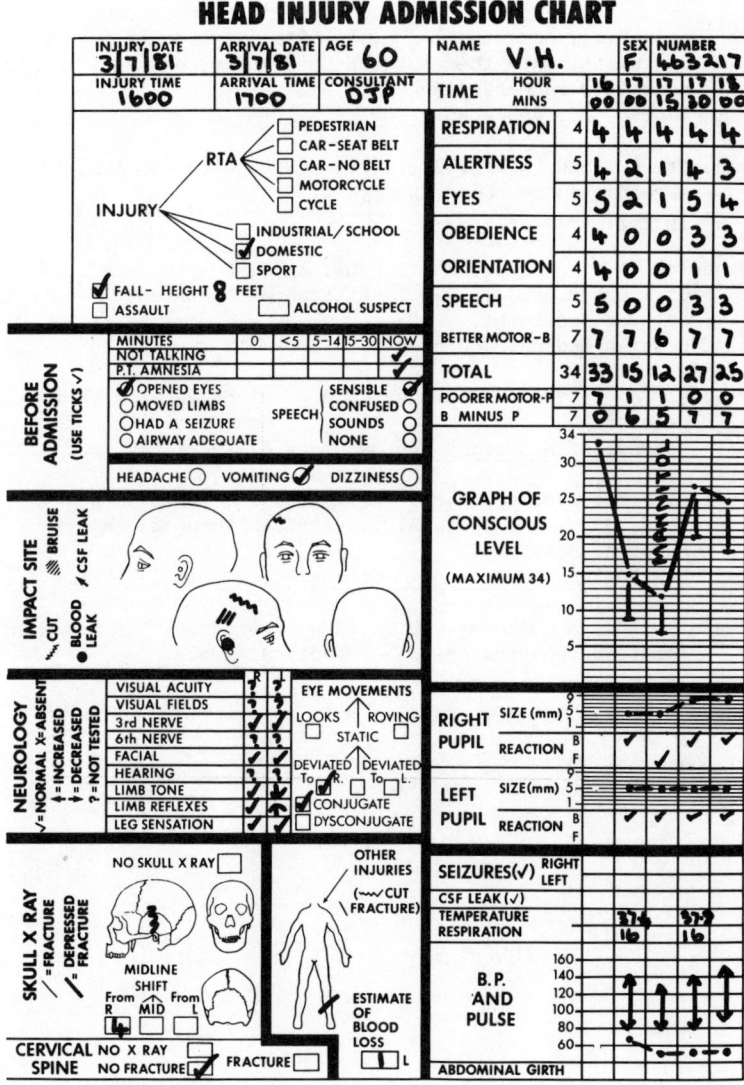

Fig. 2. The head injury observation chart used in the accident and emergency department. Medical staff complete the left half and nursing staff the right.

REFERENCES

Cranswick, T.,   Smith, B.J.,   Coulter, L.J.,   and Cowell, M.M., 1979.
    Recherche d'une echelle de coma de sensibilite optimale.
    Le Journal de l'Infirmiere de Neurochirurgie, 23, 16 - 20.

Jeffreys, R.V., and Jones, J.J.,   1981.   Avoidable factors
    contributing to the death of head injury patients in general
    hospitals in Mersey Region.
    Lancet, 2,   459 - 461.

Jennett, B., and Carlin, J., 1978.   Preventable mortality and
    morbidity after head injury.
    Injury, 10,   31 - 39.

Mendelow, A.D.,   Karmi, M.Z., Paul, K.S., Fuller, G.A., and
    Gillingham, F.J., 1979.   Extradural haematoma :   effect of
    delayed treatment.
    British Medical Journal, 1,   1240 - 1242.

Price, D.J.,   1976.   Analogue to digital conversion of conscious-
    ness.
    Journal of Neurology Neurosurgery & Psychiatry, 43, 919.

Seelig, J.M.,   Becker, D.P.,   Miller, J.D.,   Greenberg, R.P.,
    Ward, J.D., and Choi, S.C.,   1981.   Traumatic acute
    subdural hematoma.
    New England Journal of Medicine,   304.   1511- 1518.

Teasdale, G., and Jennett, B.,   1974.   Assessment of coma and
    impaired consciousness : A practical scale.
    Lancet, 2,   81 - 84

SECTION EIGHT

EMERGENCIES IN THE

GASTROINTESTINAL TRACT

Care of the Acutely Ill and Injured
Edited by D. H. Wilson and A. K. Marsden
© 1982, John Wiley & Sons Ltd.

ENDOSCOPIC REMOVAL OF FOREIGN BODIES FROM THE
UPPER GASTROINTESTINAL TRACT

P.Ventura, M.Azzola, G.Turati

1st Surgical Clinic - Emergency Endoscopy Department,
University of Milan.

ABSTRACT

Between 1976 and 1980 we have treated 24 patients with swallowed
foreign bodies which became lodged in the stomach or first part
of the duodenum. The cases and technique for removal are
described.

INTRODUCTION

The extraction of foreign bodies from the upper gastrointestinal
tract is one of the simplest and most effective applications of
operative endoscopy.

MATERIAL AND METHODS

We utilised the Olympus fiberscope GIF D2-K and TGF 2D with
different grasping forceps. All patients were premedicated with
local pharyngeal anaesthesia with lignocaine together with
i.v. diazepam.

RESULTS

Fourteen cases out of 24 underwent emergency endoscopic procedure
to remove foreign bodies from the stomach or duodenum. In four
cases a point of a dentist's drill was lodged in the stomach; in
three a nail; in two needles (one being in the stomach and the
other in the duodenal bulb). In one case the foreign body was a
gauze retained after a partial gastrectomy. In one psychologically
disturbed patient the foreign bodies were small metal fragments
collected in the stomach and duodenum.

In the thirteen who did not undergo endoscopic procedure there were
nine instances of coins or large metallic pieces (cutlery) which
were swallowed by prisoners.

DISCUSSION

Objects which are likely to wound should be removed from the
stomach or duodenum when possible - the limit of the procedure is
determined by the shape and size of the foreign body. Objects
should be seized by the instrument before withdrawal - needles

or nails are directly withdrawn into the scope.

REFERENCES

Dunkerton R.E. 1975 Fiber endoscopic removal of large foreign
  bodies from the stomach. Gastrointestinal Endoscopy 21, 196.
Gupta J.K. 1977 Removal of inadvertently swallowed endotracheal
  tube from the stomach through an esophagastomy stoma with the
  fiberoptic endoscope. Gastrointestinal Endoscopy 23, 31.

Care of the Acutely Ill and Injured
Edited by D. H. Wilson and A. K. Marsden
© 1982, John Wiley & Sons Ltd.

SURGICAL EMERGENCIES CAUSED BY POTASSIUM CHLORIDE
TABLETS.

J.Waninger and D.Waldmann

Chirurgische Universitätsklinik
Hugstetterstr.55, D-78 Freiburg

Abstract

Gastrointestinal lesions following treatment with potassium chloride tablets have been known since 1964. Hemorrhagic infarction or small bowel stenosis with ul-
ceration and perforation necessitates an emergency operation. 4 cases with lesions due to potassium chloride were
treated at the Chirurgische Universitätsklinik Freiburg
between 1977 and 1979.

Introduction

It is not a new finding that potassium chloride tablets
may cause gastrointestinal lesions. However, the few recent publications reporting individual cases of complications following treatment with potassium chloride tablets indicate that this danger is frequently overlooked.
Baker (1964) and Lindholmer (1964) reported almost at the
same time cases of small bowel ulcers with stenosis. The
last comprehensive survey by Emerson (1970) reported 414
cases of KCl-induced small bowel lesions. Since that time
73 further cases have been reported (Waninger,1981).

Pathology

The typical stenosis has a "napkin" or "pyloric-like"
appearance and the perforated ulcer looks punched out.The
mucosa is ulcerated at the site of stenosis. Histologi-
cally the submucosa shows various degrees of inflammation.
The principal location of the lesions are distal jejunum
and ileum. These areas are highly susceptible to chemical
trauma since they possess fewer mucous glands. In recent
years a total of 13 oesophageal lesions have been reported. Mouth,stomach and cecum are less often involved.

Pathophysiology

The pathophysiological mechanism is started by a high
local potassium concentration. The corrosive effect of

the potassium damages the mucosa. A spasm of the vessels
is followed by local oedema, hemorrhagic infarction and
necrosis of the bowel wall. A perforation may follow. The
potassium produces a spastic circular contraction of the
bowel wall which retains the tablet and favours the local
potassium concentration (Sundell,1971).
It is not possible in the individual case to explain why
the tablet stays at one particular place. However, a tablet may be trapped in a diverticulum or may be retained
at a relative stenosis of the oesophagus produced by the
enlargement of the right atrium in patients with mitral
stenosis (Whitney,1972).
Enteric-coated tablets pass the stomach and dissolve in
the small intestine inbetween 15 and 50 minutes. The slow-
release tablet leaks the potassium gradually in a period
of 4 to 5 hrs.

Diagnosis

The right diagnosis has rarely been made before operation.
If stenosis is present, small bowel perforation or hemorrhagic infarction may be encountered during laparotomy
and potassium may be the cause, if the patient has a history of treatment with these tablets. However, other
causes such as regional enteritis, local ischemia, a
strangulated small bowel and a nonspecific ulcer have to
be considered.

Treatment

The involved bowel has to be resected. The treatment with
potassium tablets is stopped or changed to a potassium
rich diet. 4 cases with potassium lesions were treated at
the Chirurgische Universitätsklinik Freiburg. In 3 cases
two perforations and one stenosis, a segment of bowel was
removed. One patient had a localized hemorrhagic infarction of the cecal wall. Part of the cecum was removed.

References

Baker,D.,Schrader,W.,and Hitchcock,C.,1964.Small bowel
      ulceration apparently associated with thiazide and
      potassium therapy. JAMA, 190,586.
Emerson,D.N.,1970.Potassium therapy and gastrointestinal
      lesions.Missouri Med,67.310.
Lindholmer,B.,Nyman,E.and Raf,L.,1964.Nonspecific ste-
      nosing ulceration of the small bowel. Acta Chir
      Scand,128,310.
Sundell,G.,1971.Effects of potassium tablets of different
      dissolution rates on motility pattern of small in-
      testine in the dog.Acta Pharm Suecica,8,73.
Waninger,J.und Waldmann,D.,1981.Die Kaliumtablette als Ur-
      sache chirugischer Noteingriffe.Chir Praxis,in press.
Whitney,B.,and Crozon,R.,1972.Dysphagia caused by cardiac
enlargement.Clin Radiol,23,147.

Care of the Acutely Ill and Injured
Edited by D. H. Wilson and A. K. Marsden
© 1982, John Wiley & Sons Ltd.

MANAGEMENT OF BURN INJURIES TO THE UPPER GI-TRACT
BY CORROSIVE AGENTS

H.Bartels, B.Ultsch, M.V.Clarmann[+], et al

Department of Surgery,
Department of Toxicology, Medical Center r. r. Isar
Ismaninger Str. 22, 8ooo Munchen 8o, W.Germany

ABSTRACT

Ingestion of corrosive substances presents life threatening injuries.
From our clinical material we have developed a protocol for handling
caustic burns of the upper G.I. Tract.   Our methods of management
are based on clinical and endoscopic studies; The degree of
intestinal damage should be assessed by endoscopy and, if there is
a second or third degree burn injury, emergency surgery should be
performed.   Staged reconstruction of intestinal continuity should
be done later when the patient's condition improves and the tissue
is suitable for suturing.

INTRODUCTION

Ingestion of corrosive substances produces severe injuries to the
upper GI-tract and systemic intoxication in cases of resorption.
The resulting damage is directly related to the agent ingested, its
concentration and duration of contact with the organ walls.

Superficial burns are confined only to the mucous membranes.   The
defects are replaced by reepithelisation; there is no permanent
damage.   In second degree burns the mucosa and submucosa of the
organ walls are involved.   There are erosions, ulcerations and
bleeding.   The defects are replaced by scar tissue and stricture
formation.   Third degree or transmural burns result in necrosis of
all tissue layers, maceration and acute gangreneous perforation.

The ingestion of corrosive agents presents a diagnostic and therapeutic challenge to the physician.   In the literature mostly single
cases are reported but no standardised treatment has been recommended.
Analysing our clinical data we developed a regimen for handling
caustic burns of the intestinal tract.

METHOD

Since 1973 25 patients with corrosive injuries to the upper GI-tract
were treated in the Munich Medical Center r. d. Isar.   On 23
occasions the corrosives were ingested to commit suidice, once an
alcoholic drank the agent accidentally and once a patient fell into
a bath for galvanising procedures resulting in local burns to the
body surface and swallowing of the chemical agent.

According to the classification of corrosive substances by BOSCH del MARCO (1949) the agents have been divided into fixatives (n=3), destructives (n=7), softeners (n=8) and weak substances (n=7).

Ingestion of alkali caused oesophageal burns in 100% and gastric burns in 40%, ingestion of acid oesophageal burns in 20% and gastric burns in 100%.   Only large amounts of either substances cause damage to oesophagus and stomach.   In two cases there was additional corrosion to duodenum, jejunum and after visceral perforation to spleen, liver and pancreas.

The initial signs and symptoms after ingestion of corrosives are: severe burning pain in the mouth, throat and stomach spreading rapidly over the entire abdomen, intensive thirst with great difficulty of swallowing, damage to the oropharyngeal mucous membranes and, in case of spilling, to the circumoral skin, vomiting, involuntary guarding, rigidity of the abdominal wall, rebound tenderness, hypoactive or absent bowel sounds, upper GI-bleeding and deteriorating vital signs.

Our methods of management based on clinical and endoscopical findings:

Group I: We prefer not to operate, if there is a history of ingestion but just first degree damage is found by endoscopical studies.   Therapy consists in fasting, application of antacids, antibiotics and intravenous fluids.

Group II: In case of second or third degree damage we perform a laparotomy.   The bulbus duodeni must be clamped immediately to prevent passage of corrosives into the duodenum.   If the external surface of the stomach appears normal a vigorous gastric lavage should be performed.   After closure of the laparotomy the operation can be finished without any resection procedure.

GroupIII: If the external surface of the stomach is damaged, we perform a total gastrectomy establishing the GI-continuity by an oesophago-jejunostomy provided there is no damage to the distal oesophagus.

Group IV: If the distal oesophagus is involved and an oesophageal anastomosis is prone to disrupt, a total gastrectomy, closure of the duodenal stump, closure of the distal oesophagus and cervical oesophagostomy for diversion of saliva, must be performed.

Group V: In case of total necrosis of the oesophagus in addition to gastrectomy oesophagectomy must be performed with terminal cervical oesophagostomy.

RESULTS

In the last 7 years 25 ingestions with corrosive agents were treated
following the listed regimen.   There were 10 cases of non-operative
management (Group 1), 14 patients underwent surgery, 1 patient died
in the emergency room before initiating any treatment.   The overall
mortality rate in the non-operative group was 0%, in the surgical
group 50%.

DISCUSSION

We think emergency surgery to be indicated not only in case of
complications like haemorrhage, free perforation, mediastinitis or
peritonitis after corrosive ingestion.   The extent, degree and
depth of intestinal involvement should be assessed by means of
endoscopy and in case of second or third degree damage surgery
should be performed immediately.   Staged reconstruction of
intestinal continuity can be done weeks or months later, when the
patient's condition improves and the tissue is suitable for suturing.

Our clinical results prove that the high mortality rate of caustic
burns to the upper GI-tract can be reduced by following this regimen
of treatment.

So called "first aid procedures" like application of emetics,
insertion of a stomach tube, "closed gastric lavage" and dilution
or neutralisation are not helpful.   On the contrary the use of a
stomach tube carries risks due to softening of tissue and danger
of perforation.   Gastric lavage and inducing of emesis are contra-
indicated, since perforation of the injured area, tracheobronchial
aspiration or additional damage to the oesophagus, larynx and oral
cavity by the corrosive agent may occur.   Furthermore neutralisation
with antidotes produces additional heat by chemical reaction and
probably potentiates the thermal component of burn injuries.

REFERENCES

Muhletaler, C.A.: Gastroduodenal Lesions of Ingested Acid
    AJR: 135, December 1980, 1247-1252
Allan, R.E.: Corrosive Injuries of the Stomach. Arch.Surg/Vol 100
    April 1970, 409-413
Nicosia, J.F.: Surgical Management of Corrosive Gastric Injuries
    Annals of Surgery, Vol.180. August,1977, 139-143.
Rumack, B.H.: Caustic ingestions: a rational look at diluents
    Clin Toxicology, 11. 1977. 27-34.

Care of the Acutely Ill and Injured
Edited by D. H. Wilson and A. K. Marsden
© 1982, John Wiley & Sons Ltd.

EMERGENCY OPERATIVE ENDOSCOPY IN UPPER GASTROINTESTINAL HAEMORRHAGE

L.Tognini, R.Paternollo, M.Azzola

1st Surgical Clinic, Institute of Emergency Surgery
Department of Emergency Endoscopy, University of
Milan, Italy.

ABSTRACT

The authors report their experience of emergency operative
endoscopy performed upon 551 patients out of 1302 who underwent
an endoscopic examination for haemorrhage of the upper digestive
tract between March, 1976 and December, 1980.

INTRODUCTION

The pathologic causes of haemorrhage include oesophageal varices
(16 patients), gastric ulcers (192 patients), duodenal ulcers
(69 patients), plus some other, rarer, lesions (Mallory Weiss
Syndrome, hiatus hernia, anastomotic ulcers, neoplasm etc.).

MATERIAL AND METHODS

We employed the Olympus fiberscopes GIF D2-K and TGF 2D with
different electrocoagulating tips and the Bovie model 0-4 and
EMS System 2000 electrocoagulators.   Haemostatic clips and a
Neodymium-Yag-Laser were also used.   In all cases the procedure
was performed during haemorrhage.

RESULTS

The most utilised method was electrocoagulation.
With respect to the Neodymium-Yag-Laser, the light of lasers is not
absorbed by haemoglobin - thus there is less dispersion during
bleeding.   Permanent haemostasis after coagulation is encouraged
during medical antisecretive therapy which allows scarring of the
necrosis.

In almost 90% cases haemostasis was immediately obtained; in
3.3% cases further coagulation was required and in 13% a lasting
haemostasis was not obtained - this being especially true in
lesions associated with extended gastropathies.

In bleeding oesophageal varices sclerosing procedures were
performed with immediate haemostasis in 87.5% cases - further
treatment was performed in 35% cases.   Haemostatic clips were
used in three of these cases but with poor results.

369

DISCUSSION

Our experience verifies the role of operative endoscopy - not as a primary curative procedure but merely to control the haemorrhagic complication allowing normal haemodynamic balance and an opportunity of further diagnostic screening. Haemorrhage was not controlled in many cases of haemorrhagic gastropathy where large arterial vessels were injured or where incomplete coagulation was obtained. At present we reserve electrocoagulation for the well delineated or focal haemorrhagic lesion. The results obtained by laser - photocoagulation are similar to those obtained by electrocoagulation : the advantage of easier handling has to be weighed against the cost of the instrument.

REFERENCES

Kiefhaber P., Nath G. Moritz. 1977.
Endoscopic control of massive gastrointestinal haemorrhage by irradiation with Neodymium-Yag-Laser. Progress in Surgery 15. 140-155.

Tognini L., Paternollo R. et al. 1980
L'elettrocoagulazione endoscopica in urgenza. Note di tecnica.
Urgentis Chirurgiae Commentaria, 3. 301-305.

Ghezzi C., Tognini L., Paternollo R. 1981
Emostasi endoscopica in urgenza con Neodymium-Yag-Laser nelle emorragie del tratto gastroenterico superiore.
Giornale Italiano di Gastroenterologia e Endoscopia in press.

Care of the Acutely Ill and Injured
Edited by D. H. Wilson and A. K. Marsden
© 1982, John Wiley & Sons Ltd.

OESOPHAGOGASTRIC TRANSECTION FOR THE EMERGENCY
MANAGEMENT OF BLEEDING OESOPHAGEAL VARICES   -   A SIMPLE
MECHANICAL TECHNIQUE

D. R. Osborne and K. E. F. Hobbs

Academic Department of Surgery, Royal Free Hospital,
School of Medicine, London U.K.

INTRODUCTION

Approximately one third of the patients presenting with bleeding
from oesophageal varices are not controlled by conservative measures
and require more active treatment. Because of the problems with
poor liver function, coagulation disorders and multiple blood
transfusions only the safest, fastest procedure that will stop the
bleeding should be considered.

Variceal injection, either directly or transhepatically, is
effective but requires great technical expertise and sophisticated
equipment. Emergency portosystemic shunting and transthoracic
oesophageal transection is complicated by a high mortality and
morbidity. However a recently introduced mechanical stapling device
has been used for the transection of the abdominal oesophagus
(Vankemmel 1974) with good results (Johnston 1981). We have
investigated the use of such an instrument in the management of 30
patients with uncontrolled variceal haemorrhage.

PATIENTS AND METHOD

Despite conservative treatment which included blood replacement,
intravenous vasopressin, oesophageal tamponade and in six cases
transhepatic sclerosis, thirty patients continued to bleed and
required emergency oesophageal transection. In two cases the
operation was abandoned because of dense vascular adhesions from
previous gastric surgery and an alternative treatment was used.
28 patients had emergency transection of the abdominal oesophagus
using the EEA staple gun (Autosutures UK Ltd.) 8 patients were
graded Child group A, 13 Child B and 7 Child C on the degree of
liver dysfunction. There were 16 patients with cirrhosis (5
alcoholic), 3 chronic active hepatitis, 3 primary biliary cirrhosis
and 6 patients with portal vein thrombosis. The operation has been
previously described in detail(Hobbs 1981). Briefly the oesophagogastric junction is mobilised at laparotomy. The 31 mm. diameter
staple instrument is introduced through an anterior gastrotomy and
transection with staple anastomosis performed. The procedure is kept
as simple as possible with no further devascularisation or

splenectomy. The average time taken was 60 minutes and the mean
blood loss was 500 ml.

RESULTS

The bleeding was controlled in every case as soon as the oesophagus
was transected. There were no problems with leakage or late
strictures at the anastomosis. Five of the more elderly patients,
all Child grade C died in the postoperative period from
deteriorating liver function. Only two patients of the remainder
developed postoperative encephalopathy. This was severe in only
one case; a man with acute alcoholic hepatitis, graded Child C at
surgery. Apart from one leakage from the gastrotomy, there were no
other complications.

Six patients have rebled in the follow up period. One bleeding from
fundal varices at 12 weeks required a splenectomy. Of the others
bleeding from oesophageal varices 3 eventually required mesocaval
shunts, 1 a splenectomy and gastric devascularisation and one
settled on conservative treatment. The average time of rebleeding
for the oesophageal varices was 30.8 weeks (range 19 – 50). There
were three late deaths; two from hepatic failure and one from an
unrelated malignancy.

15 of the 28 cases have survived without rebleeding for a follow-up
period of 3 – 28 months (mean 16.6). These include 7 patients
preoperatively graded Child B and two patients graded Child C.

CONCLUSIONS

Emergency oesophageal transection using the EEA staple instrument
effectively controls bleeding from oesophageal varices. It is a
safe, straightforward procedure that can be performed by any
competent surgeon and does not require sophisticated equipment.
It does not interfere with liver function and the instance of
post-operative encephalopathy is low. Re-bleeding does occur but
is rare within the first six months.

REFERENCES

HOBBS K. E. F. Portal Hypertension; in Operative Surgery and
    Management. Ed. Keene 1981. Wright P. S. G. Bristol.
JOHNSTON E. W. Bleeding oesophageal varices; the management of
    shunt rejects. A. R. C. Surg. 1981; 63: 3 – 8.
VANKEMMEL M.   Resection-anastomose de l'oesopage suscardinal
    pour rupture de varices osophiennes. Nouv. Presse. Med. 1974;
    5: 1123 – 4.

Care of the Acutely Ill and Injured
Edited by D. H. Wilson and A. K. Marsden
© 1982, John Wiley & Sons Ltd.

OESOPHAGECTOMY WITHOUT THORACOTOMY IN AN EMERGENCY FOR
ACUTE BURNS OF THE UPPER DIGESTIVE TRACT

J.G. Brun, M. Célérier, J. Ferry, Cl. DUBOST

Hôpital Fernand Widal, 200 rue du Faubourg Saint Denis
75475 PARIS Cedex 10   FRANCE

ABSTRACT

The authors describe an original procedure used in an emergency for
acute caustic burns of the upper digestive tract with visceral necrosis : through an abdominal and cervical approach an oesophageal
stripping is performed. This method, judged on 8 cases, is safer and
more successful.

INTRODUCTION
The *severity* of an acute caustic burn, is determined by the follo-
wings : *nature* of the corrosive agent, clinical examination, *endoscopy* and blood screening. If oesophagus and stomach are badly burned
with *transmural necrosis,* we beleave the *removal* is mandatory and a
real emergency.

METHODS

The procedure is performed through an *abdominal* and *cervical approach*.
Dividing the oesophagus without causing any bleeding makes its removal mandatory. *Total gastrectomy* has to be performed at the same
time. The duodenum is closed. A naso-gastric tube is inserted into
the thoraco-abdominal oesophagus, firmly secured as a stripper,
sutured into place and feds out through the abdominal wound (Fig.1)
Pulling from the abdomen results in a gentle invagination of the
oesophagus (Fig.2)
The *stripping* can be done in an almost bloodless fashion in such patients because of thrombosis in the vessels of the burned oesophagus
caused by the caustic agent. A drainage tube is inserted into the mediastinum, in the oesophageal bed, and exits through the abdominal
wall.
This technique, including terminal oesophagostomy and feeding jejunostomy, can be performed in about three hours. The drainage is removed about 10 days. Three months later, reconstruction of the digestive tract is undertaken using a *retrosternal coloplasty*.

RESULTS
In 20 months, 8 patients were treated in this fashion, with 7 succes-
ses and a death. The fatal issue, on the tenth post operative day was
related to *tracheal necrosis* by the caustic agent.

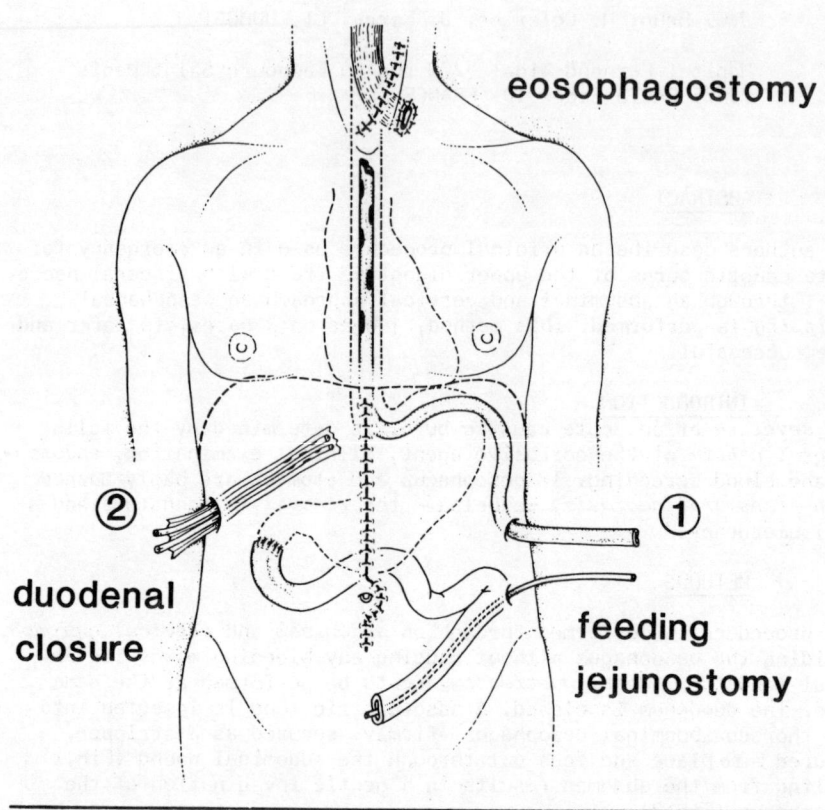

eosophagostomy

duodenal closure

feeding jejunostomy

① **mediastinal drainage**

② **abdominal drainage**

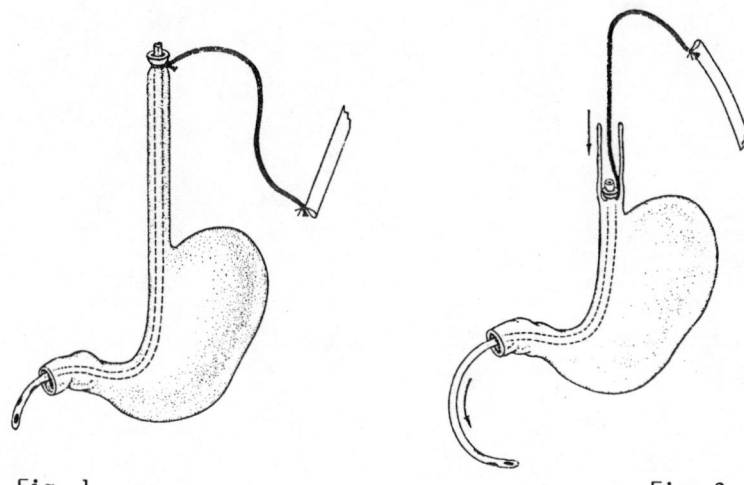

Fig. 1   Fig. 2

DISCUSSION

Since 1970, *surgery* has been performed for 68 out of the 301 patients
hospitalized in our center, in 28 cases in an emergency. *Explorato-
ries procedures* were required, for extremly serious symptoms with
8 deaths . *Total gastrectomies* were performed, in 6 cases, for delayed closed gastric perforations, with 3 survivals. *Oesophagus exclusion* performed in such condition has been judged not sufficient
because of the high risk of mediastinal empyema. *Total oeso-gastrec-
tomies* were performed in 15 cases. *Oesophagectomy with thoracotomy*
involved a high risk for patients in poor condition and generally
leaded to major septic complications as shown by its results : only
one recovery in 7 procedures.
On the contrary, *stripping of the oesophagus* without opening the
thorax has been a safer and more successful procedure in our experience.

REFERENCES
Brun J.G., Célérier M., Bessou J.P., Dubost Cl., Fournier E., Ferry J.
Bismuth Ch., Coutrot S., Pontal P.G.
Oesophagectomie sans ouverture du thorax pour brûlure caustique.
Nouv. Presse Méd., 1981, 10, 2115

Brun J.G., Célérier M., Bessou J.P., Ferry J., Dubost Cl.
Oesophagectomie sans thoracotomie. 5 observations
Nouv. Presse Méd., 1981, 10, 2365-2367.

Care of the Acutely Ill and Injured
Edited by D. H. Wilson and A. K. Marsden
© 1982, John Wiley & Sons Ltd.

OUR EXPERIENCE IN THE TREATMENT OF BLEEDING GASTRIC
AND DUODENAL ULCERS

T.Orlowski, A.Badowski, J.Domaniecki, J.Gil

Institute of Surgery, Postgraduate Medical
Education Centre, Military Medical Academy,
Warsaw, Poland.

ABSTRACT

We have treated a group of 376 patients with massive bleeding from
gastric or duodenal ulcers.   Irrespective of the volume of blood
lost we always attempted conservative treatment first.   Surgical
treatment was undertaken in 292 cases.   The overall mortality was
2%.

CLINICAL MATERIAL

A group of patients with bleeding gastric ulcers (119 cases) or
duodenal ulcers (257 cases) was treated.   The age ranged from 20
to 78 years with a mean age of 51.3 in the gastric ulcer cases and
36.5 in the duodenal ulcer cases.

The time from onset of bleeding to admission to hospital ranged from
a few hours to seven days.   In 213 cases (56.5%) this was the first
bleeding episode, in 95 cases (25.5%) the second and in 67 cases
(18%) there was a history of repeated bleeds.   Bleeding was the
presenting sign of peptic ulcer in 51 cases (13.5%).   54% cases
bled in the 3rd-4th decade of life, 26% in the 5th decade and 20%
in later years.   The mean duration of previous peptic ulcer
symptoms was 5.7 years.

On the basis of clinical signs, haemodynamic values and haematocrit
levels the estimated volume of blood lost ranged from 1500 to 3000
ml.   Only 145 patients (38.7%) arrived at hospital within 24 hours
of the onset of bleeding - in 46% of them shock was already
established at the time of admission.   Haematemesis and melaena
were present in all cases.   45.7% cases exhibited syncope -
usually during or immediately after the passage of a stool.

MANAGEMENT

Conservative treatment was always attempted in the first instance
though the surgical team remained in constant readiness should
operation be required.   In some cases thromboelastographic (TEG)
studies were performed - these demonstrated clot stability
associated with a low haematocrit and a shift towards hypercoag-
ulability indicating the possibility of spontaneous arrest of

haemorrhage and the usefulness of a conservative approach.

Initially patients were infused dextran 40, then transfused cross-matched blood - the first 1000 ml being administered within 10-20 minutes.   A gastric tube was always passed for monitoring of gastric bleeding.   Local cooling by stomach lavage with ice cold saline and gastrothrombin was used.

Shock was usually controlled within 2-6 hours with an average transfusion of 1000 - 3000 ml of blood and 1000 - 2500 ml of plasma substitutes - occasionally blood transfusions of over 5000 ml were required.   Re-bleeds occurred in about 12% cases.

Currently we perform emergency endoscopy prior to surgery.   This was undertaken on the first day in 32% cases and on the second day in 23%.   The site of bleeding was demonstrated in 329 cases (87.6%). An agreement between the operative findings and the endoscopic diagnosis was obtained in 81-100% cases.

Surgery was performed in 292 cases : in 11.6% of these for failure to respond to conservative treatment and within the first 24 hours; in 40.7% for a poor response to transfusion - within the 2nd - 4th days and in 39% for distinct re-bleeding occurring on the 5th or 6th day.   Partial gastrectomy was the operation of choice in 96.7% cases using Rydygier's method.

RESULTS

The overall mortality was 2% - deaths occurring in patients over 60 years of age treated conservatively despite the persistence or recurrence of bleeding.   No deaths occurred in patients undergoing elective surgery or emergency surgery under cover of blood transfusion.   These facts have prompted us to modify our management policy.

CONCLUSIONS

1.   Energetic conservative treatment allows sufficient control of bleeding to permit radiological or endoscopic examination. Endoscopy is a relatively safe procedure allowing establishment of the site of bleeding in most cases.
2.   The persistence or recurrence of bleeding despite conservative treatment should be an indication for operation no later than 48 hours after the onset of bleeding.   Prolongation of ineffective conservative treatment increases the operative risks and the mortality.

Care of the Acutely Ill and Injured
Edited by D. H. Wilson and A. K. Marsden
© 1982, John Wiley & Sons Ltd.

ACUTE LIVER AND BILIARY PROBLEMS

K. E. F. Hobbs

Academic Department of Surgery
Royal Free Hospital School of Medicine
London NW3, U.K.

TRAUMA

Trauma to the liver has always provided surgeons with problems of
diagnosis and management. As the number of high speed road traffic
accidents and physical assaults increases, so these problems become
more common. The diagnosis of liver trauma is often too obvious
with the severely injured, shocked patient requiring active resuscitation on arrival in hospital. Emergency laparotomy may be
necessary even before adequate resuscitation is possible. In less
severe cases, the diagnosis can be more difficult and only careful
clinical monitoring will lead the clinician to believe there is
continuing intraperitoneal haemorrhage. A four quadrant peritoneal
tap may be of value in confirming the diagnosis in these cases.

The main surgical problem with the liver is that following damage it
bleeds. Alexander Walt (1) draws attention to this very graphically
in his paper 'The mythology of hepatic trauma'. He states that the
legend of Prometheus, whose liver was eaten daily by a vulture only
to regrow overnight, was written by a poet and not a surgeon. The
author was correct in believing the liver has the potential to
regenerate rapidly following removal of part but the story failed to
take account of the inevitable haemorrhage which would have occurred.

The management of liver trauma has changed during the past few
decades. Papers published on the subject in the early 1970s
advocated an aggressive approach and young residents were very ready
to perform heroic surgical procedures on damaged livers in the
belief that they would be life saving. However in an analysis of
the outcome of liver injuries, the survival rate is 95% if the liver
alone is injured. This figure falls considerably when other organs
are injured too and unfortunately such a situation exists in about
90% of patients sustaining a liver injury. In these cases the
mortality is directly proportional to the total number of organs
injured.

In an analysis in 1978 of 1404 patients Walt (1) showed that 51% had
laparotomy alone, 38% had debridement of the injured liver, 5% had a
hemihepatectomy, 3% needed hepatic artery ligation and 0.3% required
packing to control haemorrhage. In another study in 1978 Levin (2)
and colleagues found only 8% of 546 patients needed extensive

debridement and 5% a lobectomy. Thus the current view must be to
keep any surgical procedure as simple as possible.

For the surgeon faced with uncontrollable haemorrhage, packing of
the wound and abdominal closure may be a life saving approach (3).
Such a technique is especially valuable when an inexperienced
surgeon has to treat this problem in an ill equipped centre.
Packing will control the bleeding and allow the patient to be resuscitated adequately and later transferred to a major centre for an
esperienced surgeon to carry out any further necessary surgery.

Sometimes during surgical procedures on the liver it is necessary to
clamp the hilum to control bleeding. This may be a useful technique
but it is necessary to consider how long the liver can tolerate warm
total ischaemia. Although there are reports (4) that no serious
damage occurs following total vascular occlusion for periods of an
hour, most surgeons would not want to deprive the liver of a blood
supply for more than 20 minutes at normal temperatures.

HAEMORRHAGE AND PORTAL HYPERTENSION

An acute surgical complication of chronic liver disease is haemorrhage from oesophageal varices secondary to portal hypertension.
These patients present often in a shocked state, bleeding profusely.
Initially resuscitation and diagnosis by endoscopy must be accompanied by conservative methods to control the bleeding. These
include replacement of blood, clotting products, platelets, infusion
of pitressin or somatostatin and tamponade of the bleeding vessels.
If bleeding continues or recurs, urgent occlusion of the varices by
endoscopic or percutaneous transhepatic sclerosis techniques must be
considered. Surgical ligation of the varices at thoracotomy or
laparotomy with oesophageal or gastric transection or devascularisation may be needed. Finally the complex, complicated problem of
portal decompression by some form of porta systemic vascular shunt
requires consideration. These patients are very sick and surgical
management is complicated by the liver disease. Ideally they should
be managed by a specialist unit once the acute bleeding has been
controlled (5, 6).

LIVER ABSCESS

'Never let the sun set on pus' was an aphorism taught to generations
of medical students. As soon as a possibility of a liver abscess
was considered, urgent surgery was advised, but even this carried
a very high mortality rate. Modern diagnostic techniques, especially
ultrasound, allow accurate diagnosis and localisation of liver
abscess. Acute pyogenic abscess is still complicated by a high
mortality rate but recent studies suggest needle aspiration of the
pus under ultrasound control with appropriate antibiotic cover,
especially metronidazole, may give excellent results (8). Amoebic
abscesses similarly diagnosed and treated with metronidazole can
usually be cured without formal surgical drainage.

However there is need to identify the presence of hydatid cysts in the liver before attempting needle aspiration. In this condition such an approach can kill or seriously injure the patient. Insertion of a needle almost always results in its fracture with secondary dissemination of daughter cysts throughout the peritoneal cavity and sometimes fatal anaphylactic shock. Careful ultrasound and complement fixation tests allow accurate diagnosis when formal laparotomy with careful isolation of peritoneal contents with packs or a cryofunnel (9) is needed. This instrument consists of a stainless steel funnel with a 10 cm wide base. A tube through which liquid nitrogen can be passed is fused to the base. When the liquid nitrogen flows, this is cooled and when it is placed on the cyst instant adhesion occurs. The cyst can then be opened, the membrane removed and the cavity washed out with some irritant fluid to destroy any remaining daughter cysts. Formalin, alcohol, eusol, hyperchlorite have all been used but probably saturated saline is equally effective and less potentially damaging (10). Unfortunately no drug has yet been shown to be of any value in the treatment of this condition but there is some apocryphal evidence that mebendazole (Vermox) may cure hydatid cysts if given for long periods in high doses. However more work in this field is necessary before any serious recommendations can be made (11).

THE BILIARY TRACT

Two biliary tract problems which confront the emergency surgeon are those of acute inflammation of the gall bladder and the management of jaundice due to large duct obstruction. In acute cholecystitis the main argument is should surgery be carried out in the acute situation or should the time hallowed method be followed in which the acute inflammation is allowed to settle and surgery carried out six weeks later. It is dificult to be didactic but recent studies suggest that providing the operation is carried out by an experienced surgeon under elective rather than emergency conditions the mortality and morbidity is marginally better if surgery is carried out in the early acute phase of the illness. Certainly it appears to be a more cost effective approach (12).

The management of obstruction to major biliary ducts has changed recently as a result of new diagnostic tests and methods of treatment (13). An acceptable approach to the jaundiced patient is outlined in the flow diagram (Figure 1). Decisions on the definitive treatment of the obstruction once the cause has been found must be made by clinicians according to local expertise and experience.

CONCLUSIONS

The liver is an organ which frequently produces problems for the emergency surgeon. Ideas on management have changed during the past decade because of careful studies and new diagnostic tools. As a result patient management has improved. Great damage can be done by a too aggressive, inexperienced surgical approach and the emergency surgeon should be prepared to consult with specialists before undertaking any major operation on the liver at all times except in the emergency situation. On these occasions surgery should be as

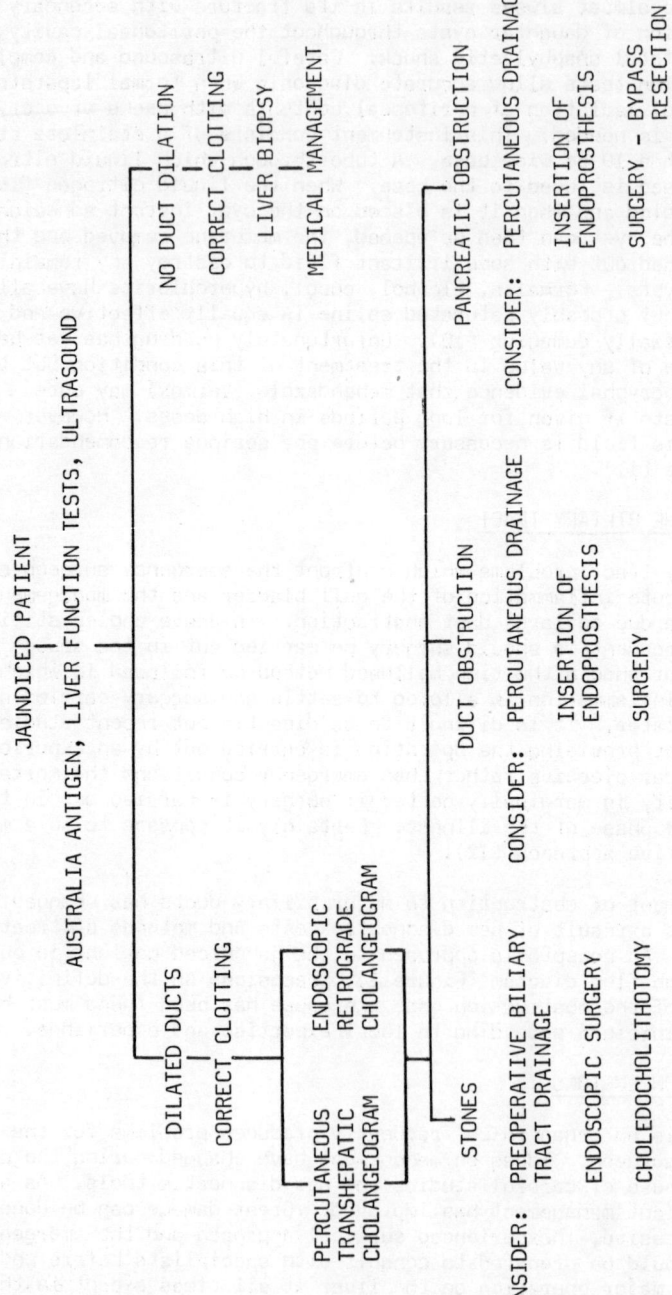

Figure 1. Flow diagram for the management of a jaundiced patient

simple as possible and designed only to control haemorrhage or save life.

REFERENCES

(1) Walt, A.J., (1978) The mythology of hepatic trauma - or Babel revisited. The American Journal of Surgery, 135, 12-18.
(2) Levin, A., Gover, P. and Nance, F.C., (1978) Surgical restraint in the management of hepatic injury: A review of charity hospital experience. The Journal of Trauma, 18, 399-404.
(3) Calne, R.Y., McMaster, P. and Pentlow, B.D. (1979) The treatment of major liver trauma by primary packing with transfer of the patient for definitive treatment. British Journal of Surgery, 66, 338-339.
(4) Huguet, C., Nordlinger, B., Galopin, J.J., Bloch, P. and Gallot, D., (1978) Normothermic hepatic vascular exclusion for extensive hepatectomy. Surgery, Gynaecology & Obstetrics, 147, 689-693.
(5) Silk, D.B.A. and Williams R. (1979) Portal hypertension, in Liver and Biliary Disease (Eds. Wright, R., Alberti, K.G.M.M., Karran, S. and Millward-Sadler, G.H.), pp 1002-1031. W.B. Saunders Company Limited, London, Philadelphia, Toronto.
(6) Hobbs, K.E.F. (1981) Portal hypertension, in Operative Surgery and Management (Ed. Keen, G.), pp 561-571. Wright P.S.G., Bristol, London, Boston.
(7) Satiani, B. and Davidson, E.D. (1978) Hepatic Abscesses: Improvement in mortality with early diagnosis and treatment. American Journal of Surgery, 135, 647-650.
(8) Perera, M.R., Kirk, A. and Noone, P. (1980) Presentation, diagnosis and management of liver abscess. Lancet, 629-632.
(9) Saidi, F. and Nazarian, I. (1971) Surgical treatment of hydatid cysts by freezing of cyst wall and instillation of 0.5 per cent silver nitrate solution. New England Journal of Medicine, 284, 1346-1350.
(10) Lewis, J.W., Koss, N. and Kerstein, M.D. (1975) A review of echinococcal disease. Annals of Surgery, April, 390-396.
(11) B.M.J. Leader: Medical treatment for hydatid disease? British Medical Journal, 8 September 1979, 563.
(12) Lancet Leader: Acute cholecystectomy for acute cholecystitis. Lancet, 1980, 2, 1120-1121.
(13) Lancet Leader: Non-invasive methods for diagnosis of jaundice. Lancet, 1979, 2, 18-20.

Care of the Acutely Ill and Injured
Edited by D. H. Wilson and A. K. Marsden
© 1982, John Wiley & Sons Ltd.

EMERGENCY CHOLECYSTECTOMY: TOWARDS GUARANTEED SAFETY

H.J. Espiner

Department of Surgery,
Bristol Royal Infirmary,
Bristol BS2 8HW

INTRODUCTION

Although cholecystectomy is a safe procedure in the management of
acute cholecystitis (Jarvinven & Hastbacka, 1980), operation is only
advised within five to seven days of the onset of symptoms, and
recent reports stress the increasing technical difficulty with
delay beyond the first week (P.A.M. Raine & A.A.Gunn, 1975 and
P.McArthur, A. Cuschievi, R.A. Sells & R. Shields, 1975).

Since 1970 a policy of cholecystectomy during the emergency admission
has been pursued regardless of the duration of the illness. This
paper presents the method evolved and the result achieved in 230
patients.

METHOD

The technique relies on two important principles. 1) no attempt is
made to identify, ligate or divide the cystic artery; this eliminates
the risk of haemorrhage during the procedure. 2) no attempt is made
to display the extra-hepatic ductal anatomy; hazardous dissection
and faulty judgment of the anatomy are thus avoided. Only one
definition is required and only one decision must be made. The
definition is "The cystic duct is that duct which unites the gall
bladder with the extra-hepatic biliary tract", and the decision
"Does the cystic duct exist?".

Dissection is begun on the fundus of the gall bladder, incising the
peritoneum at least 1cm. from the liver edge using coagulation
diathermy; a plane is developed close to the gall bladder wall and
at all times on its convexity. No cutting instrument, scissors or
knives are used and all vessels are coagulated to secure a
completely dry field. Because many of the branches of the cystic
artery are coagulated on the gall bladder wall during the dissection
from the liver bed no formal dissection of the vessel is required.
The anterior and posterior branches are frequently found in the
region of Hartmann's pouch but they are usually small vessels on the
gall bladder itself and are easily sealed by coagulation diathermy.
Any closely adherent structures such as the right hepatic artery are
avoided as dissection is conducted on the gall bladder alone. As
soon as a narrow duct is reached dissection is deemed to be complete

and the decision regarding the existence of the cystic duct can now
be made. If no narrow duct is met the surgeon is for ever aware of
the possibility that no cystic duct exists, in which case the gall
bladder may unite directly with the side of the common or any major
hepatic duct. Provided this possibility is born in mind the
dissection is safe under all circumstances of pathological
distortion. The cystic duct is opened for cholangiography and once
completed no attempt is made to dissect the duct flush with the
common duct and the latter is not usually exposed during the
procedure.

I prefer a midline epigastric incision and conduct the operation
from the left hand side of the table.

RESULTS

In the years 1970 - 1980 203 patients have undergone early
cholecystectomy during their admission for acute cholecystitis.
(64.7% female, average age 58.6 years).

Operation was carried out within seven days of the onset of symptoms
in 86 cases (average age 58.5 years) and after seven days in 117
cases (average age 58.7 years); the duration of post-operative
hospital stay for these two groups was similar with 64% and 70%
respectively being discharged within 14 days of operation. Four
patients died following surgery (overall mortality 2%); two had
the operation within seven days (2.3%) and two after seven days
(1.7%): the patients were all female and aged 83 (myocardial
infarction), 86 (broncho-pneumonia), 86 (portal pyaemia and portal
vein thrombosis) and 91 (C.V.A.). Wound infection occurred in 8.4%
of the series (5.8% of those operated on within seven days and 10.3%
in those after seven days. Other complications occurred in 13.7%
of the whole series (18.6% of those operated on within seven days
and 10.3% of those operated on after seven days). These included
one case of temporary biliary leakage, three cases of subphrenic
abscess and other non-specific problems such as urinary tract
infection, urinary retention, pulmonary embolus, D.V.T., congestive
cardiac failure, gastro-intestinal haemorrhage, severe confusion,
thrombosed haemorrhoids and myocardial infarction.

DISCUSSION

The safety of this technique is reflected in the results; there was
no incidence of duct damage in the series and no significant biliary
complication. The deaths were probably unavoidable and attributable
to the complications associated with age or the severity of the
presenting illness. The wound infection rate in those operated on
after seven days was unacceptably high but in the early part of the
series not all of the patients had been protected by intraoperative antibiotics and the group operated on after seven days
contained 34 of the 42 patients suffering from jaundice and 44 of
the 60 who had common duct explorations.

While dissection may be easy in the first 48 hours following the

onset of symptoms, and any method of cholecystectomy will be
relatively safe, as fibrosis leads to further pathological
distortion the method presented here guarantees safe dissection
provided the principles are clearly understood. When gross
inflammation has destroyed the wall of the gall bladder its
lumen will frequently be entered. This is always much safer
than entering the liver substance in an effort to avoid opening
the gall bladder: a safe plane can always be found again
with patience, and because the operative field is always
bloodless the surgeon is able to proceed with confidence.

REFERENCES

Jarvinven H.J., and Hastbacka A., 1980. Early cholecystectomy
    for acute cholecystitis: a prospective randomised study.
    Ann. Surgery, 191, 501 - 505.
Raine P.A.M., and Gunn A.A., 1975. Acute cholecystitis. Brit.
    J. Surg. 62, 697 - 700.
McArthur P., Cuschievi A., Sells R.A., and Shields R., 1975.
    Controlled clinical trial comparing early interval
    cholecystectomy for acute cholecystitis. Brit. J. Surg.
    62, 850 - 852.

Care of the Acutely Ill and Injured
Edited by D. H. Wilson and A. K. Marsden
© 1982, John Wiley & Sons Ltd.

OUR EXPERIENCE IN THE TREATMENT OF ACUTE
PANCREATITIS

T. Orlowski, A. Badowski, J. Domaniecki, J. Gil

Institute of Surgery, Postgraduate Medical
Education Centre, Military Medical Academy,
Warsaw, Poland.

ABSTRACT

We have studied 156 patients with acute pancreatitis. Initial
treatment was always conservative - in 134 patients we used
Trasylol. Where moderate or high doses of Trasylol was used
there was an improvement in the general condition with regression
of the inflammatory manifestations occurring significantly earlier.
Surgery was used in 131 cases with emergency or delayed emergency
operation in 78 cases. Twenty two patients in the series died.

CLINICAL MATERIAL

We have treated 156 patients with acute pancreatitis (A.P.) -
47 men (30%) and 109 women (70%). The age ranged from 20 to 86
years with an overall mean of 46.

The diagnosis was based on the clinical manifestations and a raised
amylase at the time of admission (256 w.u. in blood or   512
w.u. in urine). The highest serum amylase was 4096 w.u. There
was a severe course of the disease in 45.7%, moderate in 42.2% and
mild in 12%. Primary A.P. was diagnosed in 92.6% cases and the
time from the onset of symptoms to admission to the hospital ranged
from 10 hours to 5 days with an average of 48 hours.

The most frequent cause was cholecystolithiasis present in 134
patients (86%) complicated in 36 cases (27%) by common duct stones
and in 68 cases (51%) by jaundice. Alcohol abuse was reported by
12% patients. In 12 cases (7.4%) secondary A.P. followed
operations or other parts of the biliary system as an early complication.

TREATMENT AND RESULTS

Our initial management was invariably conservative involving the
following measures:

1. Inhibition of pancreatic secretion by continuous gastric
    aspiration; fasting; anticholinergic agents.
2. Energetic treatment of shock and pain.
3. Correction of electrolyte and metabolic disturbance.
4. Spasmolytic agents.

5. Antibiotics.
6. Intravenous procaine.
7. Calcium and vitamins.
8. Local hypothermia
(9. Depending upon circumstances - cardiac and Analeptic Drugs,
    Lytic mixture, hydrocortisone).

In 134 patients (86%) Trasylol was used.   As our experience grew
we increased the daily dose from 20-30 thousand units to 100-300
thousand units - recently we have used as much as 1-3 million units
daily.   The strength, frequency and duration of Trasylol therapy
was related to the clinical severity of the disease.

Nine patients, not in the Trasylol group, were treated with
5-fluorouracil.

In 90 patients (58%) regression of the systemic and local manifestations of A.P. was achieved which fact negated the necessity
for early surgery.   In the group treated with moderate and high
doses of Trasylol an improvement in general condition, regression
of inflammatory manifestations and normalisation of the biochemistry
occurred significantly earlier.   In the 5 F.U. group regression of
A.P. signs occurred within 6 days but two of the patients developed
nausea.

Surgery was performed in 131 cases (84.2%).   Emergency surgery was
undertaken in doubtful cases;   delayed emergency surgery in those
cases which had failed to respond to conservative treatment by the
3rd day and the remainder were cases operated on between 9 and 36
days after regression of the inflammation.   The operations included
cholecystectomy (93%);   bile duct exploration (73%);   choledocho-
duodenostomy (7.1%);   drainage of pseudocyst and infiltration of
pancreas with hydrocortisone, procaine and trasylol (19%).   The
peritoneal cavity was always irrigated, sometimes with lavage
drainage.   Direct surgery on the pancreas was limited to drainage
of abscesses and excision of necrotic tissue.

The overall mortality was 12% (22 patients).   In the non-Trasylol
group the mortality was 15.7%,in the low dose Trasylol group 11.5%
and in the high dose Trasylol group 4.8%.   The mortality was
greatest in those patients operated upon in the acute stage of the
disease (during the first three days).

CONCLUSIONS

1. The most frequent cause of A.P. was cholecystolithiasis.   We
   recommend that patients with gall bladder calculi be treated
   surgically before the development of this complication.
2. In cases of unquestionably proven A.P.conservative treatment
   appears justified since, in many cases, the attack abates and
   surgery can be deferred.
3. High doses of Trasylol given as part of an extensive treatment
   regime favourably influences the course of the disease.
4. Surgical treatment in the acute stage of A.P. gives the highest
   mortality.   It should be limited only to those cases of
   diagnostic uncertainty or those refractory to conservative
   treatment.

Care of the Acutely Ill and Injured
Edited by D. H. Wilson and A. K. Marsden
© 1982, John Wiley & Sons Ltd.

INCIDENCE OF DIABETES MELLITUS SECONDARY TO ACUTE
PANCREATITIS

P.Blidaru, R.Florescu and A.Blidaru

IInd Surgical Clinic, Emergency Clinical Hospital
Bucharest, Romania

ABSTRACT

The present clinical study is based on 100 patients with secondary
pancreatoprive diabetes, selected from 1050 patients admitted with a
diagnosis of acute pancreatitis and who showed no previous clinical
or biological sign of diabetes mellitus.

INTRODUCTION

Acute pancreatitis causes severe metabolic imbalance; essential in
this connection are the diabetic syndromes with hypoglycemia, hypercatabolic or hyperanabolic disturbances produced by excess glucagon or
insulin deficiency. In acute pancreatitis disorders of the antagonis-
tic insulinglucagon action, in which the feed-back system is impaired,
will lead to hypoinsulinism caused by degenerative microangiopathic
lesions, already in the incipient phase of the disease.

MATERIAL AND METHODS

The study shows that diabetes developed abruptly and irreversibly secondary to acute pancreatitis. There was a prevalence of males over
females (64% as against 36%), mean age 55 years, with chronic obstructive arteriopathies and 2nd grade obesity in many cases. The stress
of acute pancreatitis and that induced by anaesthesia and surgery may
determine the production of large quantities of hydrocortisone anti-
insulin hormones, with cellular degeneration and hypertrophy,followed
by irreversible vacuolization of Langerhans beta-cells. Of the total
100 acute pancreatitis cases, 94 were operated, and in 18 cases 2 to
4 reinterventions were performed.

RESULTS

Anaesthesia and surgical shock favour osmotic diuresis with extra-

and intracellular dehydration and accentuated hyperglycemia;corti-
sone, ACTH and saline diuretics favour diabetes mellitus. The patients with recurrent attacks of acute pancreatitis presented as a
rule an increase in glycemia, glycosuria, calcemia next to blood and
urinary high amylase levels. The stress of anaesthesia is greatly diminished by neuroleptanalgesia; surgery must be rapid with complete
haemostasis. Follow up of these patients for 5-10 years showed that
secondary pancreatoprive insulin- and sulphonamide-dependent diabetes mellitus was definitive; 7 patients developed compensated hyper-
glycemic coma, 3 patients compensated hypoglycemic coma, and 5 died
from cardiorespiratory complications. In diabetes mellitus secondary
to pancreatitis, oral hypoglycemic drugs have a temporary effect,
become inactive in superadded infections and do not exempt the diabetic from a strict diet.

DISCUSSION

Diabetes mellitus is not a disease, it is a common syndrome of
various aetiology among which acute pancreatitis that generates
irreversible destruction of the Langerhans beta-cells.

REFERENCES

Blidaru, P., 1980. Incidenţa concordanţei pancreatită acută - diabet
    zaharat pancreatopriv, Craiova District Conference on "Acute
    Pancreatitis", 4 Oct.

Blidaru,P. and Blidaru,A., 1980. Particularités du diabète sucré chez
    les malades chirurgicaux opérés en urgence, XVI Semaine Médicale
    Balkanique, Bucharest, 7-13 Sept.

Petrescu, C. and Blidaru,P., 1970. Drainage du Wirsung dans la
    pancréatitie aigue. J.chirurgie, 99, 5-6.

Suteu, I. and Blidaru,P., 1979. Our Experience in Emergency Surgery
    of Diabetics, IV Intern,Congress of Emergency Surgery,Barcelona,
    24-27 June.

Care of the Acutely Ill and Injured
Edited by D. H. Wilson and A. K. Marsden
© 1982, John Wiley & Sons Ltd.

ACUTE NEOPLASTIC OCCLUSION OF THE LARGE BOWEL

Cevese PG., D'Amico D., Frego M., Biastiato R.
Tropea A., Brunato F., Borghesi A.

Inst. of Clinica Chirurgica of Padua University
(Chief: P.G.Cevese)
Dept. of Emergency Surgery (Chief: D. D.'Amico)

SUMMARY

81 cases of complete, acute obstructions are reviewed among 905
observed neoplasm of the large bowel.   Resective criteria were
followed whenever possible (35 patients) but in 15 cases it was
necessary to proceed in several stages.   Operative mortality for
resection was 8.5% (a few higher than for elective surgery) and
19.5% after decompressive procedures alone on account of the
critical general condition.   The 5 year survival rate (39%) has
been lower than that in non-obstructed patients due to the late
stage of the disease.

INTRODUCTION

The binomial occlusion-carcinoma can often cause serious problems
in planning surgical treatment.   The most important point is
whether the primary disease should be treated together with the
acute complete obstruction or whether only an emergency procedure
be carried out on the occlusion, deferring the treatment of the
neoplasm to a more appropriate moment.   It is however controversial
whether an aggressive approach in the acute phase can favourably
influence the prognosis of the disease without significantly
aggravating the serious condition of the patient.

MATERIALS AND METHODS

During the 20 year period between 1960 and 1980 905 patients
affected with neoplasms of the colon and recum were observed at
the Surgical Clinic in the University of Padua: 81 presented acute
occlusion which required emergency surgery (recurrences and
sarcomas were not considered).   The average age was 64.   The acute
occlusion was the first sign of the disease in 27 patients while,
in the others, warning symptoms were retrospectively discovered
approximately 6 months before.   The carcinoma was in the right
colon in 16 cases and in the left colon and recum in 65 cases.
Four patients had a perforated diastasis of the cecum and a further
one a sigmoid growth perforation.   The stage, according to the
Dukes classification, was as follows:

     A=0,   B=13,   C=18,   D=34

However this classification was unable to be made in 16 patients
since only minimal surgery was carried out due to the critical
conditions.   In 46 patients the treatment consisted of an
external faecal diversion (40 cases) or intestinal by-pass alone
(6 cases) as resection was not possible.

Resection was carried out in 35 patients: primarily performed in
20 patients and as staged procedures in 15.   Three extended
resections were also carried out: a left hemicolectomy with
splenectomy, an anterior resection with ureterectomy and a Miles
with prostatectomy.

RESULTS

The resectability rate was 43% compared with 73% of the total series.
Resection was judged as curative in 31 cases and unsatisfactory in
4.   The surgical treatment included 12 post-operative deaths with
a total mortality rate of 15%: 9 deaths occurred after simple
faecal diversion and 3 after resection (respectively 2 primary and
1 staged).   The abdominal morbidity rate was 13% after decompressive
procedures and 23% after resective procedures: three anastomotic
dehiscences, two peritonitis, a colonic bleeding, a vesical and a
ureteroperineal fistula.   The 5 year survival rate was calculated
with the "life table method".   We herein report a global survival
rate of 19% (including the post-operative deaths) and of 23%
without early deaths.   Following completely curative resections
the survival rate is that of 39%.

DISCUSSION

The Carcinomas of the large bowel are complicated by obstruction
in approximately 15% of the cases.   In this series the rate of
9% is justified by the fact that only complete and acute obstructions
were considered.   The mean age was consistently high with a peak
in the 8th decade, as compared with the 7th decade of the non-
obstructed patient.   The critical condition and the advanced stage
of the tumours justify the high rate of the decompressive procedures
alone (56%).

Carcinomas of the right colon permitted, in most cases, a primary
resection (8/10) followed by primary anastomosis, while carcinomas
of the left colon and rectum allowed primary resection in half the
cases (12/25), 7 of which were associated with primary anastomosis.
The immediate results show that the mortality rate was higher after
simple derivative procedures (20%), attributable mostly to cardiopulmonary and renal complications (6 cases), to peritonitis secondary
to perforation of the caecum (2 cases) and to a perforated prestomal
hernia.

The mortality rate after resective procedures (8.5%) was not much
higher than elective resections (7.5%) and we think that the
selection process carried out on the patients played an important
role.   The early deaths were due to massive bleeding following a
right hemicolectomy, pneumonia and pelvic-peritonitis following an
extended anterior resection with caecal perforation, a generalized

peritonitis following an anterior resection with splenectomy.
In the four cases that presented with caecal perforation three
deaths occurred during the post-operative period due to abdominal
sepsis.   Primary resections carried a post-operative mortality rate
of 10%; staged procedures as 7%.   Particularly, primary
anastomosis carried a mortality rate of 2/17 (12%) and the staged
0/3 (0%), but the small number of the latter does not allow proper
evaluation.   Complications and mortality rate showed no statistical
difference between primary and staged resections, either with or
without primary anastomosis, but complications were more frequent
after resection of the colon and rectum.   The prognosis is
particularly poor following definitive surgery with a survival rate
of 7% at 5 years in all the definitive cases.   In particular, the
survival rate of 16% at 5 years for the intestinal by-pass is
undoubtedly better when compared with colostomy and caecostomy
which have a mean survival of 11% at 2 years and 0% at 3 years.
We believe that this is due not to the chosen therapy but to better
pre-operative condition and, perhaps, related to the different
biological behaviour of the disease.

The survival rate obtained after curative resections was lower than
non-obstructed patients (51%), but statistical analysis does not
show a significant difference between the two groups (P 0 25).
Therefore when a radical resection was performed occlusive
carcinomas in this series did not show the suggested higher
aggressiveness (Ragland 1971).   By separately analysing the
different parts of the large bowel we did not find a significant
difference (P 0 9) between the survival rate of the right colon
(33%) and the left colon and rectum (35%).   In relation to the
time of the resection an improved survival rate was noted on staged
resections (46%) versus primary resection (32%), even if not
statistically significant (P 0 9).   Other authors (Fielding 1974,
Clark 1975, Irvin 1977) have contrarily reported their findings by
verifying a more favourable prognosis following primary resection.
We are not, however, averse to trying an aggresive surgical approach
which we practice whenever the general condition of the patient
allows.   We feel, however, that the time interval between the
emergency colostomy and the resection does not influence the
prognosis when staged resection is performed only 2-3 weeks later.

Our conclusions are that post-operative morbidity and mortality
are correlated more with the general condition rather than the type
of intervention for they are not higher than elective surgery when
a careful selection has been carried out.   The global survival
rate is poor and even after curative procedures remains below that
registered by non-obstructed patients; we did not find a worse
prognosis by deferring the resection to a more appropriate moment
in several cases.   However these observations do not allow us to
draw any conclusions on the suspected invasive carcinoma of the
occlusive variety.

REFERENCES

Clark J., Hall A.W., Moossa A.R.: Treatment of obstructing cancer
of the colon and rectum.   Surg.Gyn.Obst. 141: 541-4. 1975.

Fielding L.P., Wells B.W.: Survival after primary and staged
resection for large bowel obstruction caused by cancer. Br.J.Surg.
61: 16-18. 1974.

Irvin T.T., Greaney M.G.: The treatment of colonic cancer
presenting with intestinal obstruction. Br.J.Surg. 64: 741-44.
1977.

Ragland J.J., Londe A.M., Spratt J.S.: Correlation of the prognosis
of obstructive colorectal carcinoma with clinical and pathological
variables. Am.J.Surg. 121: 552-6. 1971.

Care of the Acutely Ill and Injured
Edited by D. H. Wilson and A. K. Marsden
© 1982, John Wiley & Sons Ltd.

TREATMENT OF ACUTELY COMPLICATED DIVERTICULAR DISEASE
OF THE LARGE BOWEL

D'Amico D., Frego M., Biastiato R., Tropea A.,
Brunato F., Bianchera G.

Inst. of Clinical Surgery, Dept. of Emergency Surgery,
Padua University, Italy.

INTRODUCTION

Not all of the severe acute complications of diverticular disease
of the colon require emergency surgery.   There is however a high
tendency to relapse with conservative treatment with an inherent
risk of a late emergency operation attended by a greater risk in
mortality and morbidity.   Indeed the death rate ranges from 11%
to 40% in emergency surgery as compared with 5% in elective
resection and 0% - 9% with myotomies.   The trend is therefore
towards medical, dietary and elective surgical treatment.
Nevertheless urgent surgery is required in about half the cases
of acute complications.

MATERIALS AND METHODS

We studied 56 consecutive patients (31 male, 25 female) presenting
at the Surgical Clinic at Padua with complications of diverticular
disease of the descending and sigmoid colon.   Their ages ranged
from 36 to 87 years with a mean at 60 years.   Only a quarter of
them were aware of being diverticulosis victims.

The patients were considered in two groups:

Group I   "Severe Acute Diverticulitis"   (43 patients)
           e.g. walled off or intramesocolic perforation
           or peridiverticular abscess

Group II Frank peritonitis (13 patients)

Group I patients were treated conservatively with medical therapy
and rest of the affected bowel by total parenteral nutrition (TPN)
followed, after recovery, by a high residue diet.

Group II patients required urgent laparotomy -

  Three stage procedure   3 cases   (critical patients)
  Primary resection without anastomosis 6 cases (3 were faecal
  peritonitis)
          (Exteriorisation-resection in 5
          Hartmann's operation in 1)
  Single-stage primary resection plus anastomosis.(4 cases)
  - carefully selected patients with free perforation and

limited peritonitis (never faecal).   Proximal decompression
was used in every case.

RESULTS

Group I   All of the patients recovered from the acute attack but
seven did not respond to diet and presented serious recurrence.
A further four developed an organic stenosis and/or an inflammatory
mass.   These patients underwent elective resection.   The
mortality was nil but two patients suffered serious post-operative
complications.

Group II   There were two deaths following simple colostomy, suture
and drainage.   Morbidity included a subphrenic abscess and an
anastomotic dehiscence after the two stage procedures - there was
a dehiscence of the transverse loop colostomy after primary
resection with anastomosis.

DISCUSSION

There is general agreement for conservative treatment of patients
presenting with diverticulitis without generalised peritonitis.
Rest of the affected segment is fundamentally necessary.   Total
parenteral nutrition has rendered unnecessary colostomy in these
cases.   Where TPN is not practicable we favour primary resection
rather than a colostomy which ignores the persisting source of
infection.

In the first group of patients it usually is possible to achieve a
remission without surgery although only 10% of patients will be
immune to recurrence on conservative therapy (Colcock 1975,
Hollender 1978).   A high fibre diet proves effective in 90% cases
(Hyland 1980) though this figure may, in reality, be lower when
considering more seriously complicated cases - for this reason
prophylactic elective surgery after a remission may be advisable
for some patients (Rodkey 1965, Heberer 1978).

Surgical options include limited resection of the affected portion
of bowel;   left hemicolectomy or one of the varieties of myotomy
- of which latter we have no personal experience.

We do not think there were any pointers toward a more conservative
operation such as myotomy in the eleven patients operated on in
this series - in fact besides the 4 cases presenting an organic
stenosis or inflammatory mass, seven others showed serious relapses
proven at laparotomy in the form of previous infectious perforating
attacks.   The absence of mortality we report support other authors
with a mortality rate of 0% - 5% and successful results in 98%
cases (Penfold, 1973).

We are in favour of wide resection in order to remove the whole
length of bowel affected by the diverticular process and not just
the inflamed segment.

The choice of surgical procedure varies from the classical three stage to resection and primary anastomosis.

The THREE STAGE PROCEDURE reflects a conservative approach but has a high mortality in faecal peritonitis.   This is partially justified by the critical condition of the patients but it is also probable that technical factors play a role in failing to remove the source of infection.

A TWO STAGE procedure allows wide resection of the perforated segment - it may be simply carried out by exteriorisation with a double colostomy or, as this is not always practicable in low lying lesions, by Hartmann's procedure or colostomy with mucous fistula. The mortality rate of a two stage procedure varies between 8% and 10% (Hay, 1972, Hollender 1978, Hinchey 1978).   Our results of no mortality and two major complications only in the six patients treated in this group lead us to agree that exteriorisation/resection is a safe and useful procedure as it is possible to remove most or all of the tract affected by divertisulae.

The ONE STAGE procedure of primary resection and anastomosis is not widely accepted in the surgical world for emergency cases.   We feel that it has a place in carefully selected cases.

CONCLUSIONS

1. Not all acute complications of diverticular disease require emergency surgery.   Wherever possible the inflammation should be allowed to subside allowing later operative intervention under more favourable conditions.
2. Afterserious attack, elective wide resection is the safest procedure offering definitive results.
3. In the case of peritonitis we aim primarily at the removal of the lesion as an emergency.   A two stage procedure of exteriorisation/resection is to be preferred with primary anastomosis being reserved only for carefully selected cases. These procedures often result in permanent cure.

REFERENCES

Colcock B.P.,1975. Diverticular disease: proven surg.manag. Clin.Gastr. 4. 53.

Hay J.M.:1972. Les peritonites generalisees colique non traumatiques chez l'adulte. Ann Chir 26.1315.

Heberer G., Hoffman K. Bary S. 1978. Il trattamento chirurgico delle malattie infiammatorie del colon, m.di Crohn, divert-icolite. Min Chir 33. 631-642.

Hinchey E.J., Schall P.G.H., Richards G.K. 1978. Treatment of perforated diverticular disease of the colon. Adv.Surg. 12. 85-109.

Hollender L.F., Meyer C.H., Calderoli H. et al.1978. Le traitment chirurgical des sigmoidites diverticulaires compliquees. J.Chir (Paris) 115. 205-212.

Hyland J.M., Taylor I. 1980. Does a high fibre diet prevent the complications of diverticular disease? Br.J.Surg. 67. 77-79.

Penfold J.C.B. 1973. Management of uncomplicated diverticular disease by colonic resection in patients at St.Mark Hospital. Br.J.Surg. 60. 695.
Rodkey G.V., Welch C.E. 1965. Diverticulitis of the colon: evolution in concept and therapy. Surg.Clin.North Am. 1231-4 0.

Care of the Acutely Ill and Injured
Edited by D. H. Wilson and A. K. Marsden
© 1982, John Wiley & Sons Ltd.

ACUTE HAEMORRHOIDAL THROMBOSIS - INCISION OR
EMERGENCY HAEMORRHOIDECTOMY?

H.U. Schlaepfer, J.F. Ammann, H.Blessing

Surgical Department, Thurgauisches Kantonsspital
Munsterlingen, Switzerland.

INTRODUCTION

The time-honoured treatment of thrombosed haemorrhoids is incision
- a procedure presumed to be the simplest and cheapest.   Though it
may give rapid symptomatic relief the underlying problem is not
tackled and no consideration is given to complications such as
bleeding, infection or abscesses - the recurrence rate is
especially high and further incisions may be necessary.   Incision
of thombosed piles cannot thus be regarded as a radical therapy.

For these reasons W. P. Mazier (1973) proposed emergency segmental
resection for acute haemorrhoidal disease.   Since 1978 we have
performed radical haemorrhoidectomies for all cases of haemorrhoidal
thrombosis presenting at the Munsterlingen hospital.

MATERIALS AND METHODS

Between 1978 and 1980 28 patients suffering from acute thrombosed
piles underwent an emergency Milligan/Morgan resection.   There
were 20 males and 7 females with a mean age of 41.4 with an age
range from 22 to 80.   10 patients emanated from Mediterranean
countries.   Eight patients had previously received local incision
on 13 occasions, three other patients had received eight treatments
of local sclerotherapy.

All patients underwent a Milligan/Morgan resection under general
anaesthesia - according to the findings a one, two or three quadrant
open segmental haemorrhoidectomy was performed.   Post-operative
treatment consisted of "sitz baths" with camomile until secondary
wound healing.   There were no post-operative complications.

Four patients became lost to follow up;   the remaining 23 were
reviewed from 4 to 38 months with a mean follow up period of 10.8
months.

LONG-TERM RESULTS

Of the 23 patients followed up 17 were totally asymptomatic,
5 complained of occasional minor pain during defaecation (likened
to itching) but only one, female, patient experienced any major
pain.

During the follow up period there were no reports of bleeding nor of faecal or flatulent incontinence.   There was a marked lack of subjective symptomatology.

Proctological findings: In 16 cases appearances were entirely within normal limits.   Six patients showed minor pathological findings, e.g. small skin tags, anal eczema or a slightly increased sphincter tone (2 cases).   There were no cases of recurrence.

The patient referred to above was shown to have a chronic posterior fissue-in-ano together with a trans-sphincter anal fistula and increased sphincter tone.   Following re-operation by laying open of the fistula and superficial anal sphincterotomy, she, too, was relieved of pain.

DISCUSSION

In summary, 22 out of 23 patients followed after emergency haemorrhoidectomy for thrombosed piles showed excellent objective results.   We therefore believe this treatment to be now the treatment of choice.   We have shown that acute haemorrhoidectomy does not have a greater morbidity rate - the risk of infection, abscess or other complication is no higher than that for an elective operation.   There is no requirement for a patient with haemorrhoidal thrombosis to receive several incisions, each accompanied by pain, suffering and time off work when ultimately he will come to radical surgery.   We are convinced that a radical segmental resection in the acute stage must now be preferred to a more palliative incision.

REFERENCES

Eisenstat T., Salvati E.P.: The Outpatient Management of Acute
    Haemorrhoidal Disease.   Am.Soc.Col.Rec 1979. 22/5, 315-317.

Mazier W.P.: Emergency Haemorrhoidectomy. Dis. Col & Rect 1977.
    16/3. 200-205.

Morgado Nieves P.: Experience with the St.Mark's Hospital Technique
    for Emergency Haemorrhoidectomy.   Dis. Col & Rect 1977
    20/3. 197-201.

Sakulsky S.B.: Treatment of Thrombosed Haemorrhoids by Excision
    Am.J.Surg. 1970. 120. 537-540.

EDITOR'S NOTE

Herr Schlaepfer prefaced his paper with an interesting account of the early history of the Munsterlingen Hopsital.   The hopsital was founded in the eleventh century by Angela, the daughter of King Edward the Confessor (1003-1066).   As a thank-you for divine intervention for saving her from drowning after a storm on Lake Constance she founded a cloister at the spot where she reached shore - this monastery, which later became "Munsterlingen" cared for patients from them on, through the Reformation and until the present day.   The 18th century cloister block was recently renovated as a large, modern hospital.

"All of this to say that we still cherish our English origins!"

Care of the Acutely Ill and Injured
Edited by D. H. Wilson and A. K. Marsden
© 1982, John Wiley & Sons Ltd.

DIAGNOSIS AND TREATMENT OF INJURIES OF THE RECTUM
CAUSED BY FOREIGN BODIES

V. Pezzangora, R. Barina, C. Zerbinati, V. Averno,
A. Saggioro and M. Rizzo.

Umberto I Hospital, 1st Surgical Department,
Venezia-Mestre, Italy.

ABSTRACT

Injuries of the rectum caused by foreign bodies are usually easy to
diagnose. The aetiology, treatment and complications are described
in a series of 45 patients. A protocol is recommended to reduce the
morbidity resulting from these injuries.

INTRODUCTION

Rectal injuries can result from a variety of causes: road accidents,
gun shot wounds, foreign bodies. The term "foreign body" is widely
used to describe any object not normally present in the rectum. An
accurate knowledge of the anatomy of the region is essential for
evaluating the extent of the lesion and for planning prompt and
appropriate treatment.

PATIENTS

In the ten year period from 1971 to 1980, 45 patients were admitted
to our department with foreign body ano-rectal lesions sufficiently
severe to require in-patient treatment. Their ages ranged from 3
months to 76 years (mean 36 years) and the male/female ratio was
1.8: 1.0. The aetiology of the injuries is shown in Table 1.

TABLE 1

Aetiology of 45 rectal injuries caused by foreign bodies

Cause of injury	Number of patients	Percentage
Faecal foreign bodies	9	20.0
Iatrogenic causes:		
- endoscopic procedures	4	8.9
- thermometer	21	46.7
- diagnostic or therapeutic enema	5	11.1
Impalement	2	4.5
Self-inflicted injuries	3	6.7
Pneumatic injuries	1	2.2

405

In the majority of cases the diagnosis was easy, especially when the
sequence of events was known. However, in uncooperative patients,
mentally disabled people and children, the diagnosis can be difficult.
The symptoms are usually related to the severity of the lesion, which
may be a simple mucosal erosion or a complete tear of the rectal wall
with a perforation and also damage to the anal sphincter.

TREATMENT

Minimal lesions do not require surgical treatment. Only occasionally
is it necessary to apply electrocoagulation to a bleeding vessel or
to suture the mucosa for an injury caused by a thermometer. Foreign
bodies introduced by the patient rarely cause injury but great care
must be exercised in removing them. "Iatrogenic injuries" may result
from the surgical procedure used to remove the foreign body. The
treatments used for this series of patients is shown in Table II.

TABLE II

Treatment of 45 patients with rectal foreign bodies

Treatment	Number of patients	Percentage
Simple extraction of foreign body	20	46.5
Sphincter repair	4	9.3
Tamponade	3	7.0
Electrocoagulation	2	4.6
Repair of rectum	7	16.3
Laparotomy	6	14.0
Hartman's operation	1	2.3

RESULTS

In our 45 patients we had two fatalities, one due to septicaemia and
the other one to cardiogenic shock after perforation caused by a
barium enema. Post-operatively there were complications in eleven
patients (25.5%). These are described in Table III

TABLE III

Post-operative complications

Complication	Number of patients	Percentage
Dehiscence of laparotomy	1	9.0
Dehiscence of rectal repair	1	9.0
Permanent rectal incontinence	0	0
Temporary rectal incontinence	4	36.4
Subphrenic abscess	2	18.3
Prolapse of colostomy	1	9.0
Pelvic peritonitis	2	18.3

DISCUSSION

The series does not include those patients with minimal lesions that did not require surgical treatment, they were observed and treated as out-patients. For those who do require surgery, the following factors have proved to be important in reducing the mortality and complications:-

Early diagnosis

Complete definition of the lesion

Pre and post-operative antibiotic therapy

Immediate treatment of the lesion

The most difficult lesions to diagnose were those involving the retroperitoneal region. We usually practice routine recto-sigmoidoscopy using a rigid endoscope. The flexible instruments have proved to be more dangerous, especially in the presence of a perforation. This careful proctoscopic examination is useful both for determining the extent of the injury and at the same time for a thorough cleaning of the rectum. All the patients with an ano-rectal lesion receive prophylactic antibiotics. After removal of the foreign body we routinely perform a second endoscopic examination to study the appearance of the mucosa, arrest any bleeding and detect any secondary lesions caused by removal of the foreign body. This protocol for diagnosis and treatment has helped us to reduce the morbidity and mortality for our patients.

REFERENCES

BARONE, J.E. et al., 1976 Perforation and foreign bodies of the
                    rectum. Ann. Surg. 184, 601

EFTAIHA, M. et al., 1977   Principles of management of colo-rectal
                            foreign bodies. Arch. Surg. 112,691

LOWICKI, E.M., 1966   Accidental introduction of foreign body in
                            the rectum. Ann. Surg. 163, 395

THORBJARNARSON, B., 1962   Iatrogenic and related perforations of the
                            large bowel. Arch. Surg. 84, 28

Care of the Acutely Ill and Injured
Edited by D. H. Wilson and A. K. Marsden
© 1982, John Wiley & Sons Ltd.

WHAT BECOMES OF PATIENTS SUFFERING FROM NON SPECIFIC
ABDOMINAL PAIN?

B.Lukacs, Y.Flamant, J.M.Hay, J.N.Maillard.

Clinique Chirurgicale de l'hopital Louis Mourier
178 Rue des Renouillers, 92701, Colombes Cedex.

During a 21 month survey 308 adult patients were
admitted to the Surgery department of Louis Mourier Hospital
(Colombes-France) for acute abdominal pain.   All of these patients
were studied with a computer aided diagnosis program.

The predominant condition in this series was Non Specific
Abdominal Pain (N.S.A.P.).   This pathological condition was
defined as that of an adult suffering from an acute abdominal pain
for up to eight days before an emergency admission to the Surgery
department; the pain was self limiting without specific treatment
but remained unexplained at discharge.

The aim of this study was to state the results of a long
term follow up in patients discharged with such a diagnosis.
105 of these 120 patients were available to follow up one to three
years later.   The mean age was 37 years (20% over 50); the sex
distribution was equal; the mean length of hospitalisation was
6.5 days.

The original symptoms remained unexplained in 73 cases -
of which 23 suffered painful, though usually not disabling,
recurrences.   During the initial hospital evaluation, an
appendicectomy with a normal pathological examination was carried
out in 16 patients : in such cases the incidence of unexplained
painful recurrences was not significantly affected by the removal
of the appendix.

A specific cause for the initial symptoms was found in 22
cases, that is one patient out of five.   It involved the digestive
tract 17 times, the urological system 4 times, the gynaecological
system 3 times.   Only one case of cancer was found - a small
bowel lypoma.   The misdiagnosed condition affected patients over
50 more than in younger age groups (p 0.01).

This final diagnosis was usually obtained during the first
year of follow up (20 cases out of 22) through a simple out-
patient investigation.

The retrospective study of these patients records showed
that the diagnosis of the responsible condition could have been
made directly in one case out of three if the initial assessment

409

had been better programmed or interpreted.   A simultaneous
illness, probably not responsible for the initial symptoms, was
discovered twice.   Four patients died in the year following their
first admission.

We compared the initial presumptive diagnosis of computer
and clinician at admission with the definitive diagnosis established
after our follow up.   The respective efficiency of clinician and
computer appeared equivalent in dealing with N.S.A.P.

CONCLUSION

N.S.A.P. amounts to an important proportion of acute abdominal pains
admitted to an emergency surgery department.   This group of patients
should benefit by a close follow up during the year following their
first admission, as a specific underlying disease may be found, as
in our study, in one case out of five;   this is particularly true
of patients over 50 years of age.

SECTION NINE

EXPERIMENTAL RESEARCH

IN EMERGENCY CARE

Care of the Acutely Ill and Injured
Edited by D. H. Wilson and A. K. Marsden
© 1982, John Wiley & Sons Ltd.

EXPERIMENTAL RESEARCH IN EMERGENCY CARE

Editorial Overview

Andrew K. Marsden

The Accident and Emergency Department, receiving as it does, large numbers of patients, lends itself most readily to clinical and epidemiological research topics. Organizational difficulties in these areas have been largely mitigated with the advent of the microcomputer. Experimental research requires more extensive facilities but is nevertheless at the core of all advances in emergency surgery and resuscitation. The Congress was witness to a large number of free papers and poster contributions on experimental research, a selection of which are reproduced here.

Professor Stoner and his staff of the M.R.C. Trauma Unit in Manchester are making significant contributions to our understanding of the metabolic responses of the body to injury and stress. Their efforts, as we see, are supported by substantive papers from Italy.

Mr.Sharrard's session on Wound Healing contained some interesting subjects reinforced by his own speculations on future advances in this field of surgery. He likened developments in tissue trans- plantation to the gardener's practice of "taking cuttings" - he visualised a trauma unit of the future, upon being faced with a case of acute spinal cord injury,firstly requesting the appropriate segment of isolated spinal cord from the tissue bank and then treating it with enzymic "rooting" preparation and then interposing it using microsurgical techniques and finally encouraging its "take" with the help of electromagnetic radiation. Concepts more unthinkable than this a few years ago are now an established part of medical practice - perhaps an Emergency Surgery Congress in the not too distant future will hear the first successful accounts of satisfactory spinal cord regeneration!

Our present level of knowledge on aspects of research in the injured and acutely ill is admirably reviewed in Professor Wilmore's Key Note address - an encouraging and satisfying account of the State of the Art on which to conclude the Congress Proceedings.

Care of the Acutely Ill and Injured
Edited by D. H. Wilson and A. K. Marsden
© 1982, John Wiley & Sons Ltd.

METABOLIC PROBLEMS - REVIEW OF CURRENT SITUATION

H.B. STONER

MRC TRAUMA UNIT, UNIVERSITY OF MANCHESTER, MANCHESTER,U.K.

I find it very encouraging that a Congress like this should
include a session on the metabolic responses to injury. It is after
all only about 100 years since Claude Bernard started the
experimental investigation of these responses and 50 years since
Cuthbertson started us out on the detailed study of the metabolism
of the injured patient. Not only did Cuthbertson do that but he
also showed how the responses were divided into two stages, an early
one lasting hours and a later one lasting days, even weeks.
Appreciation of this is essential to understanding the effects of
trauma.

Despite the antiquity of the subject progress towards
understanding the metabolic responses to injury is very slow. We
have and are accumulating large amounts of data on the changes in
the blood, urine and tissues but the difficulty comes in interpreting
these changes and saying what they mean. It is only when we can do
that that we shall see what to do about them.

I am optimistic that we are beginning to understand certain
aspects of the responses to trauma. I think it is clear now that
the early part of the response is a neuroendocrine one and this
opens up numerous possibilities for its modulation by pharmacological
agents. It is also becoming clear that fat is the main substrate
for oxidation in both the early and later stages after severe
injuries and in severe sepsis. This occurs despite hyperglycaemia
and the provision of more than adequate amounts of carbohydrate.
The mechanism of this change in fuel is not known but is obviously
a fundamental one. A further feature of the severely injured or
septic patient to become recognised in recent years is their
reduced sensitivity to insulin. Again, this is present soon after
the injury and can persist for sometime. Since insulin is intimately
concerned in the metabolism of protein as well as of carbohydrate
and fat, this effect of injury is probably of great importance.

When we understand better what is happening in the body
after injury we shall be able to decide whether the changes are
potentially beneficial or not. From the time of John Hunter we
have tended to think that these responses have survival value.
Indeed, for the injured animal without treatment this is often the
case and attempts to correct them are often counter-productive.
However, this may no longer be true if the injuries are fully

415

treated and the fluid loss restored. It is often possible to deal fairly effectively with a metabolic disturbance, e.g. diabetes mellitus, even without fully understanding it. Unfortunately this cannot be done for the metabolic responses to injury until we have decided how far they are beneficial and, hence, which aspects of them should be promoted and which should be discouraged.

Care of the Acutely Ill and Injured
Edited by D. H. Wilson and A. K. Marsden
© 1982, John Wiley & Sons Ltd.

SUBSTRATE UTILISATION IN ACUTELY INJURED PATIENTS

R.A. Little, H.B. Stoner and K.N. Frayn

MRC Trauma Unit, University of Manchester,
Manchester, UK

ABSTRACT

Metabolic rate and respiratory exchange ratio have been measured in
patients within 6h of injury. Mean metabolic rate in the patients
was not significantly different from that in normal subjects, but
the variation between subjects was markedly increased. After severe
injuries the respiratory exchange ratio was significantly depressed,
reflecting an impairment of glucose oxidation which occurred despite
considerable hyperglycaemia.

INTRODUCTION

It is often supposed that metabolic rate is reduced in the 'ebb'
(Cuthbertson, 1942) or acute phase of the response to severe injury.
Although this has been confirmed in experimental animals, energy
production has not been measured shortly after injury in man.
Similarly there has been little study of the acute changes in
substrate utilisation after injury. Although hyperglycaemia is a
well known feature of the response, work in animals has shown that
glucose utilisation may be impaired after injury (Heath and Corney,
1973). We have now investigated these points using the technique of
indirect calorimetry in recently injured patients.

METHODS

Forty-three injured patients have been studied within 6h of their
injuries (median 2.5h) and before any definitive treatment had been
started. They have been divided into 2 groups depending on the
severity of injury, based on the Injury Severity Score (ISS) as
described by Stoner et al. (1979); 'Minor and Moderate' injuries
(ISS 4-12; 31 patients) and 'Severe' injuries (ISS 13-29; 12 patients).
Thirty-one control subjects were studied in a similar environment.
Gaseous exchange was measured using a Beckman Metabolic Measurement
Cart.

RESULTS AND DISCUSSION

The mean metabolic rate in control subjects, expressed in $kcal/m^2.h$,
was 86% of the standard value given by Fleisch (1951). The mean
values were not significantly different in the injured patients,
although the variability was significantly increased comparing each
injured group with the controls (F-test; $P<0.01$). The respiratory

TABLE 1.   Metabolic rate and substrate oxidation in injured
subjects

	Metabolic Rate[†]	Respiratory Exchange Ratio	Substrate oxidation $(g/m^2.h)$	
			Carbohydrate	Fat
Controls	86±2 (69-123)	0.84±0.03	——	—
Injured				
Minor and Moderate	92±5 (48-140)	0.86±0.02	4.7±0.6	1.3±0.2
Severe	100±10 (55-156)	0.78±0.02*	1.8±0.7*	2.9±0.4*

Results are shown as mean ± SEM, with range in parentheses
for metabolic rate. Data from Little et al. (1981)
† % of standard value (Fleisch, 1951).
* P<0.02 for difference between injured groups.

exchange ratio in the group with minor and moderate injuries was not
significantly different from that in the controls; in the severely
injured it was again not significantly different from controls, but
was significantly lower than in the other injured patients. This
difference was reflected in the calculated absolute rates of
carbohydrate and fat oxidation, the former being significantly
reduced and the latter increased in the severely injured patients
compared with those with minor and moderate injuries. This picture
was not much altered whatever assumptions were made regarding the
contribution of protein oxidation. This reduction in carbohydrate
oxidation occurred despite marked hyperglycaemia in the severely
injured (mean plasma glucose 8.4mmol/l; c.f. 6.0mmol/l in those with
minor and moderate injuries; P<0.001). Plasma insulin and free fatty
acid concentrations were similar in the two groups.

Thus, although there was no evidence for a depression of overall
metabolic rate in the injured patient, there was significant
impairment of glucose utilisation in the severely injured.

REFERENCES

Cuthbertson, D.P., 1942. Post-shock metabolic response. Lancet, 1,
    433-437.
Fleisch, A.L., 1951. Le metabolisme basal standard et sa determination
    au moyen du "Metabocalculator". Helvetia Medica Acta, 18, 23-44.
Heath, D.F., and Corney, P.L., 1973. The effects of starvation,
    environmental temperature and injury on the rate of disposal of
    glucose by the rat. Biochemical Journal, 136, 519-530.
Little, R.A., Stoner, H.B., and Frayn, K.N., 1981. Substrate
    oxidation shortly after accidental injury in man. Clinical Science.
    In press.
Stoner, H.B., Frayn, K.N., Barton, R.N., Threlfall, C.J., and
    Little, R.A., 1979. The relationships between plasma substrates
    and hormones and the severity of injury in 277 recently injured
    patients. Clinical Science, 56, 563-573.

Care of the Acutely Ill and Injured
Edited by D. H. Wilson and A. K. Marsden
© 1982, John Wiley & Sons Ltd.

INFLUENCE OF CARNITINE ON THE METABOLIC RESPONSE
TO INJURY OR SEPSIS

G.Nanni,M.Castagneto,M.Pittiruti,I.Giovannini,
P.Ronconi,A.Perla,G.Boldrini,M.T.Ramacci,
F.Maccari

Istituto di Clinica Chirurgica,Università
    Cattolica del Sacro Cuore, Roma, Italy
Centro di Studio per la Fisiopatologia dello
    Shock , C.N.R., Roma, Italy

INTRODUCTION

The physiological response to injury is characterized by
a strong neuroendocrine response which provokes marked
alterations of intermediary metabolism, such as increased
proteolysis and preferential utilization of endogenous
fuel. The qualitative aspects of adaptive response to
non-septic injury are fundamentally different from those
seen in response to a severe septic insult, which is
characterized by a decrease in peripheral utilization of
oxygen, due to impairment of oxidative metabolism
(Siegel et al., 1979).
Several recent studies have supported the contention that
a blockade in some catabolic pathway of lipidic metabolism
may be a feature of sepsis : as a possible explanation,
Border suggested that an impairment of long chain fatty
acids oxidation may occur in sepsis, due to relative
deficiency of carnitine (Border et al.,1976).

METHODS

In order to verify this hypothesis, we have studied three
groups of patients : normal controls, non-septic injury
patients, septic patients. In each study group (septic
and non-septic), half of the patients were administered
100 mg/kg/die of D,L-acetyl-carnitine, in continous i.v.

infusion (D,L-acetyl-carnitine, Sigma Tau, Italy).
Cardiovascular and respiratory measurements were carried
out in the three groups of patients : the septic patients
we have studied seemed to be in a "A" state, according to
Siegel's classification : i.e., normal stress response in
compensated sepsis ; increased cardiac index and increased
oxygen consumption. (Siegel, 1979)

RESULTS AND DISCUSSION

Figure 1 : Plasma levels of free carnitine (FC) were quite
similar in all non-treated patients, while levels of acyl-
carnitines resulting from short chain and medium chain
fatty acids (AC) were significantly decreased in septic
patients if compared to non-septic and to controls.
Therefore, AC/FC ratio was significantly lower in septics.
During Acetyl-carnitine administration, AC values showed
a threefold increase in septic patients, but a sixfold
increase in non-septics : FC levels were not significantly
affected in septic patients, while in non-septic patients
FC levels showed a twofold increase.

Fig. 1

		N	SE	N (+AC)	SE (+AC)
ACYL-CARNITINE	control	14	10.66	2.4		
	surgery	43	13.82	2.2	15	87.06	9.3
	sepsis	25	6.24	.8	17	23.6	4.4
FREE CARNITINE	control	17	36.35	2.4		
	surgery	52	41.04	2.2	18	81.04	8.9
	sepsis	31	42.67	5.6	20	52.53	4.4
AC/FC	control	14	.335	.08		
	surgery	43	.316	.03	15	1.005	.11
	sepsis	26	.22	.05	16	.385	.06

Figure 2 : Urinary excretion of FC was significantly
higher in septic if compared to controls, while non-septic
injury patients had intermediary values between controls
and septics. After acetyl-carnitine administration,
urinary excretion of FC increased significantly both in
septic and in non-septic patients.

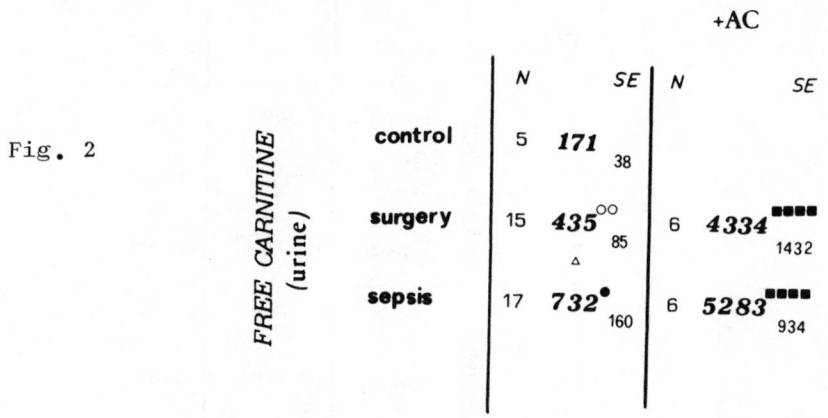

Fig. 2

These data suggest that early sepsis may be characterized
by increased utilization of acyl-carnitines : indeed, a
similar phenomenon has been reported experimentally in
starvation, hyperlipidic feeding and physical stress
(Brass and Hoppel,1978)(Ferri et al.,1978).
The importance of carnitine in the metabolism of the
septic patient is also suggested by the following observations : in our septic patients, we found significant
correlations between metabolic rate and acyl-carnitines,
between oxygen consumption and AC, between arteriovenous
oxygen difference and AC/FC ratio ; such correlations
could not be found in controls or in non-septic injury.
Figure 3-4:With regards to lipidic metabolism, we did not
find significant differences in triglycerides (TG) or in
free fatty acids (FFA) levels comparing the three groups.
Keton bodies were slightly higher in non septic and in
septic patients if compared to controls.
FFA levels were not significantly affected by acetyl-
carnitine administration, while TG decreased in treated
patients, both in non-septic and in septic patients.
We also found that AC/FC ratio did correlate with keton
bodies production in controls and in non-septic patients,

G. Nanni et al.

Fig. 3

+AC

		N		SE	N		SE
TRIGLYCERIDES	control	17	*125*	18			
	surgery	52	*129*	8	19	*100*°°	7
	sepsis	31	*130*	12	42	*103*°	9
CHOLESTEROL	control	17	*169*	15			
	surgery	52	*134*°° ▲▲▲	6	19	*126*	6
	sepsis	31	*86*°°°°	3	20	*90*	5
PHOSPHOLIPIDS	control	17	*136*	21			
	surgery	52	*135* △△	8	19	*133*	9
	sepsis	31	*120*	9	20	*122*	8

but not in sepsis. Such correlation could not be found in
treated patients.
Confirming experimental data observed during starvation
(Brass and Hoppel, 1978), our data seem to suggest that
an increase of AC/FC ratio is associated with an increased
production of keton bodies in non-septic injury, but not
in sepsis; this may be explained by an enhanced utilization
of acetyl-CoA and ketoacids in sepsis.
Figure 5 : With regards to carbohydrate metabolism, a
different behaviour was observed between sepsis and non-
septic injury. After acetyl-carnitine administration,
non-septic injury was characterized by decrease of lactate,
decrease of pyruvate, and decrease of pyruvate/lactate
ratio ; in sepsis, the pattern was opposite. Furthermore,
we found an inverse correlation between AC/FC ratio and
pyruvate in non-septic patients, while the same correlation
was direct in sepsis. These findings seem to suggest that
in septic patients an increase of AC/FC ratio is associated
with a relative impairment of pyruvate catabolism, while
in non-septic injury the increase of AC/FC ratio enhances

Fig. 4

		N	SE	+AC N	+AC SE
FFA	control	17	628 98		
	surgery	52	515 41	18	458 72
	sepsis	28	448 °° 43	17	472 38
betaOH-BUTYRATE	control	12	469 90		
	surgery	38	911 • 128 (△△)	15	769 170
	sepsis	13	578 130	14	738 128
ACETOACETATE	control	10	60.3 31		
	surgery	23	87.7 28	4	51.5 27
	sepsis	13	72.7 17	13	64.2 15

the catabolism of pyruvate and lactate.

CONCLUSIONS

In brief, our data confirm that metabolic patterns of the
septic patient are quite different, even at an early stage,
if compared to non-septic injury patients.
The metabolism of carnitines seems to be markedly affected
by the hypercatabolic state of sepsis, and it is characterized by an increased utilization of acyl-carnitines,
possibly due to increased tissue uptake, with redistribu-
tion among pools of different carnitines.
Acetyl-carnitine administration was associated with
increased lipidic metabolism, especially in septic patients,
whose energy metabolism is tightly related to endogenous
fuel. In particular, we found a direct correlation between
AC/FC ratio and keton bodies in non-septic injury, while
such correlation could not be found in septics.
The behaviour of lactate and pyruvate was different in the
two groups : while in non-septic patients acetyl-carnitine

+AC

Fig. 5

		N	SE	N	SE
PYRUVATE	control	12	*121* 16		
	surgery	39	*140* ▲ 13	15	*121* 20
	sepsis	13	*94*[oo] 16	14	*164*[□□] 55
LACTATE	control	12	*677* 70		
	surgery	38	*1638*[••] △△ 245	15	*1480* 149
	sepsis	12	*1104*[••] 140	14	*1441*[■] 122
PYR/LAC	control	12	*.196* .03		
	surgery	36	*.145*[oo] △ .02	15	*.104*[□] .03
	sepsis	12	*.100*[••] .02	14	*.246*[□□] .1

administration seemed to improve the utilization of lactate and pyruvate, in septic patients acetyl-carnitine administration was apparently associated with accumulation of pyruvate.
In conclusion, our present investigation upon carnitine metabolism in sepsis further confirms that energy metabolism of the septic patient is strictly connected to the utilization of endogenous fuel, such as FFA and ketoacids.

REFERENCES

Border et al., 1976. Multiple systems organ failure : muscle fuel deficit with visceral protein malnutrition. Surg.Clin.N.Am., 56(5),1147-1167.
Brass E.P. and Hoppel C.L.,1978. Carnitine in metabolism of the fasting rat. J.Biol.Chem.,253,2688.
Ferri L. et al.,1978. Carnitina:significato biologico e medico. Progresso Medico, 34, 1-14.
Siegel J.H. et al.,1979. Physiological and metabolic correlations in human sepsis. Surgery, 86,163-193.

Care of the Acutely Ill and Injured
Edited by D. H. Wilson and A. K. Marsden
© 1982, John Wiley & Sons Ltd.

CARDIOVASCULAR HOMOEOSTASIS AFTER INJURY IN MAN

R.A. Little, H.B. Stoner, Pamela Bithell
and Rosalind E. Atkins

M.R.C. Trauma Unit, Hope Hospital (University of
Manchester School of Medicine), Salford, U.K.

INTRODUCTION

Experimental work has shown that there is an impairment of the
cardiovascular response to a head-up tilt, and of the baro -
receptor mediated blood pressure - heart rate reflex in the
unanaesthetised rat after injury (Little, 1979; Redfern, Little
and Stoner, 1981). It is important to know if a similar
situation exists clinically, because the initial management of
the injured patient assumes normal activity of homoeostatic
reflexes. Earlier studies in man have shown that although the
pulse rate response to a deep inspiration is not affected by
injury, there is an impairment of the response to a head-up
tilt (Little, 1981) and we have now studied the responses to a
Valsalva manoeuvre shortly after injury.

METHODS

Twenty-five patients who had suffered injuries of a minor or
moderate severity (assessed by the Abbreviated Injury Scale -
Baker, O'Neill, Hadden and Long, 1974) have been studied in the
Accident and Emergency Department soon after injury (0·5 - 6h).
The patients were asked to hold a column of mercury at a height
of 20 or 40mmHg for 10sec. during expiration following a full
inspiration. The pulse was recorded with a photoelectric pulse
monitor (Lectromed, Welwyn Garden City) attached to a finger.
Twenty control subjects were studied under the same conditions.

RESULTS

In the control subjects the maximum pulse rate during
expiration was positively correlated with initial pulse rate,
and the regression line for the response at 40mmHg was
significantly elevated above that at 20mmHg, without a change
in slope. After injury, this difference was not seen, and the
lines at 20mmHg and at 40mmHg were the same as the control
20mmHg line.

On release of the expiratory strain, there was a bradycardia
and the minimum pulse rate at this time was positively
correlated with initial pulse rate. In control subjects there

was no difference in the relationship at 20mmHg and at 40mmHg.
The same was true after injury, although the regression line
(tests at 20mmHg and 40mmHg combined) was significantly
elevated above the control line, again with no change in slope.

Repeat tests on 7 patients during recovery (7-45 days after
injury - median 26 days) showed a return to a control pattern
of response.

CONCLUSIONS

The present results suggest that during the acute phase of the
response to minor and moderately severe accidental injuries in
man there is an impairment of reflex parasympathetic cardiac
control.

REFERENCES

Baker, S.P., O'Neill, B., Haddon, W., and Long, W.B., 1974.
    The injury severity score: A method for describing patients
    with multiple injuries and evaluating emergency care.
    Journal of Trauma, 14, 187-196.
Little, R.A., 1979. Effects of non-haemorrhagic injury on the
    cardiovascular response to tilting in the rat. British
    Journal of Experimental Pathology, 60, 309-313.
Little, R.A., 1981. Cardiovascular reflexes after injury. Adv.
    Physiol. Sci. Vol. 26, Homoeostasis in Injury and Shock (Eds
    Biro, Kovach, Spitzer and Stoner), pp 93-97. Budapest.
Redfern, W.S., Little, R.A., and Stoner, H.B., 1981. Resetting
    of the baroreceptor - heart rate reflex in the
    unanaesthetised rat during and following a period of hind
    limb ischaemia. Adv. Physiol. Sci. Vol. 26, Homoeostasis
    in Injury and Shock (Eds. Biro, Kovach, Spitzer and Stoner),
    pp 235-236. Budapest.

Care of the Acutely Ill and Injured
Edited by D. H. Wilson and A. K. Marsden
© 1982, John Wiley & Sons Ltd.

PaO$_2$/PAO$_2$ RATIO AS A DIAGNOSTIC AND PROGNOSTIC INDEX
IN CHEST TRAUMAS

Turetta F.   De Stefani R.   Pezzangora F.   Milanesi A.
and Cannizzaro A.

Intensive Care Unit and 1st Surgical Unit
Ospedale "Umberto 1o", MESTRE-VENICE (Italy).

ABSTRACT

The PaO$_2$/PAO$_2$ ratio has been used as a diagnostic index to determine
the size of the intrapulmonary shunt in chest trauma patients.
A good correlation has been found between these two indices.
The PaO$_2$/PAO$_2$ ratio has also proved to be a useful prognostic index
indicating the chance of survival in chest trauma victims.

INTRODUCTION

In the past the mechanical derangement of the ventilatory mechanism
was regarded as the main problem in chest injuries.   Surgical
stabilisation of the chest wall was often used as the main
therapeutic measure, especially for patients with a flail segment.

Today changes in the lung parenchyma are considered to be the
leading cause of post traumatic pulmonary insufficiency.   The
presence of hypoxaemia with normo-or hypocapnia in these patients,
even though they are breathing oxygen at a high concentration,
shows that it is not alveolar hypoventilation but a right to left
intrapulmonary shunt which takes place in the contused areas of
the lungs.

Determining the size of the shunt is therefore very important from
both a diagnostic and prognostic point of view.

Using the isoshunt diagram of Nunn (Nunn 1977) it is possible to
derive the value of the shunt, when one knows the FiO2 and the
PaO$_2$: however in order to become independent of the effects of
varying FiO2 on PAO2 it has been suggested using the PaO$_2$/PAO2
ratio as an index of respiratory efficiency (Gilbert et al. 1979).

Therefore we decided to investigate the correlation between this
ratio and the calculated shunt (Qs/Qt) in order to evaluate its
value as an indirect index of the magnitude of Qs/Qt.

MATERIALS AND METHODS

We studied the clinical records of 42 chest trauma patients without
any significant traumatic lesion elsewhere.   In all patients we
determined the PaO$_2$/PAO$_2$ ratio and in 32 we calculated also the
Qs/Qt by means of a Swan-Ganz catheter.

We performed an analysis of regression of Qs/Qt on PaO2/PAO2 and we
tested the difference between the mean PaO2/PAO2 ratio of survivors
and non-survivors by Student's "t" test.

RESULTS AND DISCUSSION

The analysis of regression of Qs/Qt on PaO2/PAO2 shows a good
correlation between the two indices (r = .715, p   .001) and
confirms that it is possible to infer the magnitude of Qs/Qt from
a single haemo-gasanalysis on arterial blood, without the need of
obtaining a mixed venous blood sample (Figure 1)

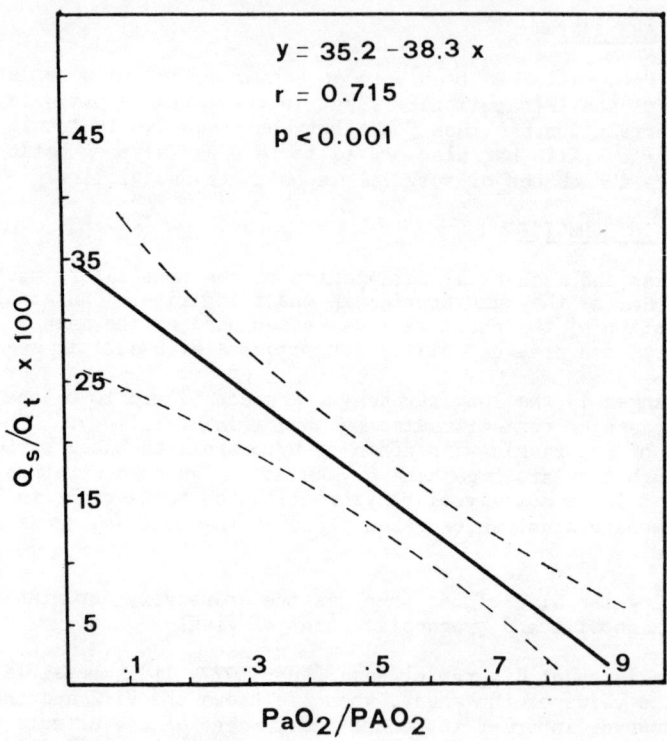

Figure 1 - Regression line of Qs/Qt on PaO2/PAO2 with
95% confidence limits (n = 32)

If we analyse the mean value of this ratio on admission in survivors
and non-survivors we find that in survivors it is significantly
higher than in non-survivors (.46 ± .09 vs. .31 ± .08, mean ± SD,
p   .001): moreover we found that a value of .28 or less is
associated with a very low probability of survival (less than 5%).
We conclude that the PaO2/PAO2 ratio is a very simple and reliable
index of Qs/Qt in chest trauma and that it can be used for the
purpose of prognosis as well.

REFERENCES

Gilbert R. Auchincloss J.H. jr. Kuppinger M. Varkey T.M. 1979.
 Stability of the arterial/alveolar oxygen partial pressure ratio.
 Critical Care Medicine. 7. 267-272.

Nunn J.F. 1977. Applied Respiratory Physiology. 2nd ed.
 Butterworths.London.

Care of the Acutely Ill and Injured
Edited by D. H. Wilson and A. K. Marsden
© 1982, John Wiley & Sons Ltd.

CHANGES IN CARDIAC OUTPUT DISTRIBUTION AFTER NON –
HAEMORRHAGIC INJURY IN THE RAT

D.W. Yates, Judith M. Hadfield and R.A. Little

M.R.C. Trauma Unit, Stopford Building, University of
Manchester Medical School, Manchester, U.K.

INTRODUCTION

Previous studies have shown a reduction in cardiac output and
changes in the distribution during the first four hours after
the non-haemorrhagic injury, bilateral hind-limb ischaemia, in
the unanaesthetised rat (Little, Yates, Reynolds and Hadfield,
1980). Although there was a marked change in the regional
distribution of cardiac output after this injury (LD_{60-80})
there were no obvious differences in the pattern of
distribution between survivors and non-survivors. We have now
studied the distribution of cardiac output at longer times
after injury in an attempt to identify such differences.

METHODS

The distribution of cardiac output was measured in 180–270g ♂
rats using ^{141}Ce labelled (New England Nuclear) 15μm diameter
microspheres injected into the left ventricle via a right
carotid artery cannula implanted one week previously (Little,
Yates, Reynolds and Hadfield, 1980). Unanaesthetised rats were
injected at different times after the end of the period of limb
ischaemia and were then left until they died or were killed
48h after injury. A 48h survival period was chosen because by
that time all the animals that were going to succumb to the
acute effects of the injury would have died (Rosenthal, 1943).
At autopsy the position of the cannula in the left ventricle
was confirmed and tissues removed, weighed and counted. Colon
temperature was measured with a thermocouple inserted 6cm from
the anus.

RESULTS AND DISCUSSION

The percentage distribution of cardiac output to the liver via
the hepatic artery was increased as expected after injury (eg:-
Ferguson, Merrill, Miller and Spitzer, 1977; Malik, Loegering,
Saba and Kaplan, 1978; Little, Yates, Reynolds and Hadfield,
1980). The increase was greatest in the rats that died although
it was still significantly raised at 48h after injury in the
survivors. The distribution to the spleen was markedly reduced
during the first 20h after injury, with no difference between

survivors and non-survivors, however there was a return to
control values by 48h. When the time interval between injection
and death was taken into account several interesting findings
emerged. For example the percentage distribution of cardiac
output to the lungs was increased in rats surviving for more
than 20h after injection, whereas distribution to the adrenals
was highest in those animals dying shortly ($< 6h$) after
injection.

Body temperature is an important determinant of cardiac output
(eg: Bullard, 1959) and as there is an impairment of thermo –
regulation and fall in temperature after injury in the rat (eg:
Stoner, 1976) some account should be taken of core temperature
at the time of injection. The percentage distribution of
cardiac output to the liver was greatest in the rats with a low
temperature ($< 30°C$) whereas that to the spleen was highest in
such animals. Diencephalon, mid brain and hind brain received
an increasing percentage distribution of cardiac output as core
temperature fell, whereas distribution to cerebral cortex and
cerebellum was less well maintained.

CONCLUSIONS

There are marked changes in the distribution of cardiac output
after injury in the unanaesthetised rat. The increased
distribution to the liver via the hepatic artery was most
marked in the animals that died after injury. Distribution to
the adrenals was greatest in animals dying 6h after injection
of the microspheres whereas distribution to the lungs was
increased in rats surviving >20h after injection. There were
suggestions that distribution to the cerebral cortex and
cerebellum was less well maintained than that to the rest of
the brain.

REFERENCES

Bullard, R.W., 1959. Cardiac output of the hypothermic rat.
    American Journal of Physiology, 196, 415-419.
Ferguson, J.L., Merrill, G.F., Miller, H.I., and Spitzer, J.J.,
    1977. Regional blood flow redistribution during early burn
    shock in the guinea pig. Circulatory Shock, 4, 317-326.
Little, R.A., Yates, D.W., Reynolds, M.I., and Hadfield, J.M.,
    1980. Changes in cardiac output and its distribution after
    non-haemorrhagic injury in the rat. British Journal of
    Experimental Pathology, 61, 421-428.
Malik, A.B., Loegering, D.J., Saba, T.M., and Kaplan, J.E.,1978
    Cardiac output and regional blood flow following trauma.
    Circulatory Shock, 5, 73-84.
Rosenthal, S.M., 1943. Experimental chemotherapy of burns and
    shock. IV. Production of traumatic shock in mice. Public
    Health Reports (Washington), 58, 1429-1436.
Stoner, H.B., 1976. Changes in the central nervous system and
    their role in the metabolic response to injury, in
    Metabolism and the Response to Injury (Eds. Wilkinson and
    Cuthbertson), pp. 179-193. Pitman Medical.

Care of the Acutely Ill and Injured
Edited by D. H. Wilson and A. K. Marsden
© 1982, John Wiley & Sons Ltd.

RESPIRATORY AND METABOLIC MANAGEMENT FOR 30 MINUTES
DURING SUCCESSFUL WARM TOTAL LIVER VASCULAR
EXCLUSION (LVE) - AN EXPERIMENTAL STUDY

Galmarini D. Tarenzi L.[*] Gattinoni L.[*] Fassati L.R.
Cantaluppi G. Zanandrea G. Rossi G. Trabucchi E.
Megevand J. Berrini C.[*] Ferrari G.[*] Pelizzola A.[*]
Pesenti A.[*] Doglia M. Fabiani M.P.

Cattedra di Chirurgia Sostitutiva dei Trapianti
d'Organo e di Organi Artificiali.

[*] Instituto di Anestesia e Rianimazione
Universita degli Studi di Milano, Via F.Sforza 35
20122 Milan, Italy.

ABSTRACT

Total normothermic liver vascular exclusion (LVE) was maintained
for 30 minutes in 6 lambs. 3 animals, in which no attempt was
made to correct the metabolic or respiratory derangements, served
as control group. All three animals died of hypotension and
arrythmia after declamping. In 3 more animals normocapnia and
normal blood pH were maintained (treated group) - all three animals
survived long term. LVE up to 30 minutes can be safely maintained
provided $PaCO_2$ and pH are kept within normal range.

INTRODUCTION

LVE allows hepatic surgery in an asanguineous field. This method
has been clinically proposed by Huguet (1976) and up to date has
received very limited application (Heaney et al.1978). This study
was designed to define a suitable respiratory and metabolic management during LVE.

METHODS

Six lambs (25-30 Kg) were anaesthetised with halothane 2% and
paralysed with pancuronium. Pulmonary artery (Swan-Ganz catheter)
and common carotid artery were cannulated. The animals were
ventilated with Servo ventilator ($F_1O_2= 0.5$; 16 b.p.m., Tidal volume
12 ml Kg^{-1}).

Distal thoracic aorta, portal triad, infrahepatic inferior vena cava
and suprahepatic inferior vena cava were isolated and then clamped
in sequence. After 30 minutes of LVE the vessels were declamped
in opposite sequence. End Tidal PCO_2 (ET PCO_2), mean pulmonary
artery (PAP) and systemic arterial pressure (AP) were continuously
recorded. Serum electrolytes, blood gases and cardiac output (CO)
were measured at 10 minute intervals before, during and after LVE.

Control group: Three animals underwent all the procedure without
any attempt to modify the metabolic or respiratory state.

Treated group: In three animals the $PaCO_2$ was maintained constant
(through end tidal PCO_2 - (ET PCO_2) - monitoring) by decreasing

V_E about 50% during LVE and by increasing V_E 50% when declamping. Two minutes before declamping 4 mEq Kg^{-1} Na HCO_3 were rapidly infused to prevent changes in blood buffer power due to $PaCO_2$ variations and to acid load from excluded emibody.

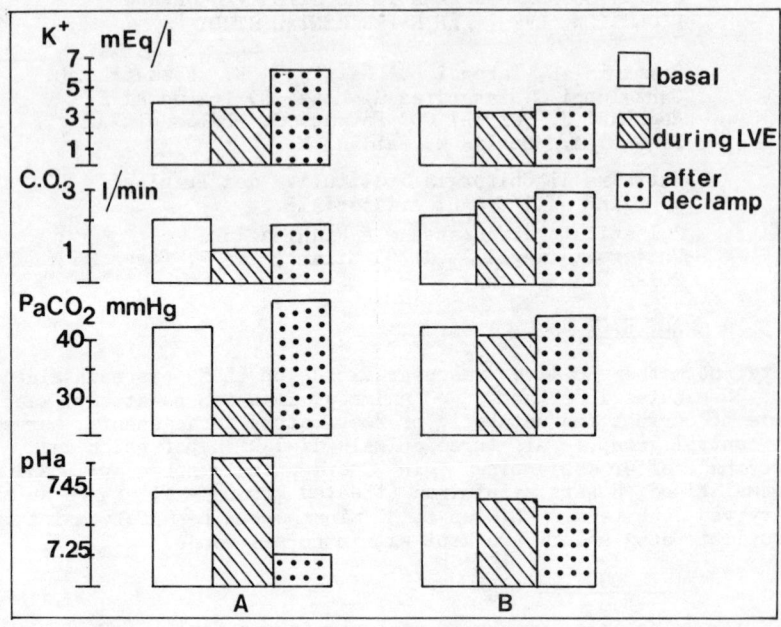

Fig. 1. - Changes in K^+, Cardiac Output (CO), $PaCO_2$, pHa in control
(A) and treated (B) groups - before, during and 30
minutes after LVE.

RESULTS

Control group: All animals died (at 10 minute-2h-5h) of hypothermia and arrythmia.

They showed a common pattern during LVE (Fig. 1a), a progressive rise in pH (from 7.45 to 7.58), decrease in $PaCO_2$ (from 35.8 to 23.5 mmHg), decrease CO (from 100 to 40 ml $Kg^{-1}min^{-1}$) and decrease in K (from 4.0 to 3.5 mEq l^{-1}).

On declamping a sudden decrease in pH(7.24)and rise in $PaCO_2$ (55mmHg) was observed; cardiac output rose up to 70 ml $Kg^{-1}min^{-1}$ and K^+ to 7.3 mEq l^{-1}.

Treated group: All three animals in the treated group survived the procedure uneventfully. The animals were sacrificed two weeks after surgery in good health. $PaCO_2$ pH and K^+ remained fairly constant throughout the procedure (Fig. 1b).

All animals survived without renal or neurological damage.

DISCUSSION

These experiments suggest that sudden variations of PCO_2, pH and K^+ rather than absolute values are life threatening.   LVE up to 30 minutes appears to be feasible and safe when $PaCO_2$ and pH are kept constant by respiratory and metabolic control.

REFERENCES

Heaney J.P. Stanton W.K. Halbert D.S. Seidel J. Vince J.:   An improved technique for vascular isolation of the liver; experimental study and case reports.   Ann.Surg. <u>163</u>. 237. 1966.

Huguet C. Gallot D. Offenstadt G. Coloigner M.:   Exclusion vasculaire totale de foie dans la chirurgie d'exerese hepatique large.   Interet et limites.   Presse Med. <u>5</u>. 1189. 1976.

Care of the Acutely Ill and Injured
Edited by D. H. Wilson and A. K. Marsden
© 1982, John Wiley & Sons Ltd.

REPAIR OF SPLENIC INJURIES IN ANIMAL
EXPERIMENTS

J.Kleinschmidt, W.L.Brückner, W.Heltzel

Surgical Policlinic of the University of Munich,
GERMANY

ABSTRACT

Experimental splenic repair and splenosis in 70 rabbits
proved possible by suture, by the Fibrin Adhesive Technique, and by a combination of both. Peritoneal splenosis
could only, however, be induced after particle suture to
the peritoneum. Tc-scans were compared to the photo-
documentation at autopsy, 4 - 12 weeks later. Histologic
evaluation has been started.

INTRODUCTION

Splenic repair by suture has been reported more than 60
years ago (Marine, 1920). Fatal sepsis after splenectomy is a major sequelae (Singer, 1973). Immunologic
impairment is being assumed (Sherman, 1980; Neilan,
1980). Immuno-protection of splenosis is controversal
in animal experiments, but seems to function in humans.

METHODS

Deliberate splenic lesions in 70 rabbits have been
treated by operations:
running suture (20); suture plus Fibrin Adhesive (10);
Fibrin Adhesive alone, after temporary clamping of the
splenic vessels (15); free intraperitoneal splenic
particles of pea-size (10); particle-suture to the
peritoneum (5); mashed splenic pastry placed onto the
stomach and the liver (5); subcutaneous particles (5);
and further 5 rabbits which died within 40 hours from
complications other than operative.

RESULTS

Only sutured particles and sutured/glued spleens did
show at autopsy, 4 - 12 weeks later. Tc-scintigrams were
positive only after splenic repair; peritoneal particles
of pea-size and less were too small to be detected by
scan. Free particles, omentum particles, and splenic

pastry were transformed into abscess-granulomata.

DISCUSSION

Splenic repair is possible (Buntain and Lynn, 1979).
Asplenia results in fatal sepsis 50 - 200 times as
often as in splenic individuals (Singer, 1973). If
splenic damage is too extensive to be sutured or glued,
autotransplantation to the peritoneal wall should be
performed (Kleinschmidt, Brückner, and Heltzel, 1981)
in order to provide, at least, partial immuno-protection
for the patient.

REFERENCES

Marine,D., and Manley,O.T., 1920. Homeotransplantation
        and Autotranplantation of the Spleen in Rabbits.
        J. Experim. Med. 32, 113 - 133
Singer, D.B., 1973. Postsplenectomy Sepsis, in:
        Perspectives in Pediatric Pathology (eds. Ro-
        senberg and Bolande), Vol.I, 285 - 311
Sherman, R., 1980. Perspectives in Management to the
        Spleen: 1979 Presidential Address.
        J. Trauma 1, 1 - 13
Buntain, W.L., and Lynn, H.B., 1979. Changing Concepts
        for the Traumatized Spleen. Surgery 5, 748-760
Neilan, B., 1980. Late sequelae of splenectomy for
        trauma. Postgraduate Medicine, Vol. 68, No. 3,
        207 - 212
Kleinschmidt,J., Brückner, W.L., and Heltzel,W., 1981.
        Scintigraphic Control after Lesion and Repair of
        the Spleen in Animal Experiment. Incontri
        Internaz. di Chirurgia, Milano. Ricerca Scient.
        ed Educaz. Permanente, Suppl. 18, L 27

Care of the Acutely Ill and Injured
Edited by D. H. Wilson and A. K. Marsden
© 1982, John Wiley & Sons Ltd.

THE VALUE OF GRAPHIC ANALYSIS OF DOPPLER WAVES
IN THE DIAGNOSIS OF THE ACUTE SCROTUM

Gavinelli M.   Anselmi A.A.   Azzoni K.

Insituto di Clinica Chirurgica 1, University of Milan,
Italy.

In entertaining the diagnosis of acute pathology of the
scrotum the difficulty often lies in differentiating between acute
torsion of the testicle and acute epididymo-orchitis.   To overcome
this problem we have turned to ultrasound examination using a
'Bidirectional Doppler Flowmeter' (the Bidirectional 80B Parks
Doppler).   The technique relies upon the interpretation of flow
waves resulting from the haemodynamic changes associated with
different pathologies.   The probe is placed in contact with the
skin in line with the testicular vessels and inclined at 45° to
the main axis such that it registers the approaching flow as
positive waves and the receding flow as negative waves.

In normal subjects there are three kinds of wave form (Figure 1)
- a positive "A" wave corresponding to systolic flow (a forward
  directed flow wave).
- a negative "B" wave corresponding to cessation of the flow with
  initial inversion during the closing of the semilunar valves
  (protodiastolic retrograde flow) and
- a positive "C" wave corresponding to the elastic arterial
  telediastolic return (forward directed flow).

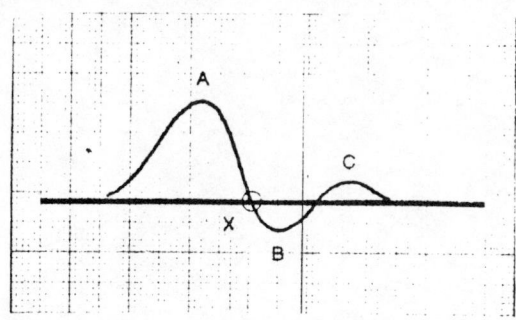

Figure 1

In recent and complete torsion of the testicle with occlusion of
the spermatic cord the flowmetry is characteristic of acute venous
stasis with an increase in duration of diastolic flow (B wave)
and the disappearance of systolic flow (A wave).

In acute epididymo orchitis the picture is characterised by
hyperaemia with a normal diastolic B wave.

The differential diagnosis can be facilitated by comparing the
flowmetry of the involved testis with that of the sound one.

REFERENCES

Austoni E. Larcher P. Patelli E. Castelli P. Redaelli A. :
"La flussimetria Doppler bidirezionale per la diagnosi delle
sindromi vascolari acute del testicolo".   Arch.st.Wrol.Nefr.
3. 183. 1979.

Levy B.J. : "The diagnosis of torsion of the testicle using the
Doppler ultrasound stethoscope". J.Wrol. 113. 63. 1975.

Milleret H. : "Doppler ultrasound diagnosis of testicular cord
torsion". J.Clin.Ultrasound 4/6. 425. 1976.

Care of the Acutely Ill and Injured
Edited by D. H. Wilson and A. K. Marsden
© 1982, John Wiley & Sons Ltd.

A NON INVASIVE COMPUTER BASED ASSESSMENT OF RESPIRATORY
CARDIOVASCULAR AND METABOLIC FUNCTION IN THE EMERGENCY
PATIENT.

Castagnetc M Giovannini I.   Boldrini G.
Sganga G. and Castiglioni G.

Instituto di Clinica Chirurgica, Universita Cattolica-
Centro di Studio per la Fisiopatologia dello Shock,
CNR, Rome.

ABSTRACT

A computer-based system for rapid non invasive assessment of
cardiorespiratory and metabolic state in the emergency and
critically ill patient has been developed and used over a five
year period.   Its main features and clinical uses are described.

INTRODUCTION

Critical illness requiring emergency surgical treatment is often
associated with profound abnormal changes of physiological
functions, whose recognition and correction may have a key role in
the successful patient management.   In modern times the surgeon is
being confronted more often than in the past with the problem of
recognizing and treating, besides the fundamental disease, the
associated physiopathological abnormalities in patients whose
clinical signs may be unreliable because of the severely ill state.
This has been determined by the recent improvements in life support
strategies at the site of accidents or during hospital transportation
which has resulted in a higher number of patients presenting in
Emergency Departments in desparate conditions.   At the same time
this has also been determined by the improvements in anaesthesia
techniques and in diagnostic and therapeutic skills that have made
the surgeon more self-confident in performing surgery on high risk
(or older age) patients with already compromised physiological
functions.

THE SYSTEM: DESCRIPTION AND APPLICATION

A method for non invasive rapid assessment of physiological
functions was developed and used in more than 700 cases over a five
year period.   According to this method (Castagneto Giovannini and
Castiglioni 1976 and Giovannini 1976) bedside collection of expired
air through a non rebreathing two-way valve and a Wright respiro-
meter is performed over a three minute period.   Arterial and right
atrial blood samples are drawn during the second half of the air
collection period.   By measuring oxygen and carbon dioxide partial
pressures in the blood and air samples and plasma pH with an
ordinary gas analyzer, a group of data is made available which,
integrated with other necessary bedside collected data, is
developed into a set of cardiorespiratory and metabolic parameters
(see the partial computer output shown in Figure 1).

441

The set of parameters can be divided into five main groups:

1) <u>Pre recorded or predictable group</u>, including information from
the past medical history, from clinical observations, from
the treatment schedule and theoretical predictable normal
basal values for some of the calculated parameters.

II) <u>Metabolic and indirect calorimetry group</u>, including oxygen
consumption (VO_2), carbon dioxide production (VCO_2),
metabolic rate (MR), respiratory quotient (RQ) and other
parameters.

III) <u>Respiratory group</u>, including ventilatory parameters, alveolar-
arterial oxygen gradient $(A-aDO_2)$, respiratory index (RI),
wasted ventilation (VD/VT), ventilatory equivalent.

IV) <u>Acid-base group</u>, including actual and standard plasma
bicarbonate, base excess, buffer base.

V) <u>Respiratory-hemodynamic and hemodynamic group</u>, including
pulmonary shunt $(\dot{Q}S/\dot{Q}T)$, overall ventilation/perfusion ratio
$(VA/\dot{Q}T)$, cardiac output (CO), cardiac work (CW), total
peripheral resistances (TPR).

Alternatively CO and related variables, that are indirectly
calculated by the Fick O_2 method, can be directly measured by the
dye dilution method together with other variables such as minute
ejection fraction, cardiac mixing time, pulmonary dispersive time
and dispersive volume; they allow important information about the
cardiac inotropic contractile state and blood volume expansion.
The system may also be implemented by use of a more sophisticated
equipment including a pneumotachograph and a mass spectrometer, in
which case metabolic, respiratory and other derived parameters are
allowed by waveform analysis of expiratory flow and gas concentrations and automated on-line computation.

Within minutes from the simple initial bedside procedure a complete
multiparametric set of information is available to integrate clinical
judgement and to yield objective guidelines for volume expansion
manoeuvres, need for cardiac inotropic and respiratory support,
use of vasodilatory agents or quantitative diagnosis of shock states.

An objective way of discriminating normal from abnormal physiopathological response and pattern evolution in time can also be
provided: in order to do it each new patient study must be
evaluated on the base of the previous experience (that is using as
comparison the patterns identified in retrospective analysis of
previous studies) by use of combined graphical, statistical and
mathematical simulation techniques.   For example Figure 2 displays
three new patients' trajectories over the 95% confidence area
calculated for previously performed studies in a statistically
based multidimensional grid.   Figure 3 shows the statistically
calculated approximate "mean tendency" areas for various categories
of patients as identified by simple use of the respiratory index
(RI) and the wasted ventilation (VD/VT).   Real time computer aided
evaluation on the basis of more complex statistical techniques
such as cluster analysis (Nanni, Jovine, Giovannini and
Castagneto 1978) is also available for the same purpose of
identifying pathophysiological states and clinical trajectories and

```
DATE      15.03.80          TIME      16.05

NAME                               SEX   M      AGE   74

              WEIGHT    75.0     HEIGHT  165    BSA   1.82

B.E.E.              1423.4680
**********************************************************
VO2           O2 consumption CC/Min.                     247.317
VCO2          CO2 production CC/Min.                     256.259
R             Exchange ratio                               1.036
VO2/M2        O2 consumption /M2                         135.616
VCO2/M2       CO2 production/M2                          140.520
T             Body temperature Celsius                    39.000
MR            Metabolic rate KCAL/M2/Hr                    41.008
MR%           MR as%of theor.basal energy expend.        126.090
MR/24Hrs      Daily energy expend KCAL/24Hrs            1794.848
KCAL.INT.     Non protein calories intake KCAL/24Hrs    1100.000
PROT.INT.     Protein intake G/24Hrs                      50.000
N.BAL.        Predicted nitrogen balance G/24Hrs          -4.018

**********************************************************
VE            Expired volume  L/Min.                      11.300
VA            Alveolar ventilation L/Min.                  7.499
VT            Tidal volume CC                            434.615
VT/KG         Normalized tidal volume CC/KG                5.795
RR            Respiratory rate  Breaths/Min.              26.000

**********************************************************
FIO2          Inspired O2 fraction                         0.210
PaO2          Arterial O2 part. pressure mmHG             73.300
SaO2          Art.O2 saturation %                         96.357
PaCO2         Art.CO2 part. pressure mmHG                 30.100
pHa           Arterial pH                                  7.540
A-a DO2       Alv.-Art.O2 Gradient mmHG                   44.220
RI            Resp.Index                                   0.603
VD/VT         Wasted ventilation %                        35.777
QS/QT         Pulmonary shunt %                           14.062
VA/QT         Ventilation/perfusion ratio                  0.905

**********************************************************
HCO3-         Actual bicarbonate(art.bl.)mEq/L            25.451
ST.HCO3-      Standard bicarbonate(art.bl.)mEq/L          27.236
B.E.          Base excess(art.bl.)mEq/L                    4.635
B.B.          Buffer base(art.bl.)mEq/L                   51.143

**********************************************************
Hct           Hematocrit     %                            35.484

**********************************************************
PvO2          Venous O2 part.pressure mmHG                38.600
SvO2          Ven.O2 saturation %                         77.585
PvCO2         Ven.CO2 part. pressure mmHG                 36.000
pHv           Venous pH                                    7.500
a-v DO2       Art.-ven.O2 content diff. CC%                2.983
CvO2          Venous O2 cont. CC%                         12.016

**********************************************************
CO            Cardiac Output L/Min.                        8.290
CI            Cardiac index L/Min./M2                      4.546
LCW           Left cardiac work KG*M/Min.                  9.395
LCWI          Left cardiac work index LCV/M2               5.152
TPR           Total peripheral resistances Din*Sec/C5    803.219
TPRI          Total periph.resist.index TPR*M2          1464.795
CVP           Central venous pressure CM H2O              -1.000
HR            Hearth rate  beats/Min.                    104.000
MBP           Mean blood pressure                         83.333

**********************************************************
```

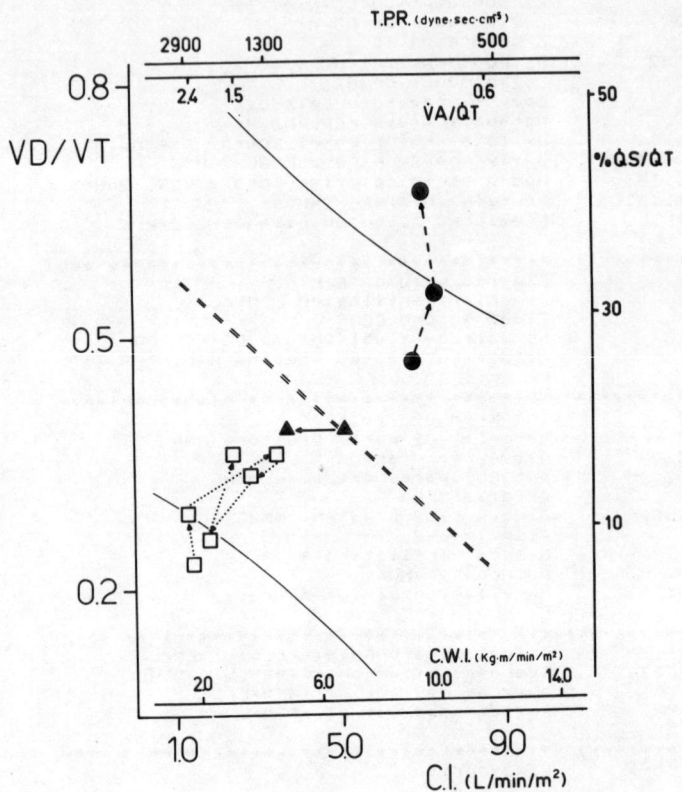

Figure 2

Trajectories of three patients compared with
previous analyses.

(From an article entitled "Functional Cardiorespiratory
Patterns in Acute Pancreatitis" by G.C. Castiglioni et al
in the publication "Controversies in Acute Pancreatitis"
reproduced by permission of Springer Verlag, Heidelberg).

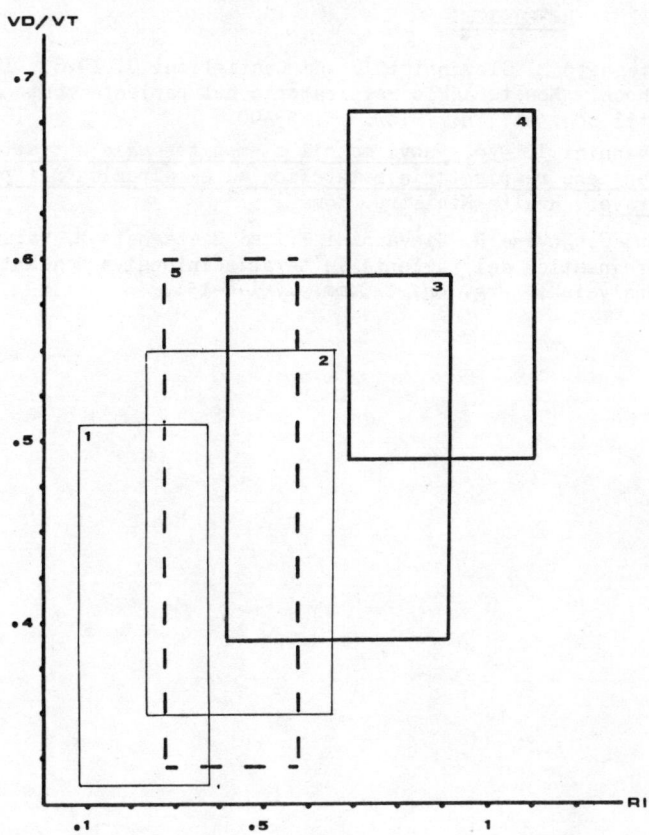

Figure 3

Mean tendency areas for patients in the following
categories:

1. Pre-operative patients
2. Post operative patients
3. Septic patients with severe cardiorespiratory
    decompensation
4. Pre-terminal patients
5. Convalescent patients

of helping in clinical decision making.

REFERENCES

Castagneto M. Giovannini I. and Castiglioni G. 1976. Il polmone da
   shock. Monitoraggio respiratorio nel paziente acuto grave.
   Atti Soc. It. Chir. Tor. 15. 53-90.

Giovannini I.1976. Nuovi metodi di monitoraggio e trattamento della
   funzione respiratoria,metabolica ed emodinamica nel paziente acuto
   grave. Health Ministry. Rome.

Nanni G. Jovine R. Giovannini I. and Castagneto M. Valutazione
   prognostica del paziente in terapia intensiva mediante "cluster
   analysis". Urg. Chir. Comm. 1. 148-151.

Care of the Acutely Ill and Injured
Edited by D. H. Wilson and A. K. Marsden
© 1982, John Wiley & Sons Ltd.

HYPOXAEMIA AFTER FRACTURES

S. S. Tachakra

Central Middlesex Hospital, Acton Lane, London N.W.10 7NS

Previously of Birmingham Accident Hospital, Bath Row,
Birmingham B15 1NA

Serial arterial blood-gas analyses showed a phase of primary
hypoxaemia in thirty-two out of fifty fracture patients (64 per cent)
without head, chest or abdominal injury. The incidence was greater
in those with shaft fractures of the femur or tibia or both, than in
those with fractured hips, and was related to the severity of injury
and the nature of the accident. Most affected subjects were already
hypoxaemic on admission to hospital: the arterial PO2 commonly fell
to between 60 and 70 millimetres of mercury, and the episode
generally lasted a few days. The hypoxaemia was generally
subclinical but four patients developed mild clinical fat-embolism.
(See figure 1) Early hypoxaemia was not found in six patients
admitted with only soft-tissue injuries. One or more subsequent
attacks of subclinical hypoxaemia, each lasting a few days, occurred
in half of those previously affected. Most episodes followed
fracture,operation or manipulation. Pulmonary thrombo-embolism
seemed responsible in two patients, but it could be excluded in
others given oral anticoagulant prophylaxis from soon after admission
(See figure 2) Pulmonary fat-embolism is the most likely explanation
of the primary episodes and could account for most of the subsequent
periods of hypoxaemia.

Random estimates on a further 50 patients showed a greater incidence
and severity of hypoxaemia in fracture patients, with associated
head, chest or abdominal injury. Under-transfusion increased the
risk of hypoxaemia in fracture patients and oxygen therapy for gross
subclinical hypoxaemia was prophylactic against clinical
fat-embolism.

From these observations, it was concluded that it is important to
realize the risks of hypoxaemia, administer oxygen to those who show
significant subclinical hypoxaemia and look for clinical
fat-embolism. Fractures need to be splinted rapidly and effectively
to avoid repeated manipulations and patients should be transfused
adequately on admission.

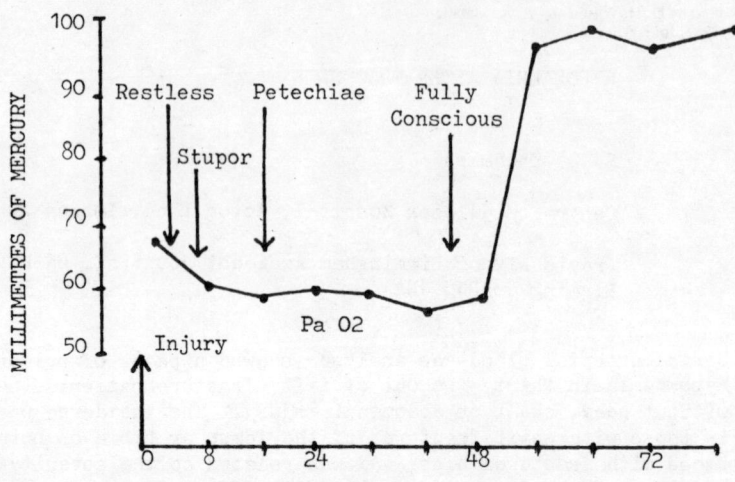

HOURS AFTER INJURY

Fig 1. Primary hypoxaemic episode after fracture of pelvis
associated with mild symptoms of fat embolism.

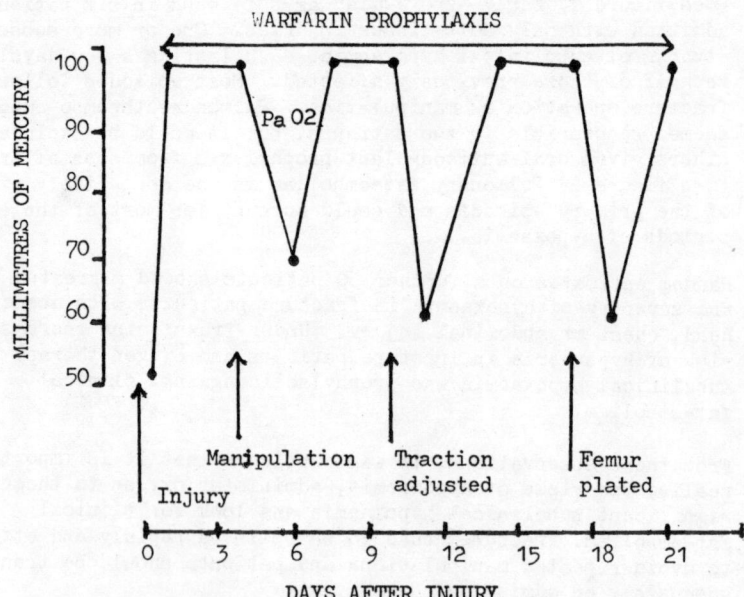

DAYS AFTER INJURY

Fig 2. Primary hypoxaemia after fracture shaft of femur.
Also three subsequent attacks, each apparently precipitated
by manipulative or surgical intervention. Note the
Warfarin prophylaxis against thromboembolism.

Reproduced by permission of the Journal of Bone and Joint Surgery,
and Churchill Livingstone.

Care of the Acutely Ill and Injured
Edited by D. H. Wilson and A. K. Marsden
© 1982, John Wiley & Sons Ltd.

INFLUENCE OF PURE VIRUS INFECTION ON WOUND HEALING

Bruckner W.L.   Mahnel H.   Kleinschmidt J.
Heltzel W. and Fonkalsrud E.W.

Munich W.Germany and Los Angeles U.S.A.

ABSTRACT

Two DNA viruses (pseudorabies and vaccinia virus) and one RNA virus
(virus Sindbis) were tested in 60 rabbits.   Skin incisions were
made on the back of the animals on both sides.   The virus solution
was inoculated into the wounds on the right side, the wounds on the
left side serving as controls.   Follow-up studies revealed that
the two DNA viruses induced pathological changes.   The rate of
disturbed wound healing depends on the concentration of the
inoculated virus solution.

INTRODUCTION

Despite an extensive search of the literature no information could
be obtained about systemic experimental studies on the influence of
viruses on wound healing, with the exception of some single reports
of clinical cases (Findlay and MacCallum 1940. Stern et al. 1959.
Foley et al 1970. Gallagher 1970).

METHODS

In our first experiments we tested the pseudorabies virus (Herpes
virus suis I, Aujeszky virus, strain Hannover II).   In our second
experiment the vaccinia virus (WHO strain Elstree) was tested.   In
our third experiment virus Sindbis (WHO strain reference) was used.
The pseudorabies virus and the vaccinia virus were tested in three
concentrations (10^6, 10^4 and 10^2 infectious units/ml) in groups of
five rabbits each.   In addition ten rabbits were used for each
virus to enable biopsies to be taken for histological evaluation.
The virus Sindbis was inoculated in five rabbits for the study of
wound healing and in five rabbits for histological studies.

Under general anaesthesia and under sterile conditions skin
incisions were made on both sides of the clipped back of the
animals.   Depending on the size of the animals five to ten wounds
were made on each side, one inch long and down to the fascia.   The
virus solution was inoculated into the wounds on the right side,
the nutrient solution into the wounds on the left as controls.

RESULTS

When pseudorabies virus and vaccinia virus were inoculated a delayed
wound healing including reddening, swelling and, in some cases,

dehiscence could be observed.   A direct correlation could be seen between the concentration of the virus solution and both the clinical onset of pathological changes and the rate of disturbed wound healing, i.e. the higher the concentration the earlier and more intense the pathological changes.   The delayed wound healing was apparently caused by the viruses since bacteriological swabs were all negative and all control wounds (118) situated close to the infected wounds did not become infected and healed well.   Upon randomising all infected wounds an average rate of impaired wound healing of 86% results.   When virus Sindbis, however, was inoculated wound healing did not appear to be disturbed.   All inoculated wounds healed at the same rate as the control wounds (i.e. within seven days).

DISCUSSION

Foley et al (1970) reported on herpes virus hominis infection of healing partial thickness burns occurring in six patients.   Two of these patients died with disseminated herpetic infection.   The viral infection may have been primary but the possibility of a reactivated infection that resulted from a post-traumatic immuno-logic defect cannot be excluded.

Gallagher (1970) gives the history of a $2\frac{1}{2}$ year old girl who had burned her right hand on an oven at six months of age.   Subsequently the hand became infected.   After this "infection" settled, a vesicular eruption later developed over the burn sites.   This happened eight or nine times during the following two years. Gallagher surmises that the "infection" that developed soon after the burn was due to herpes simplex virus rather than to bacteria.

These clinical observations can be compared with our experimental findings, since we have been using herpes virus in our studies. It is quite possible that other viruses could be incriminated in disturbed wound healing.   Therefore further studies should be undertaken.

REFERENCES

Findlay G.M. and MacCallum, F.O. 1940. Recurrent traumatic herpes. Lancet 1. 259-261.
Foley F.D. et al. 1970. Herpes virus infection in burned patients. New Engl.J.Med. 282. 652-656.
Gallagher W.F. 1970. Burn wound infection with viruses. New Engl. J.Med. 282. 1272.
Stern H. et al. 1959. Herpetic whitlow : a form of cross infection in hospitals. Lancet II. 871-874.

Care of the Acutely Ill and Injured
Edited by D. H. Wilson and A. K. Marsden
© 1982, John Wiley & Sons Ltd.

EFFECTS OF POVIDONE IODINE IN EXPERIMENTAL PERITONITIS

E.Iglesias Martinez, A.Nogues-Biau, J.Vinas Salas

Centro de cirugia experimental. ICEPU, Lleida, Spain.

ABSTRACT

We have studied the effects of Povidone Iodine in experimental
peritonitis produced in 175 Sprague-Dawley rats by the intraperitoneal injection of human E coli saline suspension.

INTRODUCTION

Povidone iodine solution has been used for intraperitoneal lavage
in peritonitis by many authors with controversial results.

MATERIALS AND METHODS

Sprague-Dawley rats weighing 200–400 g. were used.   Bacterial
peritonitis was induced by intraperitoneal injection of E Coli
grown in Trypticase Soy Broth and diluted in saline.   The
peritoneal cavities were irrigated with a 10% aqueous solution
of polyvinylpyrr olidone (PVP) iodine.

The mortality was recorded at 36 hours.

Eight specific experiments were performed as follows:-

Experiment 1: To determine the lethal dose of E Coli administered
                intraperitoneally 600 million parts of E Coli
                proved lethal.

Experiment 2: To determine the effect of intraperitoneal injection
                of neat povidone iodine in normal rats in three
                groups of ten animals receiving PVP-I.   No fatality
                occurred at doses up to 2.5 ml/kg.

Experiment 3: To determine the effect of subcutaneous injection of
                neat PVP-I.   Twenty animals were allocated to four
                groups.   No fatality occurred at volumes up to
                5 ml/kg.

Experiment 4: To determine the effect of saline on the lethal dose
                of intraperitoneal PVP-I in fifteen animals.   A
                dose of 3.5 ml/kg. of PVP-I was injected intra-
                peritoneally or subcutaneously together with 40 ml/kg.
                of saline.   With the addition of subcutaneous saline
                no mortality occurred.

Experiment 5:   To determine the effect of peritoneal lavage with undiluted PVP-I.   Ten animals underwent laparotomy during which there was peritoneal irrigation with 10 ml/kg PVP-I.   All animals died of chemical peritonitis in less than 24 hours.

Experiment 6 and 7:   To determine the effects of synchronous PVP-I and E Coli peritonitis.   Thirty five animals were allocated into four groups and each received intra-peritoneal innoculation of 2 ml. of E Coli preparation in 300 million parts/ml.   Thirty animals received 2.5 ml/kg. of various concentrations of PVP-I - undiluted; 1 in 2 and 1 in 10.   Five animals received Saline only.   The mortality decreased significantly only in the latter group.

Experiment 8:   To determine the effect of Povidone Iodine irrigation prior to E Coli peritonitis.

Forty animals were divided into four groups and pre-treated with intraperitoneal injection of 15 ml/kg. of either 1 in 2 or 1 in 100 PVP-I at 0, 1, 3 and 6 hours prior to the injection of 600 million parts of E Coli.   Pretreatment with 1:2 PVP-I increased the mortality.   The mortality disappeared when 1:100 PVP-I was injected six hours before the E Coli.

CONCLUSIONS

1. The intraperitoneal injection of PVP-I is lethal at some concentrations by producing a chemical peritonitis.
2. Sublethal doses of PVP-I increased the mortality in cases of experimental peritonitis induced by I.P. injection E Coli.
3. The prophylactic administration of 1:1000 PVP-I diminished the mortality of E Coli peritonitis but this may be a non-specific action.

REFERENCES

Lagarde M.C.   Bolton J.S.   Cohn I.   "Intraperitoneal povidone-iodine in experimental peritonitis".   Ann.Surg. 1975. 187:355.

Gilmore O.J.A.   "Intraperitoneal povidone-iodine". Lancet 1977. 2:37.

Care of the Acutely Ill and Injured
Edited by D. H. Wilson and A. K. Marsden
© 1982, John Wiley & Sons Ltd.

RESEARCH IN THE INJURED AND ACUTELY ILL:
PAST ACHIEVEMENTS AND UNSOLVED PROBLEMS

Douglas W. Wilmore

Peter Bent Brigham Hospital,
721 Huntingdon Avenue, Boston,
Massachusetts 92115, USA.

Tremendous strides have been made in understanding the pathophysiology
and biochemical derangements associated with critical illness. This
knowledge is then applied to the care of acutely ill patients. Five
major areas of interest have emerged that are important to the trauma
surgeon. These areas include shock and hemorrhage, wound healing,
post-traumatic metabolism, nutrition, and infection. Brief summaries
of work accomplished to date are included in this report.

Shock

It is well known that the administration of sodium ions in addition
to the replacement of the shed blood aids resuscitation following
severe hemorrhagic shock. The studies of Moyer, Shires, and others
have documented improved survival and decreased morbidity with
administration of lactated Ringer's in both experimental and human
hemorrhagic shock. The use of crystalloid solution has been
questioned, and randomized trials have been conducted; now reports
concerning the use of crystalloid alone versus colloid are available.
In studies from Chicago, California, and Detroit investigators have
found little physiological difference between colloid and crystalloid
resuscitation. One report suggests a slight advantage of crystalloid
over colloid resuscitation. More recently, the application of a
bedside technique for the measurement of lung water by Lewis and
associates at the University of California has documented that there
is no increase in pulmonary water when crystalloid is utilized to
resuscitate burn or traums patients. In contrast, lung water
increases markedly in the presence of septicemia, no matter what
treatment is utilized.

Cellular changes that occur following marked hypoxia and hemorrhagic
shock have been reported at an increased rate, reflecting the growth
in cellular biology. For example, it has been documented that the
ATP content in the skeletal muscle is normal following shock, although
alterations in the membrane transport of sodium and potassium do occur.
Magnesium chloride ATP ($Mg-Cl_2$-ATP) administered intravenously in
animal experiments is said to improve hepatic and renal function.
However, effects have recently been questioned by Schloerb and
colleagues who have documented a very short half-life of the substance

and a marked impermeability of membranes to this chemical. It appears, then, that this substance may not represent a panacea in terms of restoring altered energetics of the cell following prolonged hypoxia.

Pharmacologists and neurophysiologists have made tremendous contributions in the area of shock in the last several years. Because of the hypotension associated with large-dose morphine administration, the hypothesis was proposed that cardiovascular regulatory centers in the central nervous system may be sensitive to endogenous opiates. To assess the role of these substances during the shock state, animals were subjected to hemorrhagic shock and nalorphine, a morphine antagonist, was administered. The hypotension improved in a dose response manner with drug administration, and further work documented that this effect was within the central nervous system. Clinical trials have extended these observations to shock associated with sepsis, heart failure, and spinal cord transection. The hypotension associated with marked spinal cord injury, if reversed, will minimize the extent of the neurologic damage and, hence, these pharmacologic investigations may be translated into clinical care for the benefit of our patients.

Wound Healing

Research in wound healing has progressed with the use of more sophisticated techniques and the growth of cellular biology. In terms of over-all care, however, the shift by the burn surgeon toward early excision of the burn wound has been reported by Curreri and associates to reduce hospitalization and improve mortality in patients in the 20-50 year age group. Burn excision and early surface replacement have been coupled with vigorous nutritional support, respiratory therapy, and physical rehabilitation to aid the reduction in the morbidity and mortality of burn patients that has been reported over the past 10-15 years.

Once the wound is excised and donor sites are unavailable, how should the wound be covered? Investigators have proposed two alternatives.

First, epithelium taken from a patient has been cultured, and these layers of epithelial cells taken out of petri dishes several weeks later and reapplied to the graft bed. More recently, however, Burke and his associates have reported a synthetic skin substitute, which is an artificial layer covering a collagen base. The collagen base is incorporated into the underlying tissue and gradually resorbed, while the top layer can be removed at a later date and replaced with epithelium when available. The limitations in manufacture at this time have not allowed this technique to be extended to many patients, but it is hoped that this or similar methods will soon be applicable to all our patients with extensive large thermal injury.

In addition to wound coverage, an increasing quantity of information has been gained about the physiologic function of vessels supplying nutrients to the granulating wound. Aulick and associates demonstrated

that a large, open wound lacked innervation and that the blood supply
to a wound was essentially sympathectomized. Therefore, the wound
served as a large parasite, being perfused at adequate rates as long
as blood pressure is maintained. During periods of hypovolemia,
bloodflow to the wound will not change as it does in the skeletal
muscle bed and visceral tissues which are controlled by nervous
regulation from the central nervous system. In addition, these
investigators demonstrated that the wound takes up glucose and
converts it to lactate, a process which may appear inefficient but
may in fact achieve some control of bacterial invasion because of
the known bacteriostatic effect of lactic acid.

Post-Traumatic Metabolism

It is now almost 50 years since Cuthbertson and associates reported
the increased loss of nitrogen from patients following long-bone
fracture. Yet, the precise mechanisms of this post-traumatic
negative nitrogen balance remain unknown. Recently, however, Kehlet
and associates from Copenhagen have utilized epidural anesthesia in
patients undergoing elective surgical procedures. They demonstrated
that neurogenic blockade in patients undergoing hysterectomy
attenuated the hyperglycemia and cortisol response frequently seen
after operation. In addition, nitrogen balance was markedly improved
in this group of patients. Thus, stimuli arising from the wound
appear to play a major role in the initiation of the response
following operation.

Other metabolic responses have been carefully studied and categorised.
For example, using hepatic vein catheterization techniques, a marked
increase in glucose production has been quantitated. In patients
sustaining major trauma, glucose production increases to about
300 grams per day from the usual 200 grams per day observed in post-
absorptive, non-traumatized individuals. When infection occurs in
the injured subjects, glucose production rises to levels of 400 grams
per day. A portion of the glucose arises from the breakdown of
hepatic glycogen stores, but approximately one-third comes from
lactate and pyruvate which are recycled in a wound, and an additional
one-third comes from amino acids which result from skeletal muscle
breakdown.

Nutrition

Important steps have been made in the nutrition support of the
critically ill patient. The use of fat emulsion with solutions of
varied content of carbohydrate and amino acids has allowed more
specific tailoring of nutrient mixes for patients with specific
critical illness --- i.e. renal failure, hepatic failure, sepsis, etc.
Page and Ryan have popularized the catheter jejunostomy techniques.
A small catheter is placed in the upper jejunum during laparotomy
and the distal end of the tubing exited via a stab wound in the
abdominal wall. Shortly after operation, intravenous fluid is
administered through the catheter, and if tolerated, nutrient mixes

are gradually instituted. Over the next several days, two or three thousand calories can be administered to the patient via the gastrointestinal tract, thereby alleviating use of longterm intravenous infusions. This technique appears quite beneficial because of use of the gastrointestinal tract for nutrient administration, the inexpensive cost of the nutrient mix, and the low rate of complications.

A major problem still exists with patients receiving parenteral nutrition. Hepatic dysfunction remains a major complication of intravenous feeding. The specific etiology of this dysfunction is unknown, but the appropriate therapeutic response to this cholestatic jaundice is to reduce the caloric load, substitute fat for carbohydrate calories, increase the amino acid dose, convert the patient to enteral feedings if possible, or to cycle feedings, giving the caloric load at night and reduced caloric load containing amino acids during the day. Using these approaches, hepatic function tests usually improve, and this is particularly true if enteral feedings can be instituted.

Branch chain amino acids have a specific molecular configuration and are utilized as a primary fuel by skeletal muscle. Because of the marked skeletal muscle catabolism that occurs following injury and infection, it had been hoped that solutions rich in branch amino acids would diminish the rate of catabolism associated with these disease processes. Clinical trials are now in progress to evaluate this therapy. It is hoped that over the next 10 years or so more specific nutrient solutions will be available for patients with severe catabolic illnesses.

Infection

New knowledge has improved our understanding and control of infection in critically ill patients. It has been well demonstrated with extensive cancer chemotherapy that environmental control units will prevent infection in the immunologically depressed host, although these techniques have not been utilized extensively in patients following severe injury or other catabolic illnesses. The constant emphasis on isolation techniques (hand-washing, gowning, and gloving) serves as a mainstay for infection control in a busy clinical care unit. In spite of the advent of newer antibiotics, sepsis remains a major problem because of the rapid emergence of antibiotic resistant bacteria. The use of environmental control and non-specific immuno-stimulants to improve overall host responses of the critically ill patient appear to be additional methods which may be useful to aid defense mechanisms of critically ill patients. It had been hoped that nutrition would have a beneficial effect to reverse anergy associated with injury and other life-threatening illnesses. Recently it has been noted that improvement in the immunologic status of the critically ill patient is more a function of the resolution of the disease process than the nutritional state, unless the patient develops malnutrition or is severely malnourished before the onset of

illness. However, because of the interralationships between malnutrition and host defense mechanisms, it has been suggested by most
that nutritional stores be maintained through vigorous nutritional
support in the post-traumatic period.

Summary

Tremendous strides have been made in the care of patients via
research in shock and hemorrhage, wound healing, metabolism, nutrition,
and the control of infection. It is hoped that the application of
this knowledge will be translated to the bedside to aid the care of
patients with critical illness. Further research will improve our
knowledge and understanding of these and other clinical problems,
and, more important, diminish morbidity and mortality in patients
following acute illness.

459